Childhood Malnutrition

Childhood Malnutrition

Editor

Tonia Vassilakou

MDPI • Basel • Beijing • Wuhan • Barcelona • Belgrade • Manchester • Tokyo • Cluj • Tianjin

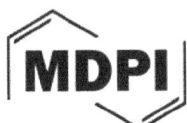

Editor
Tonia Vassilakou
University of West Attica
Greece

Editorial Office
MDPI
St. Alban-Anlage 66
4052 Basel, Switzerland

This is a reprint of articles from the Special Issue published online in the open access journal *Children* (ISSN 2227-9067) (available at: https://www.mdpi.com/journal/children/special_issues/childhood_malnutrition).

For citation purposes, cite each article independently as indicated on the article page online and as indicated below:

LastName, A.A.; LastName, B.B.; LastName, C.C. Article Title. *Journal Name* **Year**, *Volume Number*, Page Range.

ISBN 978-3-0365-2267-8 (Hbk)
ISBN 978-3-0365-2268-5 (PDF)

© 2021 by the authors. Articles in this book are Open Access and distributed under the Creative Commons Attribution (CC BY) license, which allows users to download, copy and build upon published articles, as long as the author and publisher are properly credited, which ensures maximum dissemination and a wider impact of our publications.

The book as a whole is distributed by MDPI under the terms and conditions of the Creative Commons license CC BY-NC-ND.

Contents

About the Editor vii

Preface to "Childhood Malnutrition" ix

Tonia Vassilakou
Childhood Malnutrition: Time for Action
Reprinted from: *Children* **2021**, *8*, 103, doi:10.3390/children8020103 1

Theodoros N. Sergentanis, Maria-Eleni Chelmi, Andreas Liampas, Chrysanthi-Maria Yfanti, Eleni Panagouli, Elpis Vlachopapadopoulou, Stefanos Michalacos, Flora Bacopoulou, Theodora Psaltopoulou and Artemis Tsitsika
Vegetarian Diets and Eating Disorders in Adolescents and Young Adults: A Systematic Review
Reprinted from: *Children* **2021**, *8*, 12, doi:10.3390/children8010012 5

Ioanna Kontele and Tonia Vassilakou
Nutritional Risks among Adolescent Athletes with Disordered Eating
Reprinted from: *Children* **2021**, *8*, 715, doi:10.3390/children8080715 19

Kalliopi Kappou, Myrto Ntougia, Aikaterini Kourtesi, Eleni Panagouli, Elpis Vlachopapadopoulou, Stefanos Michalacos, Fragiskos Gonidakis, Georgios Mastorakos, Theodora Psaltopoulou, Maria Tsolia, Flora Bacopoulou, Theodoros N. Sergentanis and Artemis Tsitsika
Neuroimaging Findings in Adolescents and Young Adults with Anorexia Nervosa: A Systematic Review
Reprinted from: *Children* **2021**, *8*, 137, doi:10.3390/children8020137 35

Vassiliki Diakatou and Tonia Vassilakou
Nutritional Status of Pediatric Cancer Patients at Diagnosis and Correlations with Treatment, Clinical Outcome and the Long-Term Growth and Health of Survivors
Reprinted from: *Children* **2020**, *7*, 218, doi:10.3390/children7110218 73

Lucía Fernández, Ana Rubini, Jose M. Soriano, Joaquín Aldás-Manzano and Jesús Blesa
Anthropometric Assessment of Nepali Children Institutionalized in Orphanages
Reprinted from: *Children* **2020**, *7*, 217, doi:10.3390/children7110217 99

Mónica Gozalbo, Marisa Guillen, Silvia Taroncher-Ferrer, Susana Cifre, David Carmena, José M. Soriano and María Trelis
Assessment of the Nutritional Status, Diet and Intestinal Parasites in Hosted Saharawi Children
Reprinted from: *Children* **2020**, *7*, 264, doi:10.3390/children7120264 107

Dimitrios Poulimeneas, Maria G. Grammatikopoulou, Argyri Petrocheilou, Athanasios G. Kaditis and Tonia Vassilakou
Triage for Malnutrition Risk among Pediatric and Adolescent Outpatients with Cystic Fibrosis, Using a Disease-Specific Tool
Reprinted from: *Children* **2020**, *7*, 269, doi:10.3390/children7120269 125

José Francisco López-Gil, Alba López-Benavente, Pedro Juan Tárraga López and Juan Luis Yuste Lucas
Sociodemographic Correlates of Obesity among Spanish Schoolchildren: A Cross-Sectional Study
Reprinted from: *Children* **2020**, *7*, 201, doi:10.3390/children7110201 135

Carayanni, V.; Vlachopapadopoulou, E.; Koutsouki, D.; Bogdanis, G.C.; Psaltopoulou, T.; Manios, Y.; Karachaliou, F.; Hatzakis, A.; Michalacos, S.
Effects of Nutrition, and Physical Activity Habits and Perceptions on Body Mass Index (BMI) in Children Aged 12–15 Years: A Cross-Sectional Study Comparing Boys and Girls
Reprinted from: *Children* **2021**, *8*, 277, doi:10.3390/children8040277 . . . . **147**

About the Editor

Tonia Vassilakou (Ph.D, Professor of Special Population Groups Nutrition and Public Health, Department of Public Health Policy, University of West Attica).

Tonia Vassilakou holds a degree in Food Science and Technology from the Agricultural University of Athens and she pursued her Ph.D. at the Medical School of Athens. She has been working at the Department of Nutrition and Dietetics of Harokopio University (2000–2004) and at the National School of Public Health (1988–2019). She has been a member of the National Nutrition Policy Committee since 2016 and a member of EFSA Focal Point for Greece. She is the Director of the M.Sc. Program in Public Health held by the Department of Public Health Policy, she has been teaching the subjects of Nutrition and Public Health Policy in the M.Sc. Program since 1989, and she participates as an invited lecturer in undergraduate and postgraduate courses organized by other Greek universities.

She has coordinated and participated in several research projects. Her main research interests include childhood obesity and malnutrition, food insecurity, elderly malnutrition, nutrition knowledge and dietary behavior, sustainable nutrition, food and nutrition policy, and public health policy.

Preface to "Childhood Malnutrition"

The book "Childhood Malnutrition" aims to explore every form of malnutrition, including undernutrition, hidden hunger, overweight, and obesity, in healthy infants, children, and adolescents, as well as among children suffering from various conditions. Malnutrition among children and adolescents is a major public health problem. In 2019, globally, 144 million children under the age of 5 years old were stunted, 47 million were wasted, and 38 million were overweight. Poor availability or suboptimal access to food of adequate nutritional quality, unhealthy dietary patterns or disordered eating behavior expose large population groups to the risk of being undernourished, having a poor nutritional status, or becoming overweight and/or obese. These conditions often present simultaneously and are interconnected.

A healthy diet in the early stages of life results in adequate energy and nutrient intake, and healthy weight and it is crucial for the physical, mental, and cognitive development of children and adolescents, as well as for their long-term health.

The book focuses on a plethora of issues related to childhood malnutrition, including relevant methodological considerations, dietary recommendations, health interventions, and public health policy actions.

Tonia Vassilakou
Editor

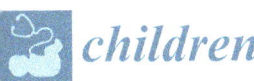

Editorial

Childhood Malnutrition: Time for Action

Tonia Vassilakou

Department of Public Health Policy, School of Public Health, University of West Attica, Athens University Campus, 196 Alexandras Ave, GR-11521 Athens, Greece; tvasilakou@uniwa.gr

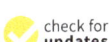

Citation: Vassilakou, T. Childhood Malnutrition: Time for Action. *Children* 2021, 8, 103. https://doi.org/10.3390/children8020103

Academic Editor: Sari A. Acra
Received: 1 February 2021
Accepted: 2 February 2021
Published: 3 February 2021

Publisher's Note: MDPI stays neutral with regard to jurisdictional claims in published maps and institutional affiliations.

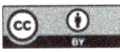

Copyright: © 2021 by the author. Licensee MDPI, Basel, Switzerland. This article is an open access article distributed under the terms and conditions of the Creative Commons Attribution (CC BY) license (https://creativecommons.org/licenses/by/4.0/).

Childhood malnutrition of every form, including undernutrition (wasting, stunting and underweight), micronutrient deficiencies, as well as overweight and obesity, consists a triple burden of disease, especially for low- and middle-income countries, and is one of the leading causes of poor health and a major impediment to personal development and achievement of full human potential worldwide [1]. Globally in 2019, 149 million children under the age of 5 years were stunted, almost 50 million wasted, 340 million suffered from micronutrient deficiencies [2] and 38,2 million were overweight and obese [3]. The nutritional needs of children and adolescents are unique and poor availability or limited access to food of adequate nutritional quality leads large population groups to undernutrition, poor nutritional status, overweight and obesity. These malnutrition forms often exist simultaneously and are interconnected [4].

Malnutrition is a global public health problem that is associated with high health care cost, and increased morbidity and mortality [5]. Approximately 45% of deaths among children under 5 years of age can be attributed to undernutrition [6]. Childhood undernutrition may result in long-term effects that are irreversible, including impaired physical growth and cognitive development [7–9]. Furthermore, undernutrition may reduce sensory-motor abilities, reproductive function and increase children's vulnerability to infections and hereditary diseases, such as diabetes [9,10]. Moreover, undernutrition causes raise of health care costs, reduction in human productivity at adulthood, and shrinkage of economic development, which can result to a long-term cycle of poverty and illness. Childhood undernutrition mostly occurs in low- and middle-income countries, mainly due to poverty, which is associated with suboptimal feeding practices, poor sanitary conditions and insufficient health care services [11–15].

While there has been some progress concerning the reduction of undernourished population from over one billion people in the 1990s to 793 million in 2015 [14], around two billion people suffer from micronutrient deficiencies or "hidden hunger" [16,17]. Regarding the situation among children, globally one-third of them are suffering from micronutrient deficiencies [18]. Hidden hunger poses a major threat to health and development of populations worldwide, particularly among children and pregnant women in low-income countries [11,19]. The health effects of micronutrient deficiency include impaired physical growth, weight loss, immune system vulnerability [19], neurological disorders, cardiovascular diseases, megaloblastic anaemia, and skin problems [18–20]. Furthermore, recent research findings on the developmental origins of disease have indicated that both fetal and infant under- and overnutrition are serious risk factors for obesity with adverse consequences throughout the life cycle [21,22].

At the same time, both in high-income and low- and middle-income countries, rates of childhood overweight and obesity are rising [3]. In the past 40 years, the obesity pandemic has changed the existing malnutrition patterns. The prevalence of obesity during childhood and adolescence has risen significantly over the last decades. Since the early 1980s, the prevalence of overweight and obesity increased rapidly, initially in high-income countries [3]. Globally, overweight and obesity prevalence is very high [3,23], especially in Europe [24]. In 2016, obesity was estimated to affect 1,9 billion persons worldwide [3]. The World Health Organization (WHO) has announced that childhood and adolescent obesity is the major public health problem and advises on actions needed to slow the progression of obesity epidemic [25]. According to the National Health and Nutrition Examination Survey (NHANES) study, the rate of obesity among adolescents in the United States has quadrupled during the last decades [26]. The etiology of obesity is multifactorial, including genetic, environmental, such as nutrition and physical activity, and socioeconomic factors [24,27–29]. Dietary shifts in recent decades, related to modern lifestyle, higher available income and increased consumption of highly processed foods, combined with low physical activity levels, are considered to contribute to this increase in obesity rates [27,29]. Unhealthy diet is the core problem of the current nutrition situation [3]. Environmental and societal factors, which originate from financial development and absence of substantial supportive policies in infrastructures and services, such as education, health, transport, urban planning, environment, climate change, agriculture, food processing, distribution and marketing, often result in changes of dietary and physical activity patterns [24,27–30].

The risk of morbidity and mortality in adult life increases among persons who are overweight or obese as children or adolescents [3,26,27,30]. It is well established that obesity and its determinants are risk factors for the main nutrition-related non-communicable diseases (NCDs), including diabetes mellitus [31], cardiovascular diseases (hypertension, coronary heart disease and stroke) [3,32] and certain cancers [3,30]. Unhealthy diet and poor nutritional status are among the most important risk factors for these diseases globally [3].

This Special Issue comprises of both research and review articles, which focus on diverse components of malnutrition among healthy and non-healthy population groups spanning high income and low- and middle-income contexts. Each of the papers provides the readers with a chance to examine a different aspect of childhood malnutrition and highlights the urgent need for design and implementation of the necessary actions and policies for its prevention and control.

Readers are encouraged to explore these articles and consider the role of malnutrition as a risk factor in their own context. Every country in the world and every population group is affected by one or more forms of malnutrition [2,4,29]. Confronting every form of malnutrition is one of the greatest global public health challenges [2,14]. A healthy diet, initiating in the early stages of life, provides adequate energy and nutrient intake, results in healthy weight, and is crucial for the physical, cognitive and mental development of children and adolescents, as well as for their long-term health [3].

Funding: This research received no external funding.

Conflicts of Interest: The author declares no conflict of interest.

References

1. Amoroso, L. The Second International Conference on Nutrition: Implications for Hidden Hunger. *World Rev. Nutr. Diet.* **2016**, *115*, 142–152.
2. United Nations International Children's Emergency Fund. The State of the World's Children 2019. *Children, Food and Nutrition: Growing Well in a Changing World.* Available online: https://www.unicef.org/reports/state-of-worlds-children-2019 (accessed on 26 January 2021).
3. World Health Organization. Obesity and Overweight. Available online: https://www.who.int/news-room/fact-sheets/detail/obesity-and-overweight (accessed on 26 January 2021).
4. Swinburn, B.A. The Global Syndemic of Obesity, Undernutrition, and Climate Change: The Lancet Commission report. *Lancet* **2019**, *393*, 791–846. [CrossRef]
5. Isanaka, S.; Barnhart, D.A.; McDonald, C.M.; Ackatia-Armah, R.S.; Kupka, R.; Doumbia, S.; Brown, K.F.; Menzies, N.A. Cost-effectiveness of community-based screening and treatment of moderate acute malnutrition in Mali. *BMJ Glob. Health* **2019**, *4*, e001227. [CrossRef] [PubMed]
6. World Health Organization. Malnutrition. Available online: https://www.who.int/en/news-room/fact-sheets/detail/malnutrition (accessed on 26 January 2021).
7. Biesalski, H.K. The 1000-Day Window and Cognitive Development. *World Rev. Nutr. Diet.* **2016**, *115*, 1–15.
8. Mkhize, M.; Sibanda, M. A Review of selected studies on the factors associated with the nutrition status of children under the age of five years in South Africa. *Int. J. Environ. Res. Public Health* **2020**, *17*, 7973. [CrossRef] [PubMed]
9. Barnett, I.; Ariana, P.; Petrou, S.; Penny, M.E.; Duc, L.T.; Galab, S.; Woldehanna, T.; Escobal, J.A.; Plugge, E.; Boyden, J. Cohort profile: The young lives study. *Int. J. Epidemiol.* **2013**, *42*, 701–708. [CrossRef] [PubMed]

10. Okiro, E.A.; Ngama, M.; Bett, A.; Cane, P.A.; Medley, G.F.; Nokes, J.D. Factors associated with increased risk of progression to respiratory syncytial virus-associated pneumonia in young Kenyan children. *Trop. Med. Int. Health* **2008**, *13*, 914–926. [CrossRef] [PubMed]
11. World Health Organization. Global Database on Child Growth and Malnutrition. Available online: http://www.who.int/nutgrowthdb/estimates/en/ (accessed on 28 January 2021).
12. Mohammed, S.H.; Habtewold, T.D.; Muhammad, F.; Esmaillzadeh, A. The contribution of dietary and non-dietary factors to socioeconomic inequality in childhood anemia in Ethiopia: A regression-based decomposition analysis. *BMC Res. Notes* **2019**, *12*, 646. [CrossRef] [PubMed]
13. Akombi, B.J.; Agho, K.E.; Merom, D.; Renzaho, A.M.; Hall, J.J. Child malnutrition in sub-Saharan Africa: A meta-analysis of demographic and health surveys (2006–2016). *PLoS ONE* **2017**, *12*, e0177338. [CrossRef]
14. Action Against Hunger. Available online: https://actionagainsthunger.ca/what-is-acute-malnutrition/underlying-causes-of-malnutrition/ (accessed on 28 January 2021).
15. Bernstein, L. The global problem of malnutrition. *Food Nutr. J.* **2017**, *2*, 159. [CrossRef]
16. Food and Agricultural Organization (FAO); International Fund for Agricultural Development (IFAD); World Food Programme (WFP). State of Food Insecurity (SOFI) in the World. 2015. Available online: http://www.fao.org/3/a-i4671e.pdf (accessed on 26 January 2021).
17. Food and Agricultural Organization (FAO). The State of Food and Agriculture (SOFA). 2013. Available online: http://www.fao.org/3/i3301e/i3301e.pdf (accessed on 26 January 2021).
18. Goedecke, T.; Stein, A.J.; Qaim, M. The global burden of chronic and hidden hunger: Trends and determinants. *Glob. Food Secur.* **2018**, *17*, 21–29. [CrossRef]
19. Perez-Escamilla, R.; Bermudez, O.; Buccini, G.S.; Kumanyika, S.; Lutter, C.K.; Monsivais, P.; Victora, C. Nutrition disparities and the global burden of malnutrition. *BMJ* **2018**, *361*, 2252. [CrossRef] [PubMed]
20. Centre for Disease Control and Prevention. Micronutrients Malnutrition. Available online: https://www.cdc.gov/nutrition/micronutrient-malnutrition/index.html (accessed on 26 January 2021).
21. Morgan, A.R.; Thompson, J.M.; Murphy, R.; Black, P.N.; Lam, W.J.; Ferguson, L.R.; Mitchell, E.A. Obesity and diabetes genes are associated with being born small for gestational age: Results from the Auckland Birthweight Collaborative study. *BMC Med. Genet.* **2010**, *11*, 125. [CrossRef] [PubMed]
22. Kim, S.Y.; Sharma, A.J.; Sappenfield, W.; Wilson, H.G.; Salihu, H.M. Association of maternal body mass index, excessive weight gain, and gestational diabetes mellitus with large-for-gestational-age births. *Obstet. Gynecol.* **2014**, *123*, 737–744. [CrossRef] [PubMed]
23. Abarca-Gómez, L.; Abdeen, Z.A.; Hamid, Z.A.; Abu-Rmeileh, N.M.; Acosta-Cazares, B.; Acuin, C.; Adams, R.J.; Aekplakorn, W.; Afsana, K.; Aguilar-Salinas, C.A.; et al. Worldwide trends in body-mass index, underweight, overweight, and obesity from 1975 to 2016: A pooled analysis of 2416 population-based measurement studies in 128.9 million children, adolescents, and adults. *Lancet* **2017**, *390*, 2627–2642. [CrossRef]
24. Rito, A.I.; Buoncristiano, M.; Spinelli, A.; Salanave, B.; Kunešová, M.; Hejgaard, T.; García Solano, M.; Fijałkowska, A.; Sturua, L.; Hyska, J.; et al. Association between Characteristics at Birth, Breastfeeding and Obesity in 22 Countries: The WHO European Childhood Obesity Surveillance Initiative—COSI 2015/2017. *Obes. Facts* **2019**, *12*, 226–243. [CrossRef] [PubMed]
25. World Health Organization. *Report of the Commission on Ending Childhood Obesity. Implementation Plan: Executive Summary*; World Health Organization: Geneva, Switzerland, 2017.
26. Golden, N.H.; Schneider, M.; Wood, C.; AAP Committee on Nutrition. Preventing Obesity and Eating Disorders in adolescents. *Pediatrics* **2016**, *138*, e20161649. [CrossRef] [PubMed]
27. Kumar, S.; Kelly, A.S. Review of Childhood Obesity: From Epidemiology, Etiology, and Comorbidities to Clinical Assessment and Treatment. *Mayo Clin. Proc.* **2017**, *92*, 251–265. [CrossRef] [PubMed]
28. Campbell, M.K. Biological, environmental, and social influences on childhood obesity. *Pediatr. Res.* **2016**, *79*, 205–211. [CrossRef] [PubMed]
29. Da Silva, J.G. Transforming food systems for better health. *Lancet* **2019**, *393*, E30–E31. [CrossRef]
30. Friedenreich, C.M.; Leitzmann, M. Physical activity, sedentary behaviour, and obesity. Established and emerging modifiable risk factors. In *World Cancer Report: Cancer Research for Cancer Prevention*; Wild, C.P., Weiderpass, E., Stewart, B.W., Eds.; International Agency for Research on Cancer (IARC): Lyon, France, 2020; pp. 101–108.
31. Lin, X.; Xu, Y.; Pan XXu, J.; Ding, Y.; Sun, X.; Song, X.; Ren, Y.; Shan, P.F. Global, regional, and national burden and trend of diabetes in 195 countries and territories: An analysis from 1990 to 2025. *Sci. Rep.* **2020**, *10*, 14790. [CrossRef] [PubMed]
32. Friedemann, C.; Heneghan, C.; Mahtani, K.; Thompson, M.; Perera, R.; Ward, A.M. Cardiovascular disease risk in healthy children and its association with body mass index: Systematic review and meta-analysis. *BMJ* **2012**, *345*, e4759. [CrossRef]

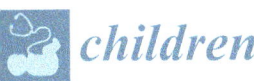

Review

Vegetarian Diets and Eating Disorders in Adolescents and Young Adults: A Systematic Review

Theodoros N. Sergentanis [1,2], Maria-Eleni Chelmi [1,3], Andreas Liampas [4], Chrysanthi-Maria Yfanti [1], Eleni Panagouli [1], Elpis Vlachopapadopoulou [5], Stefanos Michalacos [5], Flora Bacopoulou [6], Theodora Psaltopoulou [1,2] and Artemis Tsitsika [1,*]

1. MSc Program "Strategies of Developmental and Adolescent Health", 2nd Department of Pediatrics, "P. & A. Kyriakou" Children's Hospital, School of Medicine, National and Kapodistrian University of Athens, 115 27 Athens, Greece; tsergentanis@yahoo.gr (T.N.S.); mchelmi@med.uoa.gr (M.-E.C.); chrysanthiyfanti@gmail.com (C.-M.Y.); elenpana@med.uoa.gr (E.P.); tpsaltop@med.uoa.gr (T.P.)
2. Department of Clinical Therapeutics, "Alexandra" Hospital, School of Medicine, National and Kapodistrian University of Athens, 115 28 Athens, Greece
3. Clinical Psychopathology, University of Macedonia, 546 36 Thessaloniki, Greece
4. Medical School, Department of Neurology, University of Cyprus, 1678 Nicosia, Cyprus; liampasand@gmail.com
5. Department of Endocrinology-Growth and Development, "P. & A. Kyriakou" Children's Hospital, 115 27 Athens, Greece; elpis.vl@gmail.com (E.V.); stmichalakos@gmail.com (S.M.)
6. Center for Adolescent Medicine and UNESCO Chair Adolescent Health Care, First Department of Pediatrics, "Agia Sophia" Children's Hospital, School of Medicine, National and Kapodistrian University of Athens, 115 27 Athens, Greece; bacopouf@hotmail.com
* Correspondence: info@youth-health.gr; Tel./Fax: +30-2107710824

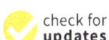

Citation: Sergentanis, T.N.; Chelmi, M.-E.; Liampas, A.; Yfanti, C.-M.; Panagouli, E.; Vlachopapadopoulou, E.; Michalacos, S.; Bacopoulou, F.; Psaltopoulou, T.; Tsitsika, A. Vegetarian Diets and Eating Disorders in Adolescents and Young Adults: A Systematic Review. *Children* 2021, *8*, 12. https://doi.org/10.3390/children8010012

Received: 30 October 2020
Accepted: 24 December 2020
Published: 28 December 2020

Publisher's Note: MDPI stays neutral with regard to jurisdictional claims in published maps and institutional affiliations.

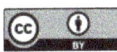

Copyright: © 2020 by the authors. Licensee MDPI, Basel, Switzerland. This article is an open access article distributed under the terms and conditions of the Creative Commons Attribution (CC BY) license (https://creativecommons.org/licenses/by/4.0/).

Abstract: Background: Eating disorders are more common among adolescents and young adults. An increase in the rates of these disorders has been reported during the last years. Meanwhile, vegetarianism is becoming more popular in these age groups. The purpose of the present paper is to evaluate the association between eating disorders and vegetarian diets in adolescents and young adults. Methods: Systematic review of related articles published in PubMed, PsycInfo and Google Scholar up to 30 May 2019. Results: A total of 20 studies (14,391 subjects) were deemed eligible for this systematic review. The majority of the studies reported significant correlations between vegetarianism and eating disorders. However, due to the cross-sectional design, a causal link between eating disorders and vegetarian status cannot be established. Conclusions: Vegetarianism seems to be associated with eating disorders. Longitudinal studies are needed to establish temporal patterns between vegetarianism and the emergence of disordered eating.

Keywords: vegetarianism; vegetarian diets; eating disorders; mental health; adolescents; young adults

1. Introduction

A vegetarian diet excludes meat, seafood and products containing both, but may include eggs and dairy [1]. Vegan diet is an extreme express of vegetarianism, excluding all animal products, namely everything based on animal origin such as additive fats [2]. Lately, there is an increasing movement toward vegetarian diets in different population groups, including adolescents (11–21 years) and young adults (up to 24 years), either due to personal initiative, ethical reasons or social factors [3]. In the United States, it has been estimated that 32% of adolescents between 8 and 18 years declare to have at least one vegetarian meal per week, while 4% of this age group is reported to completely follow vegetarian diet [3]. Concerning adults (>18 years) in the United States, the relevant rates are smaller, as 3.3% of them are recorded as vegetarians, half of them being vegans [3].

Elimination of animal products from the daily diet could potentially affect health especially that of adolescents whose development has not been yet complete. Although there is a correlation between vegetarian diet and health-related benefits, for instance regarding the decreased risk of cardiovascular disease [4,5], there is a large controversy about the effects of vegan diet on mental health [6].

Eating disorders (anorexia nervosa, bulimia nervosa and Eating Disorder Not Otherwise Specified—SCID [7]) are usually associated with restricted diets and are more commonly observed in adolescents and young adults. Vegetarianism has been increasingly considered as a way of weight control, as the diet is based in reduced animal fats [7]. In cases of eating disorders, the disorder itself leads to exclusion or restriction of specific products and different confounders and causes should be examined. According to the available literature, 45 to 54% of adolescents and young adults with anorexia nervosa followed some form of a vegetarian diet, especially females [7,8]. Additionally, in some cases (about 6%), patients have reported that they were vegetarians several years prior to the onset of their eating disorder [7]. It has been suggested that, when subjects with a suspected or diagnosed eating disorder follow a vegetarian diet, health care professionals should worry that this behavior may be used as a socially acceptable way to legitimize food avoidance [7] and avoid certain eating situations [8].

In light of the above, the aim of this systematic review was to investigate the correlation between vegetarian and vegan diets and eating disorders in adolescents and young adults.

2. Materials and Methods

2.1. Literature Search Strategy

A systematic literature search was performed on 30 May 2019 in three different databases (PubMeD, PsycInfo and Google Scholar). For the search, various terms were combined, namely vegetarian OR vegan OR vegans OR veganism OR vegetarian OR vegetarianism OR semi-vegetarian OR flexitarian OR lacto-ovo-vegetarian OR lacto-vegetarian OR lactovegetarian OR ovo-vegetarian OR fruitarian OR flexitarian, with "adolescents" OR "teenagers" OR "young adults" OR puberty OR youth OR "young adult" OR "young adults" OR "young adulthood" and anorexia OR bulimia OR "eating disorder". The reference lists of eligible papers and relevant reviews were also meticulously searched in order to include further studies reporting on vegan diet and eating disorders.

2.2. Inclusion Criteria

The eligibility criteria were based on the PICOS (Participants, Intervention, Comparison, Outcomes, Study design) acronym. Articles eligible to be included in this review were required to meet the following criteria:

1. Studies had to report on adolescents or young adults (up to 30 years of age) who follow vegetarian or vegan diet. Studies could be purely based on adolescents and young adults or include a subgroup of young adults with admixture of older individuals. At any case, the results of these two subcategories of studies were presented separately.
2. Studies had to provide data about the correlation between vegetarian/vegan diet and eating disorders.
3. Any strategy to diagnose eating disorders was deemed eligible.
4. Prospective cohorts/cross-sectional/case-control studies were included.
5. The article was written in English language.
6. There was no restriction in publication year.

2.3. Exclusion Criteria

Articles meeting the following criteria were excluded from the review:

1. Case reports
2. Review articles and medical hypotheses
3. Animal studies
4. Papers referring to subjects with low-meat consumption (i.e., not vegetarians).
5. Studies not declaring age groups

All article abstracts were screened by authors working in pairs in a blinded fashion. Those found not complying with the inclusion criteria were removed and any controversies were dealt with consensus in a meeting, in which the abstracts were reviewed.

2.4. Quality Assessment of Included Studies

All studies were rated with the Newcastle–Ottawa scale, adapted for assessing the quality of non-randomized cross-sectional studies. This scale allocates a maximum of 10 stars evaluating selection (representativeness, sample size, nonrespondents and ascertainment of exposure), comparability and outcome (assessment, statistical test) [9].

2.5. Data Collection Process

Data were extracted from each study in a structured coding scheme using Excel and included type of study, population size, gender and age distribution, population type (exclusively adolescents or young adults or a mix of them), confounders, definitions of eating habits, definitions of eating disorders and bias assessment. Data were retrieved by authors in pairs and team consensus was ensured.

2.6. Compliance with Ethics Guidelines

This article is based on previously conducted studies. The study is performed in accordance with the Preferred Reporting Items for Systematic Reviews and Meta-Analysis (PRISMA) guidelines [10].

3. Results

Study Characteristics

The literature search produced a total of 1271 results, after removal of duplicates; of them 1235 were deemed irrelevant from title and abstract, whereas 36 were evaluated in full-text. Among the latter, 16 were excluded due to various reasons and ultimately, a total of 20 studies (14.391 subjects) published between 1986 and 2019 were included in the present systematic review [7,11–29]. The PRISMA flowchart describing the successive steps in the selection of studies is presented in Figure 1. The general characteristics of the studies are presented in Table 1. Table 1 also presents the summary findings of the quality assessment (risk of bias) for the included studies; in the majority, the quality of studies was rated as low.

The majority of included studies reported a positive association between vegetarianism/veganism and eating disorders. Specifically, Bardone-Cone et al. observed that individuals with a history of eating disorder were more likely to have ever followed a vegetarian diet compared to healthy controls [7]; similarly, Zuromski et al. recorded a higher prevalence of vegetarianism amongst women with clinical diagnosis of eating pathology [16]. Likewise, in a questionnaire survey by McLean et al., female students with vegetarian dietary restraints were more likely to have a history of eating disorders [19]. In a representative community survey, Michalak et al. confirmed the association between vegetarianism and eating disorders [17]. Accordingly, a positive association between being a vegetarian and diagnosis [13] or indication (according to EAT-26 [12,15,20,21] and EAT-40 scores) [14] of an eating disorder has been reported by other researchers.

Barrack et al. observed that, despite a correlation in the univariate analysis, the association between vegetarian status and eating disorder examination scores did not persist at the multivariate analysis [18]. Notably, Timko et al. reported a trend linking semi-vegetarianism with highest levels of restraint [11].

On the other hand, a correlation between vegetarianism and eating disorders was not documented in a few studies [26,28,29], whereas an inverse association between veganism and pathological attitudes towards food was reported [27].

Regarding prognosis and features of eating disorders (lower panels of Table 1), Kadambari et al. [22] showed that vegetarian anorectics were more frequently abstainers, hyperactive, consumed large quantities of non-calorific fluid and presented higher fear of fatness versus non vegetarian anorectics. In a retrospective study, O' Connor et al. found that, as a rule, the avoidance of red meat did not predate anorexia nervosa [23]. Hansson et al. discovered that vegetarianism was more frequently present in recovered or current patients with anorexia nervosa [24]. Interestingly, Yackobovitch-Gavan et al. showed that vegetarianism (past and present) correlated with non-remission of anorexia nervosa [25].

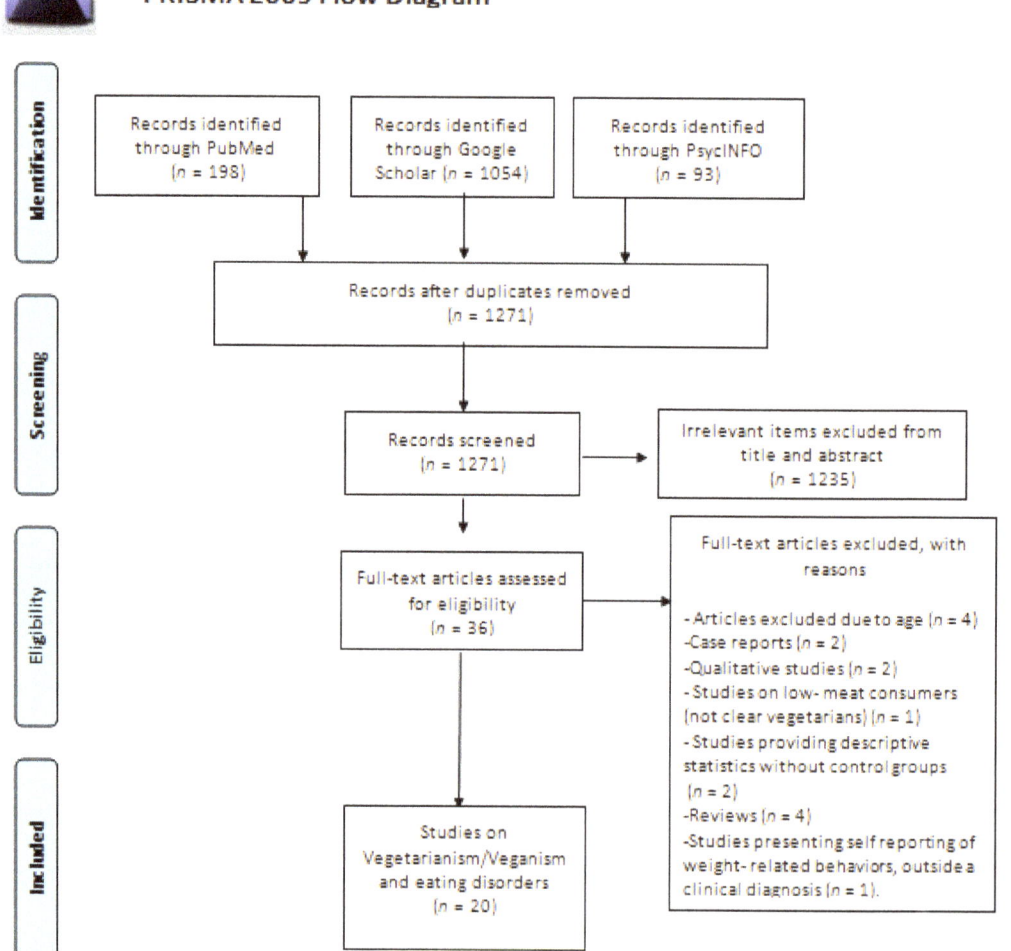

Figure 1. Successive steps in the selection of studies—PRISMA Flow Diagram.

Table 1. Characteristics of included studies. Upper panels present studies encompassing exclusively on adolescents and young adults; middle panels present studies on youth, but with admixture with older individuals; lower panels present studies on prognosis/features of eating disorders.

Author (Year)	Region, Country	Study Period	Study Design	Sample Size	Number of Vegetarians	Percentage of Males	Mean Age (SD)	Age Range	Study Population	Definition of Dietary Factor	Definition of Eating Disorders	Main Findings of the Study	Potential Cofounding Factors Assessed	NOS Quality Rating
Studies exclusively on adolescents and young adults														
Bardone-Cone 2012 [7]	USA (white 90%)	2007–2008	Case-control	160	56	0	23.61 (4.80)	16 and older	Patients seen at the University of Missouri Patients and Adolescent Specialty Clinic and university students as an additional control sample.	Self-reporting for having ever been vegetarian.	Patients seen at the University of Missouri Patients and Adolescent Specialty Clinic. clinical diagnosis (Structured Clinical Interview for DSM-IV)	Individuals with an eating disorder history were considerably more likely to ever have been vegetarian (52% vs 12%; $p < 0.001$).	None	2/10
Barrack 2019 [8]	USA (Hispanic 57%)	NR	Cross-sectional	106	5	37	18	NR	Students	Vegetarian status not explicitly defined.	Eating Disorder Examination Questionnaire (EDE-Q)	While following a vegetarian diet was associated with higher EDE-Q scores in the univariate logistic regression analysis (OR = 9.8, 95%CI: 1.0–91.4, $p < 0.05$), vegetarian status did not persist as a significant independent predictor in the multivariate regression model.	None	3/10
Bas 2005 [9]	Turkey	NR	Cross-sectional	1205	31	50	21.5 (1.9)	17–21	College students	Vegetarian status not explicitly defined.	Eating Attitude Test 26 (EAT 26)	Vegetarians presented with higher EAT-26 scores in males (17.25 ± 11.18 vs 9.38 ± 6.60, $p = 0.019$) and females (22.04 ± 13.62 vs. 11.38 ± 8.28, $p < 0.001$. Similar differences were noted in dieting and oral control, but not bulimia/preoccupation subscales.	Subgrouping on sex	4/10
Fatima 2018 [10]	Saudi Arabia	NA	Cross-sectional	120	12	0	20.7	18–23	College students	Vegetarian status not explicitly defined.	Eating Attitude Test 26 (EAT 26)	Vegetarianism in college women was not associated with disordered eating attitudes (EAT26), as the score in vegetarians (15.42 ± 11.57) did not differ versus non-vegetarians (16.07 ± 9.11), $p = 0.83$.	None	2/10

Table 1. Cont.

Author (Year)	Region, Country	Study Period	Study Design	Sample Size	Number of Vegetarians	Percentage of Males	Mean Age (SD)	Age Range	Study Population	Definition of Dietary Factor	Definition of Eating Disorders	Main Findings of the Study	Potential Cofounding Factors Assessed	NOS Quality Rating
Studies exclusively on adolescents and young adults
Fatima 2018 [20]	Saudi Arabia	From October 2017 to January 2018	Cross-sectional	314	21	17.1	NR	15-19	Adolescents students	Vegetarian status not explicitly defined.	Eating Attitude Test 26 (EAT 26)	Vegetarian adolescent girls had higher scores in the dieting ($p < 0.01$) and oral control subscales ($p = 0.01$), total EAT 26 scores (20.67 ± 13.21 vs. 13.21 ± 9.07, $p < 0.01$) than non-vegetarians.	None	2/10
Fisak 2006 [28]	USA (Caucasians 70%)	NR	Cross-sectional	256	52	0	21.07 (3.75)	NR	Undergraduate students	Vegetarians	EAT-40, EDI	No significant differences were found between vegetarians and non-vegetarians in measures of eating pathology, such as EAT-40 (67.22 ± 30.52 vs. 57.86 ± 25.84, t = 1.85), EDI-DT (17.91 ± 11.29 vs. 15.51 ± 9.73, t = 1.26) and EDI-B scores 8.92 ± 7.48 vs. 6.85 ± 6.81, t = 1.59).	None	4/10
Klopp 2003 [4]	USA (white 82%)	NR	Cross-sectional	143	30	0	19 (1)	NR	Students	Self report	Eating Attitudes Test (EAT-40) >30.	The percentage of subjects with EAT-40 score > 30 was higher in vegetarians (36.7%) vs. non-vegetarians (8.8%), $p = 0.0001$.	None	5/10
Lindeman 2000 [21]	Finland	NR	Cross-sectional	118	15	0	16.44	16-18	High school students.	Vegetarians and non-vegetarians based on food choices questionnaire (not further defined)	EAT-26 (eating attitudes test) >20	20% of the vegetarians scored >20 in EAT-26, vs. only 3.9% in non-vegetarians	None	4/10
McLean 2003 [19]	Canada	1997	Cross-sectional	596	47	0	21.5(3.9)	NR	Students	Self-report	Self report about having ever been diagnosed or treated for an eating disorder	A higher percentage of the vegetarian participants had a history of eating disorders (17.1% vs. 3.1%, $X^2 = 17.9$, $p < 0.001$). Vegetarian women had also lower self esteem.	None	4/10
Perry 2001 [13]	USA (white 48%)	1998-1999	Cross-sectional	4746	262	52	14.9	11 to 18	School students	Self report on a survey.	Previous diagnosis by a physician as having an eating disorder.	A positive association between being a vegetarian and diagnosis of an eating disorder was reported (adjusted OR = 2.72, 95%CI: 1.71-4.34)	Gender and race/ethnicity	6/10

Table 1. Cont.

Author (Year)	Region, Country	Study Period	Study Design	Sample Size	Number of Vegetarians	Percentage of Males	Mean Age (SD)	Age Range	Study Population	Definition of Dietary Factor	Definition of Eating Disorders	Main Findings of the Study	Potential Cofounding Factors Assessed	NOS Quality Rating
Studies exclusively on adolescents and young adults														
Timko 2012 [11]	USA (Caucasians 80%)	NR	Cross-sectional	486	146	23	24.94 (9.54)	The majority (69.50%, n = 338) of participants were between 18 and 25 years old.	Students, internet, local stores	FFQ	Eating attitudes test-26 (EAT-26)	Semi-vegetarians reported the highest levels of restraint, however no significant differences were noted between groups in EAT-26 scores (9.22 ± 13.39 for vegans, 10.08 ± 11.64 for vegetarians, 11.81 ± 12.23 for semi-vegetarians and 7.98 ± 8.91 for omnivores), $p = 0.052$, Kruskal-Wallis test.	None	4/10
Trautmann 2008 [13]	USA (Caucasians 86.1%)	NR	Cross-sectional	330	30	28.8	18	NR	College students	Self report	EAT-26 (Eating Attitudes Test) >20	The mean EAT-26 score of vegetarians (M = 13.21) was significantly greater than non-vegetarians (M = 8.38, $p = 0.006$).	None	4/10
Studies on adolescents and young adults, with admixture with older individuals														
Heiss 2017 [27]	NR (internet users with fluency in English language)	NR	Cross-sectional	557	357	19.6	30.59 (12.61)	NR	Internet survey targeting mostly vegans	Self-report	Eating Disorder Examination-Questionnaire (EDE-Q) global score and subscales; Eating Disorder Inventory-Drive for Thinness (EDI-DT); Binge eating scale (BES).	Vegans endorsed less pathological attitudes and behaviors towards food in terms of EDE-Q-Global (1.82 ± 1.22 vs. 2.23 ± 1.38, $p < 0.01$) and subscales, EDI-DT (3.90 ± 5.43 vs. 5.27 ± 6.13, $p = 0.05$) and similar in terms of BES (2.81 ± 4.19 vs. 3.32 ± 4.38, $p = 0.19$) versus omnivores.	None	4/10
Michalak 2012 [17]	Germany	1998/1999	Cross-sectional	4181	77	55	40	18-65	National survey	Self-report, food frequency	Computer-assisted version of the Munich Composite International Diagnostic Interview (M-CIDI)	Vegetarians displayed elevated prevalence rates for eating disorders 5.6% in completely vegetarians vs 1.2% in a non-vegetarian matched sample.	Matching on sex, age, educational level, size of the community, marital status	6/10

Table 1. Cont.

Author (Year)	Region, Country	Study Period	Study Design	Sample Size	Number of Vegetarians	Percentage of Males	Mean Age (SD)	Age Range	Study Population	Definition of Dietary Factor	Definition of Eating Disorders	Main Findings of the Study	Potential Cofounding Factors Assessed	NOS Quality Rating
Studies on adolescents and young adults, with admixture with older individuals														
Norwood 2018 [29]	Australia (79% Caucasian)		Cross-sectional	393	176	17	29.38 (13.12)	17–74	Community and students	Self reporting of vegan/vegetarian/paleo/gluten free/weight loss and unrestricted diet	5-item version of the Eating Disorder Inventory, emotional eating subscale from the Dutch Eating Behavior Questionnaire, Dieting Intentions Scale, Trait General Food Cravings Questionnaire, Brief Self-Control Scale, 21-item Depression, Anxiety and Stress Scale, Positive and Negative Affect Scale,	People following vegetarian diets (mean = 1.04) did not significantly differ from the non-restricted comparison group (mean = 1.10) regarding eating disorders.	None	4/10
Zuromski 2015 [16]	USA (white/European origin 90%)	NR	Cross-sectional	142	29	0	21.3	NR	Clinical: female patients receiving residential treatment at an eating disorder center vs. nonclinical group, denying any lifetime eating pathology.	Lifetime vegetarian in self-report	Clinical: female patients receiving residential treatment at an eating disorder center	The prevalence of lifetime vegetarianism was lowest in the nonclinical group (6.8%) and highest in the clinical group of eating pathology (34.8%), $p < 0.05$. Intermediate prevalence (17.6%) was noted in the subclinical group.	None	3/10

Table 1. *Cont.*

Author (Year)	Region, Country	Study Period	Study Design	Sample Size	Number of Vegetarians	Percentage of Males	Mean Age (SD)	Age Range	Study Population	Definition of Dietary Factor	Definition of Eating Disorders	Main Findings of the Study	Potential Cofounding Factors Assessed	NOS Quality Rating
Studies on Prognosis/features of Eating Disorders														
Hansson 2011 [24]	Sweden	August 2001–July 2002	Cross-sectional	131	NR	0	26.2 (6.5)	15–50	Eating disorders patients and controls	Vegetarians or omnivores based on food preferences questionnaire	Clinical diagnosis of anorexia or bulimia	Vegetarianism was more prevalent in recovered or current anorexic patients.	None	4/10
Kadambari 1986 [7]	UK (London area)	1968–1979	Cross-sectional	200	77	11.5	23	NR	Eating disorders patients	Self-report (vegetarianism was defined as the exclusion from the diet of food obtained by killing animals)	Clinical diagnosis	Vegetarianism characterized 45% of the anorectic population. Vegetarian anorectics were more likely to be abstainers, hyperactive and showed greater fear of fatness than nonvegetarian anorectics	None	2/10
O'Connor 1987 [5]	Australia	1982–1986	Cross-sectional	116	64	3.5	23 (6.7)	NR	Anorexia nervosa patients	Avoidance of red meat	Clinical diagnosis	54.3% patients were avoiding red meat. However, in only four (6.3%) of these did meat avoidance predate the onset of AN. The remaining 59 patients were termed pseudovegetarians and were associated with longer presence of anorexia nervosa.	None	2/10
Yackobovitch-Gavan 2009 [3]	Israel	1987–1999	Cross-sectional	91	NR	0	22–23	NR	AN patients	Vegetarians and non-vegetarians based on the Eating Disorders Family History Interview	Clinical diagnosis of AN	Vegetarianism (past and present) was correlated to non-remission of AN (OR = 0.095, 95% CI: 0.011-0.789)	None	3/10

AN: anorexia nervosa; BES: Binge Eating Scale; CI: confidence interval; EAT: Eating Attitudes Test; EDI: Eating Disorder Inventory; EDI-DT: Eating Disorder Inventory "Drive for Thinness" subscale; EDE-Q: Eating Disorder Examination-Questionnaire; NOS: Newcastle-Ottawa Scale for the assessment of quality of studies; NR: not reported; OR: odds ratio.3.2. Results of individual studies.

4. Discussion

The present systematic review is an effort to investigate the association between different types of vegetarian diet and eating disorders in adolescents and young adults. As the literature research revealed, there seems to be a correlation between vegetarianism and the presence of eating disorders [7,12–16,19,21] and particularly anorexia nervosa [22–24]. Especially for adolescents, vegetarianism and unhealthy and extreme behaviors on weight control are reported to be interconnected [13]. Females seem to be more prompt to such associations [16,17,19,20]. However, there were also studies reporting no correlation between eating disorders and vegetarianism [26,28,29].

Commenting on potential causal associations, numerous individuals with disordered eating habits and a history of vegetarianism report that the adoption of a vegetarian diet followed their disorder [7,8,17,23,30]. It seems therefore that, in a patient with an eating disorder and vegetarianism, there is a high likelihood that vegetarianism could represent a mode of restriction in eating habits, as a part of their eating disorder pathology. Perpetuation of pathology cannot be ruled out, in a vicious circle where restriction begets restriction. At any case, there is need for future prospective studies to shed light onto the aspect of temporality that is corollary for the establishment of any etiological associations.

Individuals with eating disorders might become vegetarians as a means to control weight, as a strategy of food avoidance, but also for non-weight reasons [7]. From an eating disorders perspective, subjects who are prompt to follow vegetarianism for mainly non-weight reasons (e.g., ethics, religion) could at first seem less alarming than subjects with weight-loss motives [13,18,19] and body shape worries [12], however bias in reporting the actual reasons is a concern. Specifically, in view of the stigma of eating disorders, the disclosed reason for following vegetarianism may sometimes be hard to identify in clinical practice. For a patient with an eating disorder, declaring to be a vegetarian for animal rights reasons would seem more socially acceptable and less uncomfortable than the explicit disclosure of weight loss as a motive. Social acceptability bias in this instance would denote that an eating disorder patient would purportedly prioritize animal rights/ethics when in reality the behavior could be driven by a desire to restrict.

The prevalence of reasons underlying choices of vegetarianism differ between studies. Klopp et al. [14] highlighted health/nutrition (37.5%) as the most common reason for vegetarianism, followed by weight control (18.8%) and animal ethics (14.6%). However, Bas et al. reported another context, with the most common reason being taste preferences (58.1%), followed by healthier diet (19.4%) and weight control only in 9.6% of the sample [12]. Other mechanisms have also been postulated, such as that the life experience of a mental health disorder may "sensitize" the patient towards the suffering of other beings and animals (thus eliciting vegetarianism or veganism), whereas presence of common variables underlying both vegetarianism and eating disorders (such as perfectionism, high levels of responsibility, social values) may provide another alternative explanation [17]. On the other hand, being vegetarian has been associated with positive qualities, including morality, empathy and being self-sacrificial for the greater good [31]. Concerning motivations, veganism is an entity distinct from vegetarianism, as it reflects a self-defining way of life, putting in practice ethical and moral beliefs that strongly oppose processes of treating animals in the food and animal products industry [29].

Regarding subgroups in the spectrum of semi-vegetarianism, vegetarianism and veganism, Timko et al. highlighted that semi-vegetarians had a trend towards a more restrained eating pattern [11]. Further studies are needed to differentiate between vegans, vegetarians, and semi-vegetarians.

In view of the association between vegetarianism and eating disorders, individuals who adopt a vegetarian diet should be closely examined regarding their general eating attitudes/behaviors by clinicians, to evaluate the presence of extreme weight control attitudes [13,18,19] and eating disorder chronicity [7,23,32].

The findings of the present systematic review can be inscribed into a wider perspective, regarding adverse aspects of vegetarianism in terms of mental health. A meta-analysis on 17.809 individuals, published in 2020, highlighted that vegan or vegetarian diets were associated with a higher risk of depression but with lower anxiety scores, although the synthesized studies were of low quality [33]. However, another meta-analysis, also published in 2020, indicated that there was no association between consumption of a vegetarian diet and depression or anxiety [34]. Such complex interplays between vegetarianism, eating disorders and depression would seem addressing in future studies. Eating pathology has been longitudinally associated with depression in a meta-analysis of 42 studies, that highlighted the need to identify factors that are etiological to the development of both conditions [35]. The debate regarding vegetarian diets and any effects upon mental health remains vivid and open.

Our results should be interpreted with some caution given the limitations of the synthesized studies. Firstly, most studies were of a cross-sectional design, thus cannot clarify if there is a causal relationship between vegetarianism and disorder eating. Secondly, quality ratings were low, as evidences by the Newcastle-Ottawa scale. The majority of studies were based on population-based samples, except for a few ones on clinical samples compared versus other groups [7,16,22–25]. Furthermore, a great variety of questionnaires was used. Other limitations include the lack of differentiation of eating disorder diagnoses, the scarcity of subgroup data about bulimia the small sample size in some studies, the variability in the definition of vegetarianism, and the lack of a validated measure for assessing aspects of vegetarianism or veganism. Although there was no limitation about the cultures on which studies were based, the fact that only studies in English were included in this systematic review may have actually limited synthesized evidence mainly into countries with a Western culture and lifestyle. There was paucity of data regarding subgroups of vegetarian diets, such as flexitarian, lacto-ovo-vegetarian, lacto-vegetarian, ovo-vegetarian, fruitarian and flexitarian diets that might exhibit distinct features.

5. Conclusions

In conclusion, this systematic review highlights a potential association between vegetarianism and eating disorders. Future research should focus on multi-center prospective studies in order to shed light on temporal patterns in the relationship between vegetarianism and disordered eating, although such studies would be practically demanding.

Author Contributions: Conceptualization, T.N.S. and A.T.; methodology, M.-E.C., A.L., C.-M.Y., T.P., T.N.S., A.T.; investigation, M.-E.C., A.L. and C.-M.Y.; writing—original draft preparation, M.-E.C., A.L., C.-M.Y. and E.P.; writing—review and editing, E.V., S.M., F.B., T.P., T.N.S., A.T.; visualization, E.V., S.M., F.B. and E.P.; supervision, A.T. and T.N.S. All authors have read and agreed to the published version of the manuscript.

Funding: This research received no external funding.

Data Availability Statement: Data is contained within the article.

Acknowledgments: The authors would like to thank Georgios Koulouris, Maria Kallithraka-Moschochoritou, for their help in accessing PsycInfo database and during the initial reference management of items yielded by the search algorithm.

Conflicts of Interest: The authors declare no conflict of interest.

References

1. Melina, V.; Craig, W.; Levin, S. Position of the Academy of Nutrition and Dietetics: Vegetarian Diets. *J. Acad. Nutr. Diet.* **2016**, *116*, 1970–1980. [CrossRef]
2. Appleby, P.N.; Key, T.J. The long-term health of vegetarians and vegans. *Proc. Nutr. Soc.* **2016**, *75*, 287–293. [CrossRef]
3. Segovia-Siapco, G.; Burkholder-Cooley, N.; Haddad Tabrizi, S.; Sabate, J. Beyond Meat: A Comparison of the Dietary Intakes of Vegetarian and Non-vegetarian Adolescents. *Front. Nutr.* **2019**, *6*, 86. [CrossRef]
4. Craig, W.J.; Mangels, A.R. American Dietetic Association. Position of the American Dietetic Association: Vegetarian diets. *J. Am. Diet. Assoc.* **2009**, *109*, 1266–1282.

5. Key, T.J.; Fraser, G.E.; Thorogood, M.; Appleby, P.N.; Beral, V.; Reeves, G.; Burr, M.L.; Chang-Claude, J.; Frentzel-Beyme, R.; Kuzma, J.W.; et al. Mortality in vegetarians and nonvegetarians: Detailed findings from a collaborative analysis of 5 prospective studies. *Am. J. Clin. Nutr.* **1999**, *70*, 516S–524S. [CrossRef]
6. Beezhold, B.; Radnitz, C.; Rinne, A.; DiMatteo, J. Vegans report less stress and anxiety than omnivores. *Nutr. Neurosci.* **2015**, *18*, 289–296. [CrossRef]
7. Bardone-Cone, A.M.; Fitzsimmons-Craft, E.E.; Harney, M.B.; Maldonado, C.R.; Lawson, M.A.; Smith, R.; Robinson, D.P. The inter-relationships between vegetarianism and eating disorders among females. *J. Acad. Nutr. Diet.* **2012**, *112*, 1247–1252. [CrossRef]
8. Gilbody, S.M.; Kirk, S.F.; Hill, A.J. Vegetarianism in young women: Another means of weight control? *Int. J. Eat. Disord.* **1999**, *26*, 87–90. [CrossRef]
9. Modesti, P.A.; Reboldi, G.; Cappuccio, F.P.; Agyemang, C.; Remuzzi, G.; Rapi, S.; Perruolo, E.; Parati, G.; ESH Working Group on CV Risk in Low Resource Settings. Panethnic Differences in Blood Pressure in Europe: A Systematic Review and Meta-Analysis. *PLoS ONE* **2016**, *25*, e0147601. [CrossRef]
10. Moher, D.; Liberati, A.; Tetzlaff, J.; Altman, D.G.; PRISMA Group. Preferred reporting items for systematic reviews and meta-analyses: The PRISMA statement. *PLoS Med.* **2009**, *6*, e1000097. [CrossRef]
11. Timko, C.A.; Hormes, J.M.; Chubski, J. Will the real vegetarian please stand up? An investigation of dietary restraint and eating disorder symptoms in vegetarians versus non-vegetarians. *Appetite* **2012**, *58*, 982–990. [CrossRef] [PubMed]
12. Bas, M.; Karabudak, E.; Kiziltan, G. Vegetarianism and eating disorders: Association between eating attitudes and other psychological factors among Turkish adolescents. *Appetite* **2005**, *44*, 309–315. [CrossRef] [PubMed]
13. Perry, C.L.; McGuire, M.T.; Neumark-Sztainer, D.; Story, M. Characteristics of vegetarian adolescents in a multiethnic urban population. *J. Adolesc. Health* **2001**, *29*, 406–416. [CrossRef]
14. Klopp, S.A.; Heiss, C.J.; Smith, H.S. Self-reported vegetarianism may be a marker for college women at risk for disordered eating. *J. Am. Diet. Assoc.* **2003**, *103*, 745–747. [CrossRef]
15. Trautmann, J.; Rau, S.I.; Wilson, M.A.; Walters, C. Vegetarian students in their first year of college: Are they at risk for restrictive or disordered eating behaviors? *Veg. Stud.* **2008**, *42*, 2.
16. Zuromski, K.L.; Witte, T.K.; Smith, A.R.; Goodwin, N.; Bodell, L.P.; Bartlett, M.; Siegfried, N. Increased prevalence of vegetarianism among women with eating pathology. *Eat. Behav.* **2015**, *19*, 24–27. [CrossRef]
17. Michalak, J.; Zhang, X.C.; Jacobi, F. Vegetarian diet and mental disorders: Results from a representative community survey. *Int. J. Behav. Nutr. Phys. Act.* **2012**, *9*, 67. [CrossRef]
18. Barrack, M.T.; West, J.; Christopher, M.; Pham-Vera, A.M. Disordered Eating Among a Diverse Sample of First-Year College Students. *J. Am. Coll. Nutr.* **2019**, *38*, 141–148. [CrossRef]
19. McLean, J.A.; Barr, S.I. Cognitive dietary restraint is associated with eating behaviors, lifestyle practices, personality characteristics and menstrual 79 irregularity in college women. *Appetite* **2003**, *40*, 185–192. [CrossRef]
20. Fatima, W.; Ahmad, L.M. Prevalence of disordered eating attitudes among adolescent girls in Arar City, Kingdom of Saudi Arabia. *Health Psychol. Res.* **2018**, *6*, 7444. [CrossRef]
21. Lindeman, M.; Stark, K.; Latvala, K. Vegetarianism and Eating-Disordered Thinking. *Eat. Disord.* **2000**, *8*, 157–165. [CrossRef]
22. Kadambari, R.; Cowers, S.; Crisp, A. Some correlates of vegetarianism in anorexia nervosa. *Int. J. Eat. Disord.* **1986**, *5*, 539–544. [CrossRef]
23. O'Connor, M.A.; Touyz, S.W.; Dunn, S.M.; Beumont, P.J. Vegetarianism in anorexia nervosa? A review of 116 consecutive cases. *Med. J. Aust.* **1987**, *147*, 540–542. [CrossRef] [PubMed]
24. Hansson, L.M.; Bjorck, C.; Birgegard, A.; Clinton, D. How do eating disorder patients eat after treatment? Dietary habits and eating behaviour three years after entering treatment. *Eat. Weight Disord.* **2011**, *16*, e1–e8. [CrossRef] [PubMed]
25. Yackobovitch-Gavan, M.; Golan, M.; Valevski, A.; Kreitler, S.; Bachar, E.; Lieblich, A.; Mitrani, E.; Weizman, A.; Stein, D. An integrative quantitative model of factors influencing the course of anorexia nervosa over time. *Int. J. Eat. Disord.* **2009**, *42*, 306–317. [CrossRef]
26. Fatima, W.F.R.; Suhail, N. Subclinical eating disorders and association with vegetarianism in female students of Saudi Arabia: A cross-sectional stud. *J. Nurs. Health Sci.* **2018**, *7*, 2320.
27. Heiss, S.; Coffino, J.A.; Hormes, J.M. Eating and health behaviors in vegans compared to omnivores: Dispelling common myths. *Appetite* **2017**, *118*, 129–135. [CrossRef]
28. Fisak, B., Jr.; Peterson, R.D.; Tantleff-Dunn, S.; Molnar, J.M. Challenging previous conceptions of vegetarianism and eating disorders. *Eat. Weight Disord.* **2006**, *11*, 195–200. [CrossRef]
29. Norwood, R.; Cruwys, T.; Chachay, V.S.; Sheffield, J. The psychological characteristics of people consuming vegetarian, vegan, paleo, gluten free and weight loss dietary patterns. *Obes. Sci. Pract.* **2019**, *5*, 148–158. [CrossRef]
30. Sullivan, V.; Damani, S. Vegetarianism and eating disorders—Partners in crime? *Eur. Eat. Disord. Rev.* **2000**, *8*, 263–266. [CrossRef]
31. Fox, N.; Ward, K.J. You are what you eat? Vegetarianism, health and identity. *Soc. Sci. Med.* **2008**, *66*, 2585–2595. [CrossRef] [PubMed]
32. Bakan, R.; Birmingham, C.L.; Aeberhardt, L.; Goldner, E.M. Dietary zinc intake of vegetarian and nonvegetarian patients with anorexia nervosa. *Int. J. Eat. Disord.* **1993**, *13*, 229–233. [CrossRef]

33. Iguacel, I.; Huybrechts, I.; Moreno, L.A.; Michels, N. Vegetarianism and veganism compared with mental health and cognitive outcomes: A systematic review and meta-analysis. *Nutr. Rev.* **2020**, *1*, nuaa030. [CrossRef] [PubMed]
34. Askari, M.; Daneshzad, E.; Darooghegi Mofrad, M.; Bellissimo, N.; Suitor, K.; Azadbakht, L. Vegetarian diet and the risk of depression, anxiety, and stress symptoms: A systematic review and meta-analysis of observational studies. *Crit. Rev. Food Sci. Nutr.* **2020**, *4*, 1–11. [CrossRef] [PubMed]
35. Puccio, F.; Fuller-Tyszkiewicz, M.; Ong, D.; Krug, I. A systematic review and meta-analysis on the longitudinal relationship between eating pathology and depression. *Int. J. Eat. Disord.* **2016**, *49*, 439–454. [CrossRef] [PubMed]

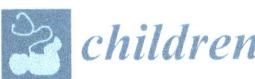

Review

Nutritional Risks among Adolescent Athletes with Disordered Eating

Ioanna Kontele and Tonia Vassilakou *

Department of Public Health Policy, School of Public Health, University of West Attica, Athens University Campus, 196 Alexandras Avenue, 11521 Athens, Greece; ioannakontele@gmail.com
* Correspondence: tvasilakou@uniwa.gr; Tel.: +30-213-2010-283

Abstract: In their attempt to achieve the optimum weight or body shape for their activity, athletes frequently use harmful weight-control practices that may lead to the development of disordered eating or eating disorders. These practices are linked to several medical and mental consequences that may be more serious in adolescent athletes, as their bodies must meet both intensive growth demands and training requirements at the same time. Among other consequences, adolescent athletes may be at nutritional risk, due to their high nutrient needs and unhealthy eating behaviors. A literature review was conducted to examine the main nutritional risks and malnutrition issues faced by adolescent athletes that present disordered eating attitudes or eating disorders. Most studies refer to adult elite athletes, however research on adolescent athletes also indicates that the most common nutritional risks that may arise due to disordered eating include energy, macronutrient and micronutrient deficiencies, dehydration and electrolyte imbalances and changes in body composition that may lead to menstrual abnormalities, and decreased bone mass density. Educational programs and early detection of disordered eating and eating disorders are crucial to avoid the emergence and ensure timely management of nutrition-related problems in the vulnerable group of adolescent athletes.

Keywords: adolescent athletes; eating disorders; disordered eating; nutritional risk; low energy availability; female athlete triad

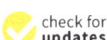

Citation: Kontele, I.; Vassilakou, T. Nutritional Risks among Adolescent Athletes with Disordered Eating. *Children* **2021**, *8*, 715. https://doi.org/10.3390/children8080715

Academic Editor: Carin Andrén Aronsson

Received: 28 June 2021
Accepted: 19 August 2021
Published: 21 August 2021

Publisher's Note: MDPI stays neutral with regard to jurisdictional claims in published maps and institutional affiliations.

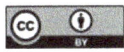

Copyright: © 2021 by the authors. Licensee MDPI, Basel, Switzerland. This article is an open access article distributed under the terms and conditions of the Creative Commons Attribution (CC BY) license (https://creativecommons.org/licenses/by/4.0/).

1. Introduction

Adolescence is the second fastest growth period after infancy and is characterized by significant alterations in body composition, metabolic and hormonal function, organ's maturation, and formation of nutrient deposits that may have an impact on future health [1]. Adolescence is also a challenging period for a person's nutrition, as adolescents are exposed to different forms of malnutrition, such as undernutrition, obesity and deficiencies of certain nutrients [2]. Moreover, adolescence is a vital time for establishing eating habits that will likely last during a person's life [3]. Even if nutritional vulnerability may not be as great as in infancy and childhood, adolescents are a nutritionally susceptible group of population, because of their high growth requirements, unhealthy eating patterns and high-risk behaviors [2]. Organized sports provide many physical, mental and cognitive benefits to young people, however adolescent athletes have very high nutritional requirements, as a result of intensive daily training in addition to their energy and nutrients needs for growth and development [4]. Adolescents who participate in sports have higher nutritional demands than their non-athletes peers of the same age, in order to meet at the same time their needs for growth and wellness, as well as for optimal sports performance [4–9].

Despite their high nutritional requirements, athletes often engage in inappropriate dietary strategies in their attempt to regulate their body weight and/or body shape, for the purpose of reaching optimal sports performance or ideal physical standards for their sport [8,10–12].

Athletes are at a higher risk of developing disordered eating than a clinical eating disorder [10,11]. Thus, they may use unhealthy weight-control practices, such as skipping meals, restrictive eating, over-exercising, dehydration techniques, vomiting, using diuretics, laxatives, or diet medications, but without fully meeting the criteria for eating disorders [8], as they are described in DSM-5 [13]. According to Sundgot-Borgen et al. (2013) and Wells et al. (2020), disordered eating behavior develops in an athlete across a spectrum. This spectrum starts from optimal nutrition (that includes healthy dieting that leads to gradual weight loss), continues to the occasional use of more intensive weight-loss methods such as short-term restrictive diets and may progress to more extreme behaviors, such as chronic energy restriction, eating nothing for one or more days (fasting), using passive or active dehydration techniques, self-induced vomiting, frequent use of diuretics, laxatives, or diet medications, and excessive exercise. This sequence may end with the presence of clinical eating disorders that fulfill the criteria of DSM-5 [8,14,15]. According to Wells et al. (2020), "individual athletes can move back and forth along the spectrum of eating behavior at any point in time over their career and within different stages of a training cycle" [8].

Disordered eating prevalence is higher among adolescent elite athletes compared to their non-athlete peers and it may affect athletes of any gender, sport type or level of competition [16,17]. It is estimated that up to 45% of adolescent athletes develop disordered eating attitudes, especially females in aesthetic and weight-sensitive sports [16,18–33]. Disordered eating etiology is multi-factorial, as socio-cultural, psychological, family, biological and genetic factors interrelate [14]. Moreover, in athletic population, risk factors that are also associated with the development of disordered eating are high competitiveness, starting sport-specific training in young age, weight class rules and pressures from the sport environment to attain a certain body weight or shape [14]. Weight pressures in the sports environment include the comments from coaches, judges or teammates regarding weight and body shape, requirements for specific weight or body shape to compete, the revealing nature of the training or competition uniform and the perception that low weight gives performance advantages [34,35]. Although athletes from any sport may experience the above mentioned pressures, it seems that athletes from aesthetic and weight-class sports experience higher risk to develop disordered eating due to weight pressures [33,34,36]. Regardless of the severity of disordered eating, health and performance consequences are serious and they increase as disordered eating attitudes turn into a clinical eating disorder [8]. The health effects of disordered eating depend on various factors, such as the person's age, other health problems and body composition prior to the weight loss initiation, as well as the duration, volume and rate of energy restriction and purging behaviors [14,25]. Physiological and medical complications affect most of the body systems, including the cardiovascular, gastrointestinal, endocrine, skeletal, renal, reproductive, and central nervous systems, and may also be linked to psychological stress and depression [16,37,38]. Disordered eating attitudes may also cause negative effects on sport performance due to low energy availability, excessive body fat and lean mass loss, fluids' and electrolytes' imbalance, that may increase illness and injury risk, cause limitations in quality and consistency of training and impair recovery after training or injuries [39–42]. These effects depend also on the duration and the severity of disordered eating [43]. Long-term consequences are also possible, but the research regarding the possible damages on health, that may last or arise many years after the initiation of disordered eating behaviors, is very scarce. One possible consequence is the long-term maintenance of the disorder. Sundgot-Borgen et al. (2012) reported that just 72% of former elite athletes with eating disorders during their athletic career had recovered after 15–20 years [44]. Moreover, athletes with long-term inadequate energy and nutrient intake as well as menstrual disturbances during the growth period of adolescence, may never achieve an optimal peak bone mass, resulting in greater risk of development of osteopenia or osteoporosis later in life [45]. Growth retardation is also possible but studies on elite young athletes show a catch-up effect for bone and body mass growth when energy intake becomes normal [46,47]. Finally, there is the hypothesis of greater cardiovascular disease risk later in life, due to endothelial dysfunction, which has been found in female athletes suffering from amenorrhea and energy deficiency [48–50].

During the past two decades, there has been a plethora of published studies that have examined the potential harmful consequences of disordered eating attitudes among athletes. However, research has focused primarily on adult (mainly college-age) elite female athletes [11,51–56]. Less studies have examined the health consequences, and especially those related to the nutritional status, of disordered eating behaviors in adolescent elite and non-elite athletes. The present article aims to review the existing literature on the common nutritional risks and malnutrition issues faced by adolescent athletes that present disordered eating or eating disorders and, to emphasize the value of nutritional interventions regarding the prevention and early treatment of disordered eating in adolescents participating in sports.

2. Materials and Methods

An electronic search of the international literature was carried out, using three different databases (PubMeD/MEDLINE® (United States National Library of Medicine (NLM), Bethesda, MD, USA), PsycInfo (American Psychological Association, Washington, DC, USA) and Google Scholar (Google, Mountain View, CA, USA) in order to track relevant observational studies, reviews, systematic reviews and meta-analyses published until May 2021. The keywords that were used in our search include the following: "adolescent athlete", "high school athlete", "nutritional risk", "malnutrition", "undernutrition", "nutritional deficiencies", "low energy availability", "dehydration", "disordered eating", "eating disorder", "female athlete triad". All articles were reviewed for relevance. Included studies had to provide data about the correlation between disordered eating or eating disorders and specific nutritional risks.

For the scope of our review, "adolescents" were considered males and females aged 10 to 19 years, according to WHO definition [2]. Under this condition, articles that defined in detail the age of the studied population or mentioned that the sample consisted of high-school athletes were included. Studies involving only adult athletes (>19 years of age) and college-age athletes were excluded, as well as studies not declaring age groups. Moreover, a small number of studies included both adolescents and adults, but our review presents only the results regarding adolescents.

Moreover, the review includes articles regarding adolescents that participate in various organized sports in elite or non-elite level. Articles regarding participation in recreational activities have been excluded. Articles of adolescents who did not systematically participate in sports were also excluded.

Finally, articles that were written in non-English languages and those that had no full text available were excluded. There was no restriction regarding the year of publication.

3. Results

Adolescent athletes are more vulnerable than adult athletes to the physical consequences of disordered eating attitudes, due to their high energy and nutrient requirements [4,5]. Their sport performance is compromised, but also normal growth, development and maturation may be impaired [5,40,42].

Nutritional risks that may arise due to disordered eating include energy, macronutrient and micronutrient deficiencies, dehydration, electrolyte imbalances, menstrual irregularities, and decreased bone mass density [37,38,40]. Moreover, disordered eating is associated with the development of the "Female Athlete Triad" and the "Relative Energy Deficiency in Sport Syndrome (RED-S)" [41,42].

The present electronic search retrieved 463 articles. After thorough examination of article abstracts and full-texts, a final number of 34 articles considered eligible to be included in the present review. Twenty-eight of them were articles of original researches, four were reviews and two were clinical reports. The majority (19 articles) examined mainly the association between disordered eating and "Female Athlete Triad" or bone mineral density, 15 articles discussed "low energy availability", three articles examined nutrient deficiencies of athletes with disordered eating and five articles presented the topic of dehydration and electrolyte imbalances due to disordered eating. Some articles examined more than one of the above-mentioned issues.

3.1. Low Energy Availability

"Energy Availability" is the amount of dietary energy available for other body functions after exercise training, and it is calculated by subtracting the energy expended during exercise from the dietary energy intake [57]. Energy availability is usually adjusted to fat-free mass (FFM), since the majority of energy is spent by FFM [57]. Energy availability for optimal bodily function is normally 45 kcal per kg of FFM per day [57], but in adolescents, who are still growing and developing, it may be much higher [48]. Low energy availability (LEA) refers to an imbalance between the energy intake that a person ingests from foods compared to the energy expenditure for exercise, allowing inadequate energy quantity to support the necessary human physiological functions required to maintain optimal health [42]. Although there is no specific cut-off point for energy that defines LEA, it seems that in the case that energy availability falls below 30 kcal/kg FFM/day, the human body tends to reestablish energy balance and prolong survival, but reproductive and skeletal health are impaired [57–59]. Moreover, energy availability of 30 kcal/kg FFM/day is just below the average resting metabolic rate (RMR) of healthy adults [57].

Athletes are often in LEA status due to increased energy expenditure for exercise or due to low energy intake from food that is not enough to cover their high exercise energy demands [58]. LEA may occur unintentionally due to lack of knowledge regarding the best practices to balance the amount of daily energy needed for training and normal physiological functions by the athletes [60]. However, LEA may also occur due to intentional decreased energy intake as noticed in the cases of disordered eating, such as food restriction, vomiting, stimulants or laxatives use, in an attempt to control body weight [61].

Low energy availability (whether intentional or unintentional) may cause health impairment and lead to several medical complications, including problems in the function of cardiovascular, endocrine, reproductive, and skeletal systems, since, as a response to LEA, physiological processes lower the amount of energy utilized for cellular maintenance, thermoregulation, growth, and reproductive function [37,62]. LEA is also a common cause of menstrual dysregulation and amenorrhea in adolescent female athletes [63,64], and it is considered the underlying cause of the "Female Athlete Triad" [37,48] as well as the "Relative Energy Deficiency in Sport Syndrome" (RED-S) [41]. Health effects of LEA, especially amenorrhea and imbalance in bone remodeling, are critical for female adolescent athletes, because the development and maturation of the reproductive system, and the attainment of peak bone mass density is achieved during this period [14]. "Female Athlete Triad" and low bone mineral density are further discussed in Section 3.3.

Many surveys have investigated the prevalence and consequences of LEA in adolescent athletes. A study of 36 elite competitive adolescent female figure skaters in the USA found that 25% of the athletes scored above cut-off score in disordered eating screening test (EAT-40) and reported lower than recommended energy intakes [65]. In a study in Brazil, 91.7% of adolescent female tennis players fulfilled the criteria for disordered eating and/or low energy availability. The average energy availability of the athletes was 31.17 kcal/kg FFM/day, while 87.5% were found to have energy availability less than 45 kcal/kg FFM/day and 33.3% below 30 kcal/kg FFM/day [66]. In another study of 77 adolescent female swimmers also in Brazil, all the athletes who consumed less than 30 kcal/kg FFM/day presented disordered eating behaviors [67]. Moreover, Wood et al. (2021) found that female adolescent endurance runners with a high level of cognitive dietary restraint reported lower energy consumption than runners without dietary restraint [68]. Low energy availability has also been reported in 36% of female high-school athletes of various sports [69], in adolescent female acrobatic gymnasts, where the average energy intake was 32.8 ± 9.4 kcal/kg FFM/day [70], in female adolescent elite football players in Germany, with 53% of them reporting energy availability of less than 30 kcal/kg lean body mass/day [71] and in female and male high-school cross-country runners in the USA, with

30% and 60% respectively meeting the criteria for LEA [72]. It is worth to mention that, although adolescent female athletes may be considered at a greater risk of inadequate energy intake [67] and the research investigating adolescent male athletes is relatively sparse, studies of male adolescents have demonstrated that they are also at risk for disordered eating and low energy availability [42,73,74].

Although athletes lower their energy intake to achieve weight loss, LEA has been correlated with higher body fat percentage and decreased resting metabolic rate (RMR) [75,76]. In a study of 353 young athletes in Germany, female athletes with LEA had higher body fat mass than females with normal energy availability [75], while a study of 42 gymnasts in the USA showed that energy deficits are associated with higher body fat percentage [76]. These findings are possibly explained due to an adaptive reduction in RMR of the athletes with low energy intake [76], and higher leptin concentrations [75]. LEA has also been associated with decreased RMR in studies among adult male and female athletes [77,78].

In conclusion, it seems that LEA is frequent among adolescent male and female athletes in various sports and that it is often correlated to disordered eating behaviors.

3.2. Macronutrient and Micronutrient Deficiencies

Low energy availability is often accompanied by low macronutrient and micronutrient intakes [58]. In athletes, reduced intakes of macronutrients may cause decrease of the physiological ability for bone formation, muscle mass maintenance, damaged tissue repair, and injury recovery [58]. Glycogen stores may not be properly replaced during time periods of intensive activity training if carbohydrate intake is inadequate [79]. At the same time, protein requirements may rise, because body protein stores may be used as alternative energy source [58]. Micronutrients are also required for the formation of bones and muscular tissue, the replenishment of red blood cells, and the provision of co-factors for the regulation of energy-producing metabolic pathways [58]. Athletes who consume less than required calories or restrict certain food groups from their diet, in an attempt to control their body weight, may undergo low nutrient intakes, which may result to ineffective use of energy intake regarding health maintenance and provision of adequate energy for physical activity [58,80,81].

Studies that have examined nutrient intakes of adolescent athletes with disordered eating are very scarce. Costa et al. (2013) found that adolescent athletes with disordered eating behaviors presented lower protein and calcium intakes, while 70% of them had carbohydrate intake below the recommended levels [67]. Wood et al. (2021) found that female adolescent endurance runners that intentionally restricted their dietary intakes had lower carbohydrate intake than runners with normal eating attitudes [68]. Higher scores in the Eating Attitudes Test 26 (EAT26 screening tool) were also associated with lower micronutrient intakes in a study of 21 adolescent competitive female figure skaters [82].

Even though data on nutrient deficiencies in this population group are limited, it is expected that athletes who restrict their energy intake or specific food groups, as well as those that use purging behaviors, will be deficient in a number of essential nutrients.

3.3. Low Bone Mass Density

Adolescence is a critical period for bone growth, acquisition and maturation, as the greatest rate of bone mass formation occurs during puberty. Almost 90% of peak bone mass density (BMD) is achieved by 18 years of age, and 25% of bone mass is formed during the two years around menarche [83]. Bone mass that is formed during the years of childhood and adolescence is important for the achievement of peak bone mass density of the person and the prevention of osteoporosis later in adulthood [84]. Achievement of optimal BMD during adolescence depends on adequate nutrition, including overall adequate energy availability, intakes of certain nutrients (especially vitamin D and calcium), and regular weight-bearing physical activity [48,62]. Increased risk of low BMD has been linked to several factors, such as low body weight, over-exercise, dietary restrictions and menstrual irregularities (late menarche, oligomenorrhea, amenorrhea) [83,85].

In athletic populations, menstrual abnormalities and low bone mass density are associated to low energy availability as a result of decreased energy intake or over-exercise [37]. Energy intake is considered a more crucial factor for the formation of bone mass than certain nutrients (calcium and vitamin D), since energy restriction causes hormonal profile changes resulting to decreased calcium absorption and increased calcium mobilization in the bones [86].

Athletes with disordered eating behaviors may experience low energy availability, which disrupts the normal cycle of menstruation, and, eventually, results to imbalance in bone remodeling that may lead to osteopenia or osteoporosis [37]. The three interrelated conditions of amenorrhea, osteoporosis, and disordered eating have been recognized as the syndrome of "Female Athlete Triad", which was first described in 1992 [37,40]. In 2007, the American College of Sports Medicine revised its position statement regarding the triad suggesting that each one of the three clinical conditions comprises the pathological end of a spectrum of interrelated, subclinical conditions between health and disease. Therefore the three conditions were renamed to (a) menstrual function, (b) bone mineral density, and (c) energy availability, to more appropriately depict the entire spectrum, which may vary from excellent health to sickness in each component [37]. Each one of the triad components may exist independently, but it seems that the emphasis on weight loss and low energy intake may initiate a cycle where all three diseases occur in sequence [43]. "Female Athlete Triad" is particularly harmful during adolescence, as the achievement of maximum bone mass density, as well as the development and maturation of the reproductive system, take place at this age [14,48].

The "Female Athlete Triad" syndrome affects female athletes of any sport type and competition level [62]. The prevalence of the full syndrome in adolescent female athletes seems to be relatively low and ranges from 1.2% to 4.2% [20,24,66]. Yet, a much greater percentage of female adolescent athletes may present with 1 or 2 components of the triad [19,20,24,60,66,69,87]. In studies of adolescent athletes, prevalence of disordered eating ranges from 18.2% to 91.7%, prevalence of menstrual irregularities is found between 18.8% and 48.0%, and prevalence of low bone mass ranges between 15.4% to 42.1% [19,20,24,60,66,69,87].

The assessment of menstrual abnormalities prevalence among adolescents involves a number of challenges, as it is common for girls during their first year after menarche to experience amenorrhea and oligomenorrhea [88]. Yet, the results of studies among adolescent athletes show that menstrual irregularities are quite common in this group and are linked to disordered eating and low energy availability [19,20,25,60,89–91]. Moreover, several studies in adolescent athletes have found a correlation between low bone mass and both disordered eating and menstrual dysfunction [20,25,68,90–94].

Weimann et al. (2000) studied 22 female adolescent elite gymnasts in Germany and found that female gymnasts experienced delayed menarche, bone formation retardation, and reduced height potential, while their nutritional intake was insufficient [89]. Beals (2002) investigated the nutritional status, eating behavior and menstruation of 23 nationally ranked female adolescent volleyball players. Their average caloric intake was lower than their average calorie expenditure, while 17% reported past or present amenorrhea, 13% past or present oligomenorrhea and 48% irregular menstrual cycles. Almost half of the athletes reported actively "dieting" [60]. Nichols et al. (2007) examined the association of disordered eating and menstruation irregularities among 423 high-school athletes and found that athletes with oligomenorrhea and amenorrhea consistently reported higher levels of dietary restriction and higher scores on disordered eating scales (EDE-Q) than eumenorrheic athletes, while athletes with disordered eating were more than twice as likely to report oligo/amenorrhea than athletes without disordered eating behavior [19]. In another study of 170 female athletes, Nichols et al. (2006) found that athletes with oligomenorrhea and amenorrhea had significantly lower trochanter BMD values compared to athletes with regular menses. Moreover, among athletes with disordered eating, those who reported pathological behaviors had lower BMD for all bone sites compared to those who reported normal eating behaviors [20]. Barrack et al. (2010) found that female adolescent runners whose bone turnover was elevated had lower body mass index, less menstrual cycles during the past year, and lower than the recommended energy intakes compared to those with normal bone turnover [92]. Thein-Nissenbaum et al. (2011) studied 311 female high-school athletes and found that athletes reporting disordered eating attitudes were twice more likely to suffer an injury and to experience menstrual irregularities during the season than those who reported normal eating behavior. Moreover, aesthetic and endurance sports athletes who reported disordered eating were eight and three times, respectively, more likely to suffer an injury than athletes from the same sports who reported normal eating behaviors [25]. These findings were similar with the results reported by Rauh et al. (2010), who found that female athletes from 6 high schools in California reporting disordered eating were nearly three times more likely to experience menstrual disorders than their counterparts who reported normal eating behaviors. Moreover, disordered eating, menstrual irregularities and low BMD were linked to musculoskeletal injuries [90]. A study on female and male adolescent runners by Tenforde et al. (2015) found that the main risk factors for decreased BMD Z-scores in girls were current menstrual irregularities, menarche at a later age, lower fat free mass, and lower milk consumption. In boys, lower BMD Z-scores were associated with lower body mass index (BMI) Z-scores, as well as with the belief that thinness improves performance in sports [93]. In a study of 320 adolescent female athletes, Thralls et al. (2016) found that underweight was linked to a greater likelihood of menstrual abnormalities and low BMD. In fact, athletes whose BMI was lower than the 5th percentile for their age were nine times more likely to report menstrual abnormalities and had lower BMD compared to those whose BMI was between the 50th and 85th percentile [91]. A study of 390 elite female athletes in Japan found that among adolescent female athletes, the risk of stress fractures was increased by 12.9 times in those with secondary amenorrhea, 4.5 times in those with low BMD for the whole body, and by 1.1 times in those with a low ratio of actual body weight to ideal body weight [94]. Finally, a recent study on 40 adolescent female endurance runners in the USA found that the athletes with elevated cognitive dietary restriction exhibited significantly lower BMD Z-scores in lumbar spine compared to the athletes with normal eating behavior [68].

It seems that there is substantial amount of scientific evidence regarding bone mineral density imbalances in athletes. It can be assumed that low bone mineral density in adolescent athletes is correlated in a direct way to disordered eating attitudes (such as low consumption of energy or certain nutrients) as well as in an indirect way as a result of disordered eating consequences, such as low energy availability and menstrual irregularities.

3.4. Dehydration

Athletes in weight-sensitive sports often use hypohydration and dehydration techniques in an attempt to lose weight and, thus, obtain a perceived advantage in a competition or compete in a lower weight category [95]. Common dehydration practices used by athletes include restriction of fluid intake, spitting, vomiting, use of diuretics and/or laxatives, steam baths, saunas, and wearing nonporous suits to increase sweat production [14,96].

It is estimated that up to 67% of athletes participating in weight-class sports (e.g., Taekwondo, wrestling, boxing) try to lose weight with various dehydration practices [97]. Most studies focus on adult athletes. In a study of 2532 high-school wrestlers, 2% reported weekly use of laxatives, diet pills, or diuretics, while the same percentage reported at least weekly self-induced vomiting to lose weight. Fasting and various dehydration methods were the primary techniques used for rapid weight loss [98]. In a study of 4746 adolescent athletes it was found that, compared to athletes of non-weight-related sports, males participating in a weight-related sport were more likely to report vomiting, laxative and diuretic use during past week and past year, while females participating in a weight-related sport were more likely to report vomiting and laxative use during past week and past year [74]. A more recent study of 1138 elite adolescent athletes in Germany indicated that passive or active dehydration practices (e.g., sauna, exercise in sweatsuits) were the most commonly used methods to control weight [33]. The ATHENA program, that was conducted in a sample of 1668 female team sport athletes of 18 high schools in the USA found that 4% of the athletes had used vomiting, 1% diuretics and 1% laxatives during the past 3 months, while 14% had not eaten for one or more days, in order to cause rapid weight loss [22].

Maintaining adequate fluid balance during exercise is crucial for dehydration prevention and maintenance of normal cardiovascular and thermoregulatory functions required for effective exercise performance [99]. Sport performance and health may be affected by hydration status, which refers to body water content as well as to body electrolytes concentration [100]. A dehydrated person's lower blood volume may compromise thermoregulatory capacity during exercise, resulting in poor performance [100,101]. With high-intensity exercise, dehydration causes decreased strength, power, and endurance [102–104] as well as increased body temperature and higher susceptibility to heat illness [96]. Moreover, electrolyte concentration changes caused by dehydration are likely to be detrimental to muscular function, resulting in muscle mass loss and decreased strength and power [101]. Hypohydration has an impact on muscle metabolism by hastening glycogen depletion, and central nervous system function by lowering motivation and effort [100]. Therefore, athletes who practice severe energy or fluid restriction to lose weight may suffer unfavorable repercussions such as loss of lean tissue, hormonal disturbances, and performance impairment [95,101].

In adults, dehydration of at least 2% of body weight has been linked to a reduction in endurance and work capacity [99]. It is unclear how much dehydration impacts adolescent endurance performance [99]. Unlike adults, we still do not know the hypohydration level that is associated with adverse athletic performance and negative health effects in young athletes [100].

Dehydration and electrolyte imbalances have been thoroughly studied in sports, as they result in serious health and performance problems. Unfortunately, it seems that adolescent athletes with disordered eating often use harmful weight control techniques that cause detrimental imbalances regarding hydration status.

4. Discussion

The scope of the present review is to present the available literature evidence regarding the main nutritional risks and challenges faced by adolescent athletes who adopt disordered eating behaviors in their attempt to control their body weight, aiming to meet the ideal physical standards for their sport. During the last 20 years a great deal of research has been implemented regarding the health and performance consequences of disordered eating and eating disorders in adult athletes. This work has resulted in a number of guidelines and position papers, such as the International Olympic Committee (IOC) consensus statements on Relative Energy Deficiency in Sport [41,42]. The amount of research regarding the vulnerable group of adolescent athletes is limited, and it is focused mainly on the prevalence of disordered eating as well as the prevalence of the "Female Athlete Triad".

As it was mentioned earlier, athletes have a higher risk of developing disordered eating than a clinical eating disorder [10,11]. Moreover, clinical interviews are necessary to examine the prevalence of clinical eating disorders, according to the specific diagnostic criteria [13]. Most studies on adolescents use questionnaires that can assess symptoms associated with eating disorders rather than clinical interviews [16]. This is the reason that the majority of studies presented in this review discuss the associations between disordered eating behaviors (and not eating disorders) and their consequences.

According to the present literature review, the most well documented consequences of disordered eating regarding the nutritional status of adolescent athletes are low energy availability and low bone mass density. Nutrient deficiencies and fluids' and electrolytes' imbalances due to disordered eating have also been studied to a lesser extent.

Low energy availability is well documented in studies of adolescents, as well as adult athletic populations. The prevalence of disordered eating is considered to be higher among athletes who participate in weight-sensitive sports, such as aesthetic and endurance sports, as well as in weight-class sports [11,18,19,25,33], but some studies in adolescent athletes show that athletes from non-weight-sensitive sports may also use pathogenic weight control behaviors [16,22]. Respectively, low energy availability is also present in adolescent athletes of weigh-sensitive sports [65,70], as well as of non-weight-sensitive sports [66,71].

Studies from various countries and different sports agree that adolescent athletes, who report disordered eating attitudes, consume less than the required energy through their nutrition plan [65,66] and that athletes that choose unhealthy ways to control their weight have lower energy availability than athletes who don't engage in unhealthy behaviors [67,68]. Using the commonly agreed limit of 30 kcal/kg FFM/day, studies have found that 30% to 60% of athletes experience low energy availability [66,69–72]. It seems that a significant number of athletes do not consume enough energy, necessary not only to cover their training demands, but most importantly for the maintenance of their normal physiological functions. This situation may cause medical complications in several body systems and impair growth and maturation [10,37,62]. There is a great amount of research evidence regarding health consequences of LEA, especially in adult female athletes. The most predominant complications concern the function of endocrine system, including the disruption of the hypothalamic-pituitary-gonadal axis that causes functional hypothalamic amenorrhea [42]. Moreover, endocrine system is affected regarding thyroid function and secretion of various hormones, such as insulin, cortisol, growth hormone and appetite-regulating hormones (leptin, ghrelin, adiponectin and peptide YY) [42,59,63,105,106]. It has also been hypothesized that functional hypothalamic amenorrhea and the alterations in hormone secretion may also cause detrimental consequences on future pregnancies [105,107]. LEA has also been associated with increased susceptibility to upper respiratory tract and gastrointestinal tract infections [108].

The research regarding LEA in male athletes is limited and it appears that men's physiology is characterized by a greater resilience in LEA regarding the effects on endocrine system and bone metabolism [109,110], probably because women's energy demands are associated to gestation. Nevertheless, there are studies suggesting that adult male athletes may also develop suppression of the reproductive function known as exercise hypogonadal male condition [105]. Male athletes in LEA state are also expected to have reduced testosterone [42,93], leptin and insulin [110] as well as reduced skeletal muscle protein and muscle glycogen stores [109,111,112]. Another significant finding is that male athletes who restrict their energy intake have negative psychological effects and high risk of bulimic symptomatology [111,113]. A less studied effect of disordered eating in sports is the "result" of these methods regarding the desired reduction in body weight and fat percentage of the athletes. Two studies demonstrated that low energy availability was correlated with higher body fat percentage and decreased resting metabolic rate [75,76]. Metabolic adaptations that are physiologically expected to occur after a period of low energy availability will probably cause a decline in BMR and a weight loss plateau, that may lead the athlete in further caloric restriction to continue losing weight. This vicious cycle may continue and lead to long-term state of low energy availability, as well as to the development of an eating disorder [114]. Athlete's RMR and body composition may be further negatively affected by macronutrients and micronutrients deficiencies. Adolescent athletes that use unhealthy weight control methods have lower than recommended intakes of carbohydrates, protein, calcium, and iron [67,68,82]. Moreover, low energy intake is expected to be associated with low intakes of other nutrients too [58]. These nutrient deficiencies, along with athlete's increased requirements due to growth and training, may cause physiological inefficiency to repair muscles after training or create new muscle mass effectively [58]. Muscle mass may be further depleted when glycogen stores are exhausted due to low carbohydrate intake [58,79]. These findings suggest that athletes' efforts to control their body weight by unhealthy methods do not provide athletic performance benefits. Moreover, they may even result to the opposite than desired results, leading to muscle mass decrease and body fat increase. Therefore, athletes should be discouraged from using unhealthy weight-loss methods in order to achieve the desired body composition.

Furthermore, nutrient deficiencies along with dehydration and electrolyte imbalances are detrimental to athletic performance [4,7,100]. In both children and adults, maintaining fluids' and electrolytes' balance is critical for athletic performance and thermoregulation [115], as dehydration causes abnormalities in cardiovascular and thermoregulatory functions, decreases in strength, power and endurance and raised susceptibility to heat illness [96,99,101–104]. Unfortunately, dehydration techniques such as use of diuretics and laxatives, vomiting, steam baths, saunas and exercise in sweatsuits are used by a large number of athletes to lose weight. However, the number of studies investigating this topic on adolescent athletes is small [22,33,74,98].

The "Female Athlete Triad", that leads, as a sequence, from low energy availability to menstrual irregularities and, finally, to suboptimal bone mineral density is probably the most well documented consequence of disordered eating in sports [37,48,63,88]. Since the development of the reproductive system and the peak bone mass density achievement occur during adolescence, the consequences of the triad are particularly severe for female adolescent athletes [14,48,83,84]. Even in the case of normal menstruation, poor diet and low BMI are more likely to be associated with low bone mass density or musculoskeletal injuries than with normal diets [48]. Athletes that use unhealthy weight control methods are at increased risk to develop low bone mass density, as they usually face simultaneously a number of risk factors, such as low energy availability, menstrual irregularities, underweight and calcium deficiency [83,85].

The triad may affect female athletes from all sports and competition levels [62]. Athletes from weight sensitive sports may be at a greater risk for delayed menarche and bone maturation due to their disordered eating attitudes used to control their body weight [25,89], but adolescent athletes from non-weight-sensitive sports may also present menstrual abnormalities [60]. Many studies of female adolescent athletes of various levels demonstrate that disordered eating is associated with the development of menstrual problems, low bone mineral density and musculoskeletal injuries [19,20,25,68,90–92].

Although the "Female Athlete Triad" is a syndrome that concerns only females, there is growing evidence that male athletes (especially from weight-class sports), may also experience the underlying causes of low energy availability, as they engage in unhealthy weight control behaviors [42,73,74]. These practices also cause low bone mineral density in males [93], as long as other health and performance consequences of disordered eating [43,53,73]. In 2014, the "International Olympic Committee" (IOC), considering the fact that male athletes are also affected by disordered eating and low energy availability, introduced the term of "Relative Energy Deficiency in Sport" (RED-S) [41]. The RED-S Syndrome refers to "impaired physiological function including, but not limited to, metabolic rate, menstrual function, bone health, immunity, protein synthesis, cardiovascular health, caused by relative energy deficiency" [41].

5. Conclusions

Eating disorders and disordered eating are serious conditions with complex and multifactorial etiology that affect mental and physical health. Regardless of gender, age, body size, culture, socioeconomic background, or athletic ability, disordered eating can strike any athlete of any sport at any time [8].

Adolescent athletes, as any person with disordered eating, are at increased risk to develop several nutritional and medical problems, which are associated with the use of unhealthy behaviors to change or control their weight. Malnutrition, such as energy and nutrient deficiencies, is expected to develop due to inadequate food consumption, as well as purging behaviors. Adolescent athletes are more exposed to nutritional risks, as their bodies are attempting to balance their increased needs for growth and training, at the same time. Data on the long-term consequences of disordered eating among adolescent athletes are sparse. Nevertheless, it might be the case that some problems linked to their poor nutritional status, such as low bone mineral density, will remain stable during their adult life.

Prevention and early diagnosis of eating disorders and disordered eating is crucial. The "Ad Hoc Research Working Group on Body Composition, Health and Performance", under the auspices of the IOC Medical Commission in its position statement suggests specific measures in order to decrease the percentage of athletes who use unhealthy weight-loss methods and suffer from disordered eating. Specifically, the suggested measures are: educational programs against extreme dieting and disordered eating, taking into serious consideration the athletes who are trying to lose weight or change their body composition, modification of weight-related regulations in weight-class sports and development of concrete "does not start" (DNS) criteria to protect athlete's health [14]. Prevention programs should be initiated as early as at 9–11 years of age [14].

Prevention educational programs should focus on adolescent athletes and their parents, as well as their coaches. The programs' topics may include understanding of physical development during adolescence, information on balanced nutrition for health and performance, healthy ways to control body weight, health and performance effects of unhealthy weight control methods, body composition assessment techniques, avoidance of negative comments and pressure on body weight in the context of sports and family environment, and information on professionals who may advice athletes on nutrition and eating disorders [8,10,14].

Moreover, the regular use of eating disorders (ED) screening tools as a part of the regular medical monitoring could be another useful preventive measure in order to detect eating disorders at an early stage [40]. In case of diagnosis of an eating disorder, the treatment protocol recommended by the treatment team (consisting of a doctor, a psychologist and a dietitian) should be implemented and the training program should be modified according to the athlete's condition [8,10].

Future research could focus more on long-term effects of disordered eating in athletic populations, as the majority of studies present its direct consequences in health and performance, leaving a knowledge gap regarding the nutritional and health problems that athletes may face after completion of their athletic life. Longitudinal studies on adolescent athletes will be of great importance, especially regarding the consequences that may arise in adult life. Furthermore, there is a need for additional research on specific nutrient deficiencies, as well fluids and electrolytes' imbalances, in correlation to disordered eating. Use of nutritional intake assessment tools and clinical interviews, in combination with ED screening tools, will be useful for this purpose. Finally, interventional studies in adolescent athletes are also extremely necessary, so that prevention and treatment protocols may be issued and applied in various sports, as it is already happening in college-age and adult athletes.

Author Contributions: Conceptualization, I.K. and T.V.; methodology, I.K. and T.V.; investigation, I.K.; writing—original draft preparation, I.K.; writing—review and editing, I.K. and T.V.; visualization, I.K.; supervision, T.V. All authors have read and agreed to the published version of the manuscript.

Funding: This research received no external funding.

Institutional Review Board Statement: Not applicable.

Informed Consent Statement: Not applicable.

Data Availability Statement: Not applicable.

Conflicts of Interest: The authors declare no conflict of interest.

References

1. Sawyer, S.M.; Afifi, R.A.; Bearinger, L.H.; Blakemore, S.-J.; Dick, B.; Ezeh, A.C.; Patton, G.C. Adolescence: A Foundation for Future Health. *Lancet* **2012**, *379*, 1630–1640. [CrossRef]
2. Delisle, H.; World Health Organization. *Nutrition in Adolescence: Issues and Challenges for the Health Sector: Issues in Adolescent Health and Development*; WHO: Geneva, Switzerland, 2005; ISBN 978-92-4-159366-3.

3. Prentice, A.M.; Ward, K.A.; Goldberg, G.R.; Jarjou, L.M.; Moore, S.E.; Fulford, A.J.; Prentice, A. Critical Windows for Nutritional Interventions against Stunting. *Am. J. Clin. Nutr.* **2013**, *97*, 911–918. [CrossRef]
4. Desbrow, B.; McCormack, J.; Burke, L.M.; Cox, G.R.; Fallon, K.; Hislop, M.; Logan, R.; Marino, N.; Sawyer, S.M.; Shaw, G.; et al. Sports Dietitians Australia Position Statement: Sports Nutrition for the Adolescent Athlete. *Int. J. Sport Nutr. Exerc. Metab.* **2014**, *24*, 570–584. [CrossRef]
5. Bingham, M.E.; Borkan, M.; Quatromoni, P. Sports Nutrition Advice for Adolescent Athletes: A Time to Focus on Food. *Am. J. Lifestyle Med.* **2015**, *9*, 398–402. [CrossRef]
6. Purcell, L.K. Sport Nutrition for Young Athletes. *Paediatr. Child Health* **2013**, *18*, 200–202. [CrossRef]
7. Berg, E.K. Performance Nutrition for the Adolescent Athlete: A Realistic Approach. *Clin. J. Sport Med.* **2019**, *29*, 345–352. [CrossRef]
8. Wells, K.R.; Jeacocke, N.A.; Appaneal, R.; Smith, H.D.; Vlahovich, N.; Burke, L.M.; Hughes, D. The Australian Institute of Sport (AIS) and National Eating Disorders Collaboration (NEDC) Position Statement on Disordered Eating in High Performance Sport. *Br. J. Sports Med.* **2020**, *54*, 1247–1258. [CrossRef] [PubMed]
9. Unnithan, V.B.; Baxter-Jones, A.D.G. The Young Athlete. *Nutr. Sport* **2000**, *7*, 429–441.
10. Bonci, C.M.; Bonci, L.J.; Granger, L.R.; Johnson, C.L.; Malina, R.M.; Milne, L.W.; Ryan, R.R.; Vanderbunt, E.M. National Athletic Trainers' Association Position Statement: Preventing, Detecting, and Managing Disordered Eating in Athletes. *J. Athl. Train.* **2008**, *43*, 80–108. [CrossRef] [PubMed]
11. Sundgot-Borgen, J.; Torstveit, M.K. Prevalence of Eating Disorders in Elite Athletes Is Higher than in the General Population. *Clin. J. Sport Med. Off. J. Can. Acad. Sport Med.* **2004**, *14*, 25–32. [CrossRef]
12. Reardon, C.L.; Hainline, B.; Aron, C.M.; Baron, D.; Baum, A.L.; Bindra, A.; Budgett, R.; Campriani, N.; Castaldelli-Maia, J.M.; Currie, A.; et al. Mental Health in Elite Athletes: International Olympic Committee Consensus Statement. *Br. J. Sports Med.* **2019**, *53*, 667–699. [CrossRef] [PubMed]
13. American Psychiatric Association. *Diagnostic and Statistical Manual of Mental Disorders*, 5th ed.; American Psychiatric Association: Washington, DC, USA, 2013; ISBN 978-0-89042-555-8.
14. Sundgot-Borgen, J.; Meyer, N.L.; Lohman, T.G.; Ackland, T.R.; Maughan, R.J.; Stewart, A.D.; Müller, W. How to Minimise the Health Risks to Athletes Who Compete in Weight-Sensitive Sports Review and Position Statement on Behalf of the Ad Hoc Research Working Group on Body Composition, Health and Performance, under the Auspices of the IOC Medical Commission. *Br. J. Sports Med.* **2013**, *47*, 1012–1022. [CrossRef] [PubMed]
15. Sundgot-Borgen, J.; Torstveit, M.K. Aspects of Disordered Eating Continuum in Elite High-Intensity Sports. *Scand. J. Med. Sci. Sports* **2010**, *20* (Suppl. 2), 112–121. [CrossRef] [PubMed]
16. Martinsen, M.T.; Sundgot-Borgen, J. Higher Prevalence of Eating Disorders among Adolescent Elite Athletes than Controls. *Med. Sci. Sports Exerc.* **2013**, *45*, 1188–1197. [CrossRef]
17. Mancine, R.P.; Gusfa, D.W.; Moshrefi, A.; Kennedy, S.F. Prevalence of Disordered Eating in Athletes Categorized by Emphasis on Leanness and Activity Type—A Systematic Review. *J. Eat. Disord.* **2020**, *8*, 47. [CrossRef]
18. Jankauskiene, R.; Baceviciene, M. Body Image and Disturbed Eating Attitudes and Behaviors in Sport-Involved Adolescents: The Role of Gender and Sport Characteristics. *Nutrients* **2019**, *11*, 3061. [CrossRef] [PubMed]
19. Nichols, J.F.; Rauh, M.J.; Barrack, M.T.; Barkai, H.-S.; Pernick, Y. Disordered Eating and Menstrual Irregularity in High School Athletes in Lean-Build and Nonlean-Build Sports. *Int. J. Sport Nutr. Exerc. Metab.* **2007**, *17*, 364–377. [CrossRef]
20. Nichols, J.F.; Rauh, M.J.; Lawson, M.J.; Ji, M.; Barkai, H.-S. Prevalence of the Female Athlete Triad Syndrome among High School Athletes. *Arch. Pediatr. Adolesc. Med.* **2006**, *160*, 137–142. [CrossRef]
21. Pernick, Y.; Nichols, J.F.; Rauh, M.J.; Kern, M.; Ji, M.; Lawson, M.J.; Wilfley, D. Disordered Eating among a Multi-Racial/Ethnic Sample of Female High-School Athletes. *J. Adolesc. Health Off. Publ. Soc. Adolesc. Med.* **2006**, *38*, 689–695. [CrossRef]
22. Ranby, K.W.; Aiken, L.S.; MacKinnon, D.P.; Elliot, D.L.; Moe, E.L.; McGinnis, W.; Goldberg, L. A Mediation Analysis of the ATHENA Intervention for Female Athletes: Prevention of Athletic-Enhancing Substance Use and Unhealthy Weight Loss Behaviors. *J. Pediatr. Psychol.* **2009**, *34*, 1069–1083. [CrossRef] [PubMed]
23. Rosendahl, J.; Bormann, B.; Aschenbrenner, K.; Aschenbrenner, F.; Strauss, B. Dieting and Disordered Eating in German High School Athletes and Non-Athletes. *Scand. J. Med. Sci. Sports* **2009**, *19*, 731–739. [CrossRef]
24. Schtscherbyna, A.; Soares, E.A.; de Oliveira, F.P.; Ribeiro, B.G. Female Athlete Triad in Elite Swimmers of the City of Rio de Janeiro, Brazil. *Nutr. Burbank Los Angel. City Calif.* **2009**, *25*, 634–639. [CrossRef] [PubMed]
25. Thein-Nissenbaum, J.M.; Rauh, M.J.; Carr, K.E.; Loud, K.J.; McGuine, T.A. Associations between Disordered Eating, Menstrual Dysfunction, and Musculoskeletal Injury among High School Athletes. *J. Orthop. Sports Phys. Ther.* **2011**, *41*, 60–69. [CrossRef]
26. Toro, J.; Galilea, B.; Martinez-Mallén, E.; Salamero, M.; Capdevila, L.; Mari, J.; Mayolas, J.; Toro, E. Eating Disorders in Spanish Female Athletes. *Int. J. Sports Med.* **2005**, *26*, 693–700. [CrossRef] [PubMed]
27. Van Durme, K.; Goossens, L.; Braet, C. Adolescent Aesthetic Athletes: A Group at Risk for Eating Pathology? *Eat. Behav.* **2012**, *13*, 119–122. [CrossRef]
28. Heradstveit, O.; Hysing, M.; Nilsen, S.A.; Bøe, T. Symptoms of Disordered Eating and Participation in Individual- and Team Sports: A Population-Based Study of Adolescents. *Eat. Behav.* **2020**, *39*, 101434. [CrossRef] [PubMed]
29. Sundgot-Borgen, J. Eating Disorders, Energy Intake, Training Volume, and Menstrual Function in High-Level Modern Rhythmic Gymnasts. *Int. J. Sport Nutr.* **1996**, *6*, 100–109. [CrossRef]

30. Nordin, S.M.; Harris, G.; Cumming, J. Disturbed Eating in Young, Competitive Gymnasts: Differences between Three Gymnastics Disciplines. *Eur. J. Sport Sci.* **2003**, *3*, 1–14. [CrossRef]
31. Okano, G.; Holmes, R.A.; Mu, Z.; Yang, P.; Lin, Z.; Nakai, Y. Disordered Eating in Japanese and Chinese Female Runners, Rhythmic Gymnasts and Gymnasts. *Int. J. Sports Med.* **2005**, *26*, 486–491. [CrossRef]
32. Donti, O.; Donti, A.; Gaspari, V.; Pleksida, P.; Psychountaki, M. Are They Too Perfect to Eat Healthy? Association between Eating Disorder Symptoms and Perfectionism in Adolescent Rhythmic Gymnasts. *Eat. Behav.* **2021**, *41*, 101514. [CrossRef]
33. Giel, K.E.; Hermann-Werner, A.; Mayer, J.; Diehl, K.; Schneider, S.; Thiel, A.; Zipfel, S. Eating Disorder Pathology in Elite Adolescent Athletes. *Int. J. Eat. Disord.* **2016**, *49*, 553–562. [CrossRef] [PubMed]
34. Reel, J.J.; Petrie, T.A.; SooHoo, S.; Anderson, C.M. Weight Pressures in Sport: Examining the Factor Structure and Incremental Validity of the Weight Pressures in Sport—Females. *Eat. Behav.* **2013**, *14*, 137–144. [CrossRef] [PubMed]
35. Anderson, C.M.; Petrie, T.A.; Neumann, C.S. Effects of Sport Pressures on Female Collegiate Athletes: A Preliminary Longitudinal Investigation. *Sport Exerc. Perform. Psychol.* **2012**, *1*, 120–134. [CrossRef]
36. Byrne, S.; McLean, N. Elite Athletes: Effects of the Pressure to Be Thin. *J. Sci. Med. Sport* **2002**, *5*, 80–94. [CrossRef]
37. Nattiv, A.; Loucks, A.B.; Manore, M.M.; Sanborn, C.F.; Sundgot-Borgen, J.; Warren, M.P.; American College of Sports Medicine. American College of Sports Medicine Position Stand. The Female Athlete Triad. *Med. Sci. Sports Exerc.* **2007**, *39*, 1867–1882. [CrossRef] [PubMed]
38. Female Athlete Issues for the Team Physician: A Consensus Statement—2017 Update. *Med. Sci. Sports Exerc.* **2018**, *50*, 1113–1122. [CrossRef] [PubMed]
39. El Ghoch, M.; Soave, F.; Calugi, S.; Dalle Grave, R. Eating Disorders, Physical Fitness and Sport Performance: A Systematic Review. *Nutrients* **2013**, *5*, 5140–5160. [CrossRef]
40. Joy, E.; Kussman, A.; Nattiv, A. 2016 Update on Eating Disorders in Athletes: A Comprehensive Narrative Review with a Focus on Clinical Assessment and Management. *Br. J. Sports Med.* **2016**, *50*, 154–162. [CrossRef]
41. Mountjoy, M.; Sundgot-Borgen, J.; Burke, L.; Carter, S.; Constantini, N.; Lebrun, C.; Meyer, N.; Sherman, R.; Steffen, K.; Budgett, R.; et al. The IOC Consensus Statement: Beyond the Female Athlete Triad—Relative Energy Deficiency in Sport (RED-S). *Br. J. Sports Med.* **2014**, *48*, 491–497. [CrossRef]
42. Mountjoy, M.; Sundgot-Borgen, J.; Burke, L.; Ackerman, K.E.; Blauwet, C.; Constantini, N.; Lebrun, C.; Lundy, B.; Melin, A.; Meyer, N.; et al. International Olympic Committee (IOC) Consensus Statement on Relative Energy Deficiency in Sport (RED-S): 2018 Update. *Int. J. Sport Nutr. Exerc. Metab.* **2018**, *28*, 316–331. [CrossRef] [PubMed]
43. Torstveit, M.K.; Sundgot-Borgen, J. Eating Disorders in Male and Female Athletes. In *The Encyclopaedia of Sports Medicine*; John Wiley & Sons, Ltd.: Hoboken, NJ, USA, 2013; pp. 513–525. ISBN 978-1-118-69231-8.
44. Sundgot-Borgen, J.; Danielsen, K.; Klungland-Torstveit, M. Female Former Elite Athletes Suffering from Eating Disorders during Their Career. A 15–20 Year Follow-Up. *Med. Sci. Sports Exerc.* **2012**, *44*, 267–958.
45. Soric, M.; Misigoj-Durakovic, M.; Pedisic, Z. Dietary Intake and Body Composition of Prepubescent Female Aesthetic Athletes. *Int. J. Sport Nutr. Exerc. Metab.* **2008**, *18*, 343–354. [CrossRef] [PubMed]
46. Caine, D.; Lewis, R.; O'Connor, P.; Howe, W.; Bass, S. Does Gymnastics Training Inhibit Growth of Females? *Clin. J. Sport Med. Off. J. Can. Acad. Sport Med.* **2001**, *11*, 260–270. [CrossRef] [PubMed]
47. Roemmich, J.N.; Sinning, W.E. Weight Loss and Wrestling Training: Effects on Nutrition, Growth, Maturation, Body Composition, and Strength. *J. Appl. Physiol.* **1997**, *82*, 1751–1759. [CrossRef] [PubMed]
48. Kelly, A.K.W.; Hecht, S.; Fitness, C. The Female Athlete Triad. *Pediatrics* **2016**, *138*, e20160922. [CrossRef]
49. Soleimany, G.; Dadgostar, H.; Lotfian, S.; Moradi-Lakeh, M.; Dadgostar, E.; Movaseghi, S. Bone Mineral Changes and Cardiovascular Effects among Female Athletes with Chronic Menstrual Dysfunction. *Asian J. Sports Med.* **2012**, *3*, 53–58. [CrossRef]
50. Hoch, A.Z.; Papanek, P.; Szabo, A.; Widlansky, M.E.; Schimke, J.E.; Gutterman, D.D. Association between the Female Athlete Triad and Endothelial Dysfunction in Dancers. *Clin. J. Sport Med. Off. J. Can. Acad. Sport Med.* **2011**, *21*, 119–125. [CrossRef]
51. Beals, K.A.; Hill, A.K. The Prevalence of Disordered Eating, Menstrual Dysfunction, and Low Bone Mineral Density among US Collegiate Athletes. *Int. J. Sport Nutr. Exerc. Metab.* **2006**, *16*, 1–23. [CrossRef]
52. Greenleaf, C.; Petrie, T.A.; Carter, J.; Reel, J.J. Female Collegiate Athletes: Prevalence of Eating Disorders and Disordered Eating Behaviors. *J. Am. Coll. Health J ACH* **2009**, *57*, 489–495. [CrossRef]
53. Dipasquale, L.; Petrie, T.A. Prevalence of Disordered Eating: A Comparison of Male and Female Collegiate Athletes and Nonathletes. *J. Clin. Sport Psychol.* **2013**, *7*, 186–197. [CrossRef]
54. Anderson, C.M.; Petrie, T.A.; Neumann, C.S. Psychosocial Correlates of Bulimic Symptoms among NCAA Division-I Female Collegiate Gymnasts and Swimmers/Divers. *J. Sport Exerc. Psychol.* **2011**, *33*, 483–505. [CrossRef] [PubMed]
55. Anderson, C.; Petrie, T.A. Prevalence of Disordered Eating and Pathogenic Weight Control Behaviors among NCAA Division I Female Collegiate Gymnasts and Swimmers. *Res. Q. Exerc. Sport* **2012**, *83*, 120–124. [CrossRef]
56. Sundgot-Borgen, J. Prevalence of Eating Disorders in Elite Female Athletes. *Int. J. Sport Nutr.* **1993**, *3*, 29–40. [CrossRef] [PubMed]
57. Loucks, A.B. Energy Balance and Energy Availability. In *The Encyclopaedia of Sports Medicine*; John Wiley & Sons, Ltd.: Hoboken, NJ, USA, 2013; pp. 72–87. ISBN 978-1-118-69231-8.
58. Manore, M.; Cialdella-Kam, L.; Loucks, A. The Female Athlete Triad: Components, Nutrition Issues, and Health Consequences. *J. Sports Sci.* **2007**, *25* (Suppl. 1), S61–S71. [CrossRef]

59. Ihle, R.; Loucks, A.B. Dose-Response Relationships between Energy Availability and Bone Turnover in Young Exercising Women. *J. Bone Miner. Res. Off. J. Am. Soc. Bone Miner. Res.* **2004**, *19*, 1231–1240. [CrossRef]
60. Beals, K.A. Eating Behaviors, Nutritional Status, and Menstrual Function in Elite Female Adolescent Volleyball Players. *J. Am. Diet. Assoc.* **2002**, *102*, 1293–1296. [CrossRef]
61. Brown, A.; Jones, S.W.; Rowan, H. Baby-Led Weaning: The Evidence to Date. *Curr. Nutr. Rep.* **2017**, *6*, 148–156. [CrossRef]
62. Souza, M.J.D.; Nattiv, A.; Joy, E.; Misra, M.; Williams, N.I.; Mallinson, R.J.; Gibbs, J.C.; Olmsted, M.; Goolsby, M.; Matheson, G.; et al. 2014 Female Athlete Triad Coalition Consensus Statement on Treatment and Return to Play of the Female Athlete Triad: 1st International Conference Held in San Francisco, California, May 2012 and 2nd International Conference Held in Indianapolis, Indiana, May 2013. *Br. J. Sports Med.* **2014**, *48*, 289. [CrossRef]
63. Ackerman, K.E.; Misra, M. Amenorrhoea in Adolescent Female Athletes. *Lancet Child Adolesc. Health* **2018**, *2*, 677–688. [CrossRef]
64. Thein-Nissenbaum, J.; Hammer, E. Treatment Strategies for the Female Athlete Triad in the Adolescent Athlete: Current Perspectives. *Open Access J. Sports Med.* **2017**, *8*, 85–95. [CrossRef] [PubMed]
65. Dwyer, J.; Eisenberg, A.; Prelack, K.; Song, W.O.; Sonneville, K.; Ziegler, P. Eating Attitudes and Food Intakes of Elite Adolescent Female Figure Skaters: A Cross Sectional Study. *J. Int. Soc. Sports Nutr.* **2012**, *9*, 53. [CrossRef]
66. De Oliveira Coelho, G.M.; de Farias, M.L.F.; de Mendonça, L.M.C.; de Mello, D.B.; Lanzillotti, H.S.; Ribeiro, B.G.; de Abreu Soares, E. The Prevalence of Disordered Eating and Possible Health Consequences in Adolescent Female Tennis Players from Rio de Janeiro, Brazil. *Appetite* **2013**, *64*, 39–47. [CrossRef]
67. Da Costa, N.F.; Schtscherbyna, A.; Soares, E.A.; Ribeiro, B.G. Disordered Eating among Adolescent Female Swimmers: Dietary, Biochemical, and Body Composition Factors. *Nutrition* **2013**, *29*, 172–177. [CrossRef]
68. Wood, K.L.; Barrack, M.T.; Gray, V.B.; Cotter, J.A.; Van Loan, M.D.; Rauh, M.J.; McGowan, R.; Nichols, J.F. Cognitive Dietary Restraint Score Is Associated with Lower Energy, Carbohydrate, Fat, and Grain Intake among Female Adolescent Endurance Runners. *Eat. Behav.* **2020**, *40*, 101460. [CrossRef]
69. Hoch, A.Z.; Pajewski, N.M.; Moraski, L.; Carrera, G.F.; Wilson, C.R.; Hoffmann, R.G.; Schimke, J.E.; Gutterman, D.D. Prevalence of the Female Athlete Triad in High School Athletes and Sedentary Students. *Clin. J. Sport Med. Off. J. Can. Acad. Sport Med.* **2009**, *19*, 421–428. [CrossRef]
70. Silva, M.-R.G.; Silva, H.-H.; Paiva, T. Sleep Duration, Body Composition, Dietary Profile and Eating Behaviours among Children and Adolescents: A Comparison between Portuguese Acrobatic Gymnasts. *Eur. J. Pediatr.* **2018**, *177*, 815–825. [CrossRef] [PubMed]
71. Braun, H.; von Andrian-Werburg, J.; Schänzer, W.; Thevis, M. Nutrition Status of Young Elite Female German Football Players. *Pediatr. Exerc. Sci.* **2018**, *30*, 157–167. [CrossRef] [PubMed]
72. Matt, S.A.; Barrack, M.T.; Gray, V.B.; Cotter, J.A.; Van Loan, M.D.; Rauh, M.J.; McGowan, R.; Nichols, J.F. Adolescent Endurance Runners Exhibit Suboptimal Energy Availability and Intakes of Key Nutrients. *J. Am. Coll. Nutr.* **2021**, 1–8. [CrossRef] [PubMed]
73. Defeciani, L. Eating Disorders and Body Image Concerns Among Male Athletes. *Clin. Soc. Work J.* **2016**, *44*. [CrossRef]
74. Vertalino, M.; Eisenberg, M.E.; Story, M.; Neumark-Sztainer, D. Participation in Weight-Related Sports Is Associated with Higher Use of Unhealthful Weight-Control Behaviors and Steroid Use. *J. Am. Diet. Assoc.* **2007**, *107*, 434–440. [CrossRef]
75. Koehler, K.; Achtzehn, S.; Braun, H.; Mester, J.; Schaenzer, W. Comparison of Self-Reported Energy Availability and Metabolic Hormones to Assess Adequacy of Dietary Energy Intake in Young Elite Athletes. *Appl. Physiol. Nutr. Metab.* **2013**, *38*, 725–733. [CrossRef] [PubMed]
76. Deutz, R.C.; Benardot, D.; Martin, D.E.; Cody, M.M. Relationship between Energy Deficits and Body Composition in Elite Female Gymnasts and Runners. *Med. Sci. Sports Exerc.* **2000**, *32*, 659–668. [CrossRef]
77. Melin, A.; Tornberg, Å.B.; Skouby, S.; Møller, S.S.; Sundgot-Borgen, J.; Faber, J.; Sidelmann, J.J.; Aziz, M.; Sjödin, A. Energy Availability and the Female Athlete Triad in Elite Endurance Athletes. *Scand. J. Med. Sci. Sports* **2015**, *25*, 610–622. [CrossRef] [PubMed]
78. Woods, A.L.; Garvican-Lewis, L.A.; Lundy, B.; Rice, A.J.; Thompson, K.G. New Approaches to Determine Fatigue in Elite Athletes during Intensified Training: Resting Metabolic Rate and Pacing Profile. *PLoS ONE* **2017**, *12*, e0173807. [CrossRef]
79. Burke, L.M. Carbohydrate Needs of Athletes in Training. In *The Encyclopaedia of Sports Medicine*; John Wiley & Sons, Ltd.: Hoboken, NJ, USA, 2013; pp. 102–112. ISBN 978-1-118-69231-8.
80. Manore, M.M. Dietary Recommendations and Athletic Menstrual Dysfunction. *Sports Med.* **2002**, *32*, 887–901. [CrossRef]
81. Woolf, K.; Manore, M. B-Vitamins and Exercise: Does Exercise Alter Requirements? *Int. J. Sport Nutr. Exerc. Metab.* **2006**, *16*, 453–484. [CrossRef]
82. Ziegler, P.; Hensley, S.; Roepke, J.B.; Whitaker, S.H.; Craig, B.W.; Drewnowski, A. Eating Attitudes and Energy Intakes of Female Skaters. *Med. Sci. Sports Exerc.* **1998**, *30*, 583–586. [CrossRef]
83. Barrack, M.T.; Rauh, M.J.; Barkai, H.-S.; Nichols, J.F. Dietary Restraint and Low Bone Mass in Female Adolescent Endurance Runners. *Am. J. Clin. Nutr.* **2008**, *87*, 36–43. [CrossRef]
84. Golden, N.H.; Schneider, M.; Wood, C.; Adolescence, C.O.; Obesity, S.O. Preventing Obesity and Eating Disorders in Adolescents. *Pediatrics* **2016**, *138*, e20161649. [CrossRef]
85. Barrack, M.T.; Rauh, M.J.; Nichols, J.F. Prevalence of and Traits Associated with Low BMD among Female Adolescent Runners. *Med. Sci. Sports Exerc.* **2008**, *40*, 2015–2021. [CrossRef]

86. Christo, K.; Prabhakaran, R.; Lamparello, B.; Cord, J.; Miller, K.K.; Goldstein, M.A.; Gupta, N.; Herzog, D.B.; Klibanski, A.; Misra, M. Bone Metabolism in Adolescent Athletes With Amenorrhea, Athletes With Eumenorrhea, and Control Subjects. *Pediatrics* **2008**, *121*, 1127–1136. [CrossRef] [PubMed]
87. Skorseth, P.; Segovia, N.; Hastings, K.; Kraus, E. Prevalence of Female Athlete Triad Risk Factors and Iron Supplementation Among High School Distance Runners: Results From a Triad Risk Screening Tool. *Orthop. J. Sports Med.* **2020**, *8*, 2325967120959725. [CrossRef]
88. Javed, A.; Tebben, P.J.; Fischer, P.R.; Lteif, A.N. Female Athlete Triad and Its Components: Toward Improved Screening and Management. *Mayo Clin. Proc.* **2013**, *88*, 996–1009. [CrossRef]
89. Weimann, E.; Witzel, C.; Schwidergall, S.; Böhles, H.J. Peripubertal Perturbations in Elite Gymnasts Caused by Sport Specific Training Regimes and Inadequate Nutritional Intake. *Int. J. Sports Med.* **2000**, *21*, 210–215. [CrossRef] [PubMed]
90. Rauh, M.J.; Nichols, J.F.; Barrack, M.T. Relationships among Injury and Disordered Eating, Menstrual Dysfunction, and Low Bone Mineral Density in High School Athletes: A Prospective Study. *J. Athl. Train.* **2010**, *45*, 243–252. [CrossRef] [PubMed]
91. Thralls, K.J.; Nichols, J.F.; Barrack, M.T.; Kern, M.; Rauh, M.J. Body Mass-Related Predictors of the Female Athlete Triad Among Adolescent Athletes. *Int. J. Sport Nutr. Exerc. Metab.* **2016**, *26*, 17–25. [CrossRef] [PubMed]
92. Barrack, M.T.; Van Loan, M.D.; Rauh, M.J.; Nichols, J.F. Physiologic and Behavioral Indicators of Energy Deficiency in Female Adolescent Runners with Elevated Bone Turnover. *Am. J. Clin. Nutr.* **2010**, *92*, 652–659. [CrossRef] [PubMed]
93. Tenforde, A.S.; Fredericson, M.; Sayres, L.C.; Cutti, P.; Sainani, K.L. Identifying Sex-Specific Risk Factors for Low Bone Mineral Density in Adolescent Runners. *Am. J. Sports Med.* **2015**, *43*, 1494–1504. [CrossRef] [PubMed]
94. Nose-Ogura, S.; Yoshino, O.; Dohi, M.; Kigawa, M.; Harada, M.; Hiraike, O.; Onda, T.; Osuga, Y.; Fujii, T.; Saito, S. Risk Factors of Stress Fractures Due to the Female Athlete Triad: Differences in Teens and Twenties. *Scand. J. Med. Sci. Sports* **2019**, *29*, 1501–1510. [CrossRef]
95. Committee on Sports Medicine and Fitness Promotion of Healthy Weight-Control Practices in Young Athletes. *Pediatrics* **2005**, *116*, 1557–1564. [CrossRef]
96. Carl, R.L.; Johnson, M.D.; Martin, T.J.; Fitness, C. Promotion of Healthy Weight-Control Practices in Young Athletes. *Pediatrics* **2017**, *140*. [CrossRef]
97. Oppliger, R.A.; Landry, G.L.; Foster, S.W.; Lambrecht, A.C. Bulimic Behaviors among Interscholastic Wrestlers: A Statewide Survey. *Pediatrics* **1993**, *91*, 826–831.
98. Kiningham, R.B.; Gorenflo, D.W. Weight Loss Methods of High School Wrestlers. *Med. Sci. Sports Exerc.* **2001**, *33*, 810–813. [CrossRef]
99. Petrie, H.J.; Stover, E.A.; Horswill, C.A. Nutritional Concerns for the Child and Adolescent Competitor. *Nutr. Burbank Los Angel. City Calif.* **2004**, *20*, 620–631. [CrossRef] [PubMed]
100. Meyer, F.; Volterman, K.A.; Timmons, B.W.; Wilk, B. Fluid Balance and Dehydration in the Young Athlete: Assessment Considerations and Effects on Health and Performance. *Am. J. Lifestyle Med.* **2012**, *6*, 489–501. [CrossRef]
101. Rankin, J.W. Weight Loss and Gain in Athletes. *Curr. Sports Med. Rep.* **2002**, *1*, 208–213. [CrossRef]
102. Jones, L.C.; Cleary, M.A.; Lopez, R.M.; Zuri, R.E.; Lopez, R. Active Dehydration Impairs Upper and Lower Body Anaerobic Muscular Power. *J. Strength Cond. Res.* **2008**, *22*, 455–463. [CrossRef]
103. Judelson, D.A.; Maresh, C.M.; Anderson, J.M.; Armstrong, L.E.; Casa, D.J.; Kraemer, W.J.; Volek, J.S. Hydration and Muscular Performance: Does Fluid Balance Affect Strength, Power and High-Intensity Endurance? *Sports Med.* **2007**, *37*, 907–921. [CrossRef]
104. Hayes, L.D.; Morse, C.I. The Effects of Progressive Dehydration on Strength and Power: Is There a Dose Response? *Eur. J. Appl. Physiol.* **2010**, *108*, 701–707. [CrossRef] [PubMed]
105. Logue, D.M.; Madigan, S.M.; Melin, A.; Delahunt, E.; Heinen, M.; Donnell, S.-J.M.; Corish, C.A. Low Energy Availability in Athletes 2020: An Updated Narrative Review of Prevalence, Risk, Within-Day Energy Balance, Knowledge, and Impact on Sports Performance. *Nutrients* **2020**, *12*, 835. [CrossRef]
106. De Souza, M.J.; Koltun, K.J.; Williams, N.I. The Role of Energy Availability in Reproductive Function in the Female Athlete Triad and Extension of Its Effects to Men: An Initial Working Model of a Similar Syndrome in Male Athletes. *Sports Med.* **2019**, *49*, 125–137. [CrossRef] [PubMed]
107. Maïmoun, L.; Georgopoulos, N.A.; Sultan, C. Endocrine Disorders in Adolescent and Young Female Athletes: Impact on Growth, Menstrual Cycles, and Bone Mass Acquisition. *J. Clin. Endocrinol. Metab.* **2014**, *99*, 4037–4050. [CrossRef] [PubMed]
108. Drew, M.; Vlahovich, N.; Hughes, D.; Appaneal, R.; Burke, L.M.; Lundy, B.; Rogers, M.; Toomey, M.; Watts, D.; Lovell, G.; et al. Prevalence of Illness, Poor Mental Health and Sleep Quality and Low Energy Availability Prior to the 2016 Summer Olympic Games. *Br. J. Sports Med.* **2018**, *52*, 47–53. [CrossRef]
109. Areta, J.L.; Taylor, H.L.; Koehler, K. Low Energy Availability: History, Definition and Evidence of Its Endocrine, Metabolic and Physiological Effects in Prospective Studies in Females and Males. *Eur. J. Appl. Physiol.* **2021**, *121*, 1–21. [CrossRef]
110. Koehler, K.; Hoerner, N.R.; Gibbs, J.C.; Zinner, C.; Braun, H.; De Souza, M.J.; Schaenzer, W. Low Energy Availability in Exercising Men Is Associated with Reduced Leptin and Insulin but Not with Changes in Other Metabolic Hormones. *J. Sports Sci.* **2016**, *34*, 1921–1929. [CrossRef]
111. Fagerberg, P. Negative Consequences of Low Energy Availability in Natural Male Bodybuilding: A Review. *Int. J. Sport Nutr. Exerc. Metab.* **2018**, *28*, 385–402. [CrossRef]

112. Kojima, C.; Ishibashi, A.; Tanabe, Y.; Iwayama, K.; Kamei, A.; Takahashi, H.; Goto, K. Muscle Glycogen Content during Endurance Training under Low Energy Availability. *Med. Sci. Sports Exerc.* **2020**, *52*, 187–195. [CrossRef] [PubMed]
113. Petrie, T.; Galli, N.; Greenleaf, C.; Reel, J.; Carter, J. Psychosocial Correlates of Bulimic Symptomatology among Male Athletes. *Psychol. Sport Exerc.* **2014**, *15*, 680–687. [CrossRef]
114. Wasserfurth, P.; Palmowski, J.; Hahn, A.; Krüger, K. Reasons for and Consequences of Low Energy Availability in Female and Male Athletes: Social Environment, Adaptations, and Prevention. *Sports Med. Open* **2020**, *6*, 44. [CrossRef]
115. Arnaoutis, G.; Kavouras, S.A.; Angelopoulou, A.; Skoulariki, C.; Bismpikou, S.; Mourtakos, S.; Sidossis, L.S. Fluid Balance During Training in Elite Young Athletes of Different Sports. *J. Strength Cond. Res.* **2015**, *29*, 3447–3452. [CrossRef] [PubMed]

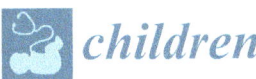

Review

Neuroimaging Findings in Adolescents and Young Adults with Anorexia Nervosa: A Systematic Review

Kalliopi Kappou [1,†], Myrto Ntougia [1,†], Aikaterini Kourtesi [1], Eleni Panagouli [1], Elpis Vlachopapadopoulou [2], Stefanos Michalacos [2], Fragiskos Gonidakis [3], Georgios Mastorakos [4], Theodora Psaltopoulou [1,5], Maria Tsolia [1], Flora Bacopoulou [6], Theodoros N. Sergentanis [1,5,‡] and Artemis Tsitsika [1,*,‡]

1. MSc "Strategies of Developmental and Adolescent Health", 2nd Department of Pediatrics, "P. & A. Kyriakou" Children's Hospital, School of Medicine, National and Kapodistrian University of Athens, 115 27 Athens, Greece; kappouk5@gmail.com (K.K.); myntou@gmail.com (M.N.); kourtesikaterina@yahoo.com (A.K.); elenpana@med.uoa.gr (E.P.); tpsaltop@med.uoa.gr (T.P.); mariantsolia@gmail.com (M.T.); tsergentanis@yahoo.gr (T.N.S.)
2. Department of Endocrinology-Growth and Development, "P. & A. Kyriakou" Children's Hospital, 115 27 Athens, Greece; elpis.vl@gmail.com (E.V.); stmichalakos@gmail.com (S.M.)
3. First Department of Psychiatry, Medical School, National and Kapodistrian University of Athens, Eginition Hospital, 115 28 Athens, Greece; frgonid@med.uoa.gr
4. Unit of Endocrinology, Diabetes Mellitus and Metabolism, Aretaieion Hospital, School of Medicine, National and Kapodistrian University of Athens, 115 28 Athens, Greece; gmastorak@med.uoa.gr
5. Department of Clinical Therapeutics, "Alexandra" Hospital, School of Medicine, National and Kapodistrian University of Athens, 115 28 Athens, Greece
6. Center for Adolescent Medicine and UNESCO Chair Adolescent Health Care, First Department of Pediatrics, "Agia Sophia" Children's Hospital, School of Medicine, National and Kapodistrian University of Athens, 115 27 Athens, Greece; bacopouf@hotmail.com
* Correspondence: info@youth-health.gr; Tel./Fax: +30-210-771-0824
† The two first authors contributed equally to this manuscript.
‡ The two senior authors contributed equally to this manuscript.

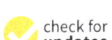

Citation: Kappou, K.; Ntougia, M.; Kourtesi, A.; Panagouli, E.; Vlachopapadopoulou, E.; Michalacos, S.; Gonidakis, F.; Mastorakos, G.; Psaltopoulou, T.; Tsolia, M.; et al. Neuroimaging Findings in Adolescents and Young Adults with Anorexia Nervosa: A Systematic Review. *Children* **2021**, *8*, 137. https://doi.org/10.3390/children8020137

Academic Editor: Tonia Vassilakou

Received: 31 December 2020
Accepted: 3 February 2021
Published: 12 February 2021

Publisher's Note: MDPI stays neutral with regard to jurisdictional claims in published maps and institutional affiliations.

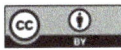

Copyright: © 2021 by the authors. Licensee MDPI, Basel, Switzerland. This article is an open access article distributed under the terms and conditions of the Creative Commons Attribution (CC BY) license (https:// creativecommons.org/licenses/by/ 4.0/).

Abstract: Background: Anorexia nervosa (AN) is a serious, multifactorial mental disorder affecting predominantly young females. This systematic review examines neuroimaging findings in adolescents and young adults up to 24 years old, in order to explore alterations associated with disease pathophysiology. Methods: Eligible studies on structural and functional brain neuroimaging were sought systematically in PubMed, CENTRAL and EMBASE databases up to 5 October 2020. Results: Thirty-three studies were included, investigating a total of 587 patients with a current diagnosis of AN and 663 healthy controls (HC). Global and regional grey matter (GM) volume reduction as well as white matter (WM) microstructure alterations were detected. The mainly affected regions were the prefrontal, parietal and temporal cortex, hippocampus, amygdala, insula, thalamus and cerebellum as well as various WM tracts such as corona radiata and superior longitudinal fasciculus (SLF). Regarding functional imaging, alterations were pointed out in large-scale brain networks, such as default mode network (DMN), executive control network (ECN) and salience network (SN). Most findings appear to reverse after weight restoration. Specific limitations of neuroimaging studies in still developing individuals are also discussed. Conclusions: Structural and functional alterations are present in the early course of the disease, most of them being partially or totally reversible. Nonetheless, neuroimaging findings have been open to many biological interpretations. Thus, more studies are needed to clarify their clinical significance.

Keywords: anorexia nervosa; neuroimaging; magnetic resonance imaging; diffusion tensor imaging; single photon emission computed tomography; magnetic resonance spectroscopy

1. Introduction

Anorexia nervosa (AN) is a serious mental disorder affecting predominantly adolescent girls and young adult women. Although relatively rare, it is the third most common chronic disease during adolescence [1,2]. It is characterized by a significantly low body weight, an intense fear of gaining weight, a disturbed perception of one's body image and a persistent lack of recognition of the seriousness of the condition [3]. Patients display marked treatment resistance or no response to treatment, frequent medical complications and a substantial risk of death. [4] The two designated subtypes of the disease are the restricting type (R—AN), which describes presentations in which weight loss is accomplished primarily through food restriction and/or excessive exercise and the binge eating/purging type (BP—AN), which is characterized by recurrent episodes of binge eating or purging behavior. The restricting subtype is associated with an earlier age of onset, a better prognosis, and a greater likelihood of crossover to the other subtype [3].

Coexisting psychiatric disorders include bipolar, depressive and anxiety disorders, as well as obsessive and compulsive disorder (OCD) (especially among those with the restrictive subtype) and alcohol and other substance use disorder (especially among those with the binge/purging subtype) [3]. The underlying mechanisms that drive anorectic patients to deprive themselves of food while being hungry and emaciated are not yet fully understood. Current knowledge suggests that the disease is an interface between genetic and biological predispositions, environmental and sociocultural influences, and psychological traits [5].

Compared to other mental health disorders, the number of neuroimaging studies in AN is relatively small, although the literature is rapidly growing. Structural magnetic resonance imaging (MRI) has been long used to investigate volumetric differences between AN patients and healthy controls (HC). The first systematic review of structural MRI studies in AN patients was that by Van den Eynde et al. who did not find clear evidence for global grey matter (GM) and white matter (WM) volume reductions, and unraveled only preliminary findings for regionally reduced GM [6]. Systematic reviews and meta-analyses that followed have reported significant global reductions in GM and WM volumes as well as significant increase in cerebrospinal fluid (CSF) [7–9]. In a recent meta-analysis, adolescent patients showed greater reduction in GM volume than adults (7.6% vs. 3.7%) [10]. Similarly, WM was also significantly reduced in both adolescent and adult patients, on average 3.2% and 2.2% respectively, while CSF was conversely increased by 15%. These findings seem to normalize after long-term recovery, especially for the adult population, while for adolescents data are scarce [7,10]. Regional volume decreases have also been detected, more pronounced in the cingulate cortex, the supplementary motor area (SMA) and the amygdala [11]. On the other hand, studies in adult patients have demonstrated increased GM volumes in the insula and orbitofrontal cortex (OFC) [12–14].

While MRI identifies volumetric changes, magnetic resonance spectroscopy (MRS), provides information about the metabolism of brain tissues. Proton-MRS or Phosphorus-MRS offers various data regarding membrane composition and functionality, neuronal consistence and glial cells integrity, through the measurement of various metabolites such as choline (Cho) and total choline-containing metabolites (tCho), glutamate/glutamine (Glx), N-acetyl-aspartate (NAA), myo-Inositol (mI), total creatine compounds (tCr) and ethanolamine containing metabolites. In line with structural MRI studies, GM seems to be more affected than WM and these molecular changes could be identified before structural alterations become apparent, providing the benefit of early intervention [15,16].

In parallel with structural neuroimaging, researchers have further investigated functional brain processes to elucidate the causative underpinning of the disease. One of the most frequently used brain imaging techniques is functional magnetic resonance imaging (fMRI). Altered activation of the amygdala and insula has been consistently observed in patients with AN during passive viewing of visual food stimuli [17]. With regard to taste stimuli, most studies conclude to increased activation in reward-related regions [18,19]. In addition, fMRI studies utilizing body image related tasks have reported alterations of the precuneus, the inferior parietal lobe, the prefrontal cortex (PFC), the insula and the amygdala [20]. A recent systematic review of fMRI studies has provided evidence of impaired cognitive flexibility and social cognition skills in adolescent patients [21].

These published papers have reported considerable inconsistencies which could be attributed to differences in study design, selection of the stimuli or task and to the cognitive abilities of the participants. An approach to potentially overcome these inconsistencies is the investigation of resting-state functional connectivity (RSFC). With this technique potential biases stemming from the effort to perform a task are diminished, although unwanted thoughts, emotional status and ruminations could potentially affect RSFC [22]. The first RSFC study in AN adult patients was conducted by Cowdrey et al., who found increased RSFC between the default mode network (DMN) and the precuneus and the dorsolateral prefrontal cortex (dlPFC) when comparing patients with controls [23]. In a recent systematic review of fMRI studies, functional alterations were encountered in areas and networks related to the main symptoms of the disease, such as impaired cognitive control and body image disturbances [24]. These functional alterations are in line with data emerging from electroencephalography studies, showing decreased electrical activity in frontal and parietal-occipital regions during cognitive tasks. Likewise, altered electrical activity in fusiform gyrus and parahippocampal gyrus is demonstrated during resting-state paradigms [25].

On the other hand, fMRI is unable to identify and evaluate more precisely the functionality of brain neurotransmitters. For that purpose, single-photon emission computed tomography (SPECT) has been used. This three-dimensional nuclear medicine imaging technique provides information about regional cerebral blood flow (rCBF), showing alterations in perfusion and thus, evaluating brain functionality [26]. Moreover, by injecting radionuclides that selectively attach to receptors, specific information about neurotransmission can be provided. In particular, the serotonin neuronal system has been extensively studied, as it is believed to play a crucial role in the pathophysiology of AN, being involved in many cognitive features of patients and, therefore, providing possible therapy targets [26–28].

In recent years, the micro-architecture of WM axons connecting the abovementioned areas has been further explored by using diffusion tensor imaging (DTI). Four indices of diffusion are commonly used: fractional anisotropy (FA), mean diffusivity (MD), axial diffusivity (AD) and radial diffusivity (RD). Monzon et al. were the first to systematically review the limited at that time literature on DTI studies in AN [29]. They reported alterations in a range of WM structures of the limbic system as well as the fronto-occipital fiber tracts. In a more recent systematic review, Gaudio et al. concluded that patients with AN showed mainly WM microstructure abnormalities in thalamo-cortical tracts and occipital-parietal-temporal-frontal tracts [30]. The researchers were not able to draw a clear conclusion whether these alterations persist after recovery or not. To our knowledge, three meta-analyses have been published so far. In the first one, the quantitative voxel-based meta-analysis identified decreased FA in the posterior areas of the corpus callosum, the left superior longitudinal fasciculus (SLF) II and the left precentral gyrus as well as increased FA in the right corticospinal projections and lingual gyrus [31]. In the second one, Meneguzzo et al. identified two clusters of decreased FA, in the left corona radiata and in the left thalamus [32]. Finally, more recently, Zhang et al. analyzed DTI studies using tractbased spatial statistics (TBSS) and reported lower FA in the corpus callosum and the cingulum [33].

The aim of this paper is to systematically review current literature concerning structural and functional brain alterations in patients with AN, focusing on adolescents and young adults. Building on previous findings, our principal objective is to identify the main areas, networks and circuits that are vulnerable to the effects of the disease, while making an effort to disambiguate between effects of starvation and alterations possibly contributing to the pathogenesis of the disease.

The Adolescent Brain

AN has its peak incidence between 13–18 years old [5]. Neuroimaging studies in adolescent patients at the early stages of the disease can provide the clinicians with valuable information with regard to early biomarkers before the effects of malnutrition become apparent. Nonetheless, the interpretation of findings is particularly challenging, as adolescence is a period of profound morphological and functional changes. In fact, adolescence is a very active period regarding neurodevelopment. A hallmark of the brain transformations is synaptic pruning, a highly specific process that has been speculated to help with the "rewiring" of brain connections into adult-typical patterns [34]. On the other hand, myelin production escalates during adolescence, leading to acceleration of speed and efficiency of information flow across distant brain regions [35]. In specific areas such as the PFC, myelin continues to increase until early adulthood, delaying maturation [36]. The combination of dendritic pruning and increased myelination of WM tracts results in the developmental "thinning" of the neocortex, a decline in thickness of outer layers of the brain that play an important role in high order functions [34]. Animal studies have shown that the abovementioned changes are critically driven by sex hormones [37]. Functional brain organization undergoes significant changes as well, shifting from a local connectivity pattern to a more distributed architecture [38,39]. In addition, the interconnectivity of core neurocognitive networks continues to change throughout adolescence, becoming other stronger or weaker. The net result of these developmental changes likely is the attainment of mature functional networks, optimally capable of supporting cognitive and behavioral demands [40]. Summarizing, we could suppose that the ongoing developing brain may be substantially vulnerable to the effects of starvation, which could disrupt the normal development. Understanding the normal developmental processes is critical for the interpretation of alterations observed in adolescent neuroimaging.

2. Materials and Methods

2.1. Search Strategy Criteria

The present systematic review was performed in accordance with the Preferred Reporting Items for Systematic Reviews and Meta-Analyses (PRISMA) guidelines [1]. A systematic and comprehensive search of PubMed, EMBASE and CENTRAL was carried out for papers published between database inception and October 2020. We used the following search algorithm: brain AND ("anorexia nervosa") AND ("computed tomography" OR CT OR SPECT OR "SPECT-CT" OR "magnetic resonance imaging" OR MRI OR "functional MRI" OR "functional magnetic resonance tomography"). End-of-search date was set at 5 October 2020. Further article identification through reference lists of full text examined papers completed the research.

2.2. Selection Criteria

The eligibility criteria were based on the PICOS (Participants, Intervention, Comparison, Outcomes, Study design) acronym. To be included in the review, studies had to fulfill the following criteria: (i). written in English language; (ii). investigated participants aged between 10 and 24 years old with a current diagnosis of AN; (iii). were of case-control, cross-sectional or longitudinal design; (iv). excluded patients with a comorbid psychiatric disorder other than depression, anxious disorder or OCD; (v). excluded participants taking psychotropic medications other than antidepressants or anti-anxiety medications. Regarding fMRI studies, only resting-state fMRI studies were included, while task-based or stimuli-based fMRI papers were excluded due to space limitations. Due to the lack of sufficient papers using the same methodological approach, a meta-analysis was not performed.

2.3. Quality Assessment and Data Extraction

Two authors (KPK and MSN) independently screened titles and abstracts from retrieved papers and analyzed full-text articles that met the eligibility criteria. Disagreements were resolved through consensus. The quality of the final studies was assessed by using the Newcastle–Ottawa scale. Two reviewers independently performed data extraction as follows: study design, demographic information (age, gender), sample size, age (mean age, age range), Body Mass Index (mean BMI), AN subtype, criteria for diagnosis, illness duration, co-morbidity and medication, scanning method and data analysis method. For DTI studies in particular, hydration status before neuroimaging was extracted as well.

2.4. Search Results and Selection of Studies

The search strategy yielded 857 articles, 33 of which met the inclusion criteria. The PRISMA flow diagram (Figure 1) shows selection and exclusion of studies.

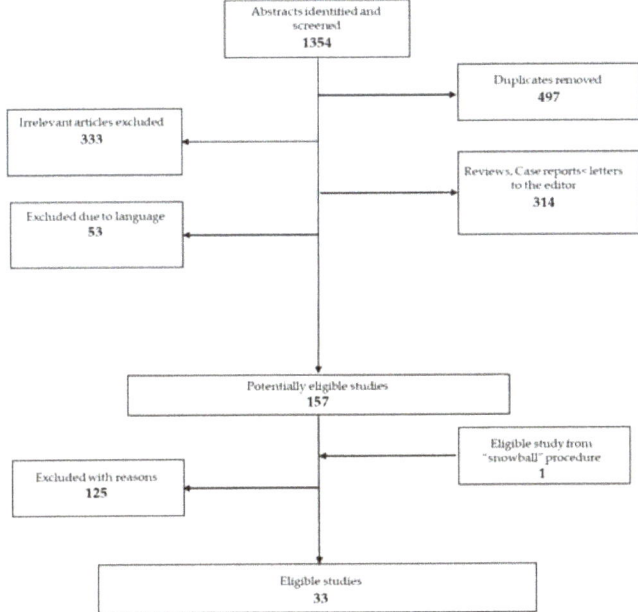

Figure 1. PRISMA flow chart.

2.5. Compliance with Ethics Guidelines

This article consists a review of previously conducted studies, which complies with the PRISMA guidelines [41].

3. Results

3.1. Study Characteristics

Selection of studies is presented in the flow chart (Figure 1); full-text studies excluded due to various reasons (n = 125) are presented in Supplemental Table S1. Overall, the 33 eligible studies included 587 participants with a current diagnosis of AN and 663 HC. Of the 33 studies, 31 were cross-sectional (9 also had a longitudinal follow-up) and 2 were longitudinal studies. Eighteen studies were conducted in a sample of exclusively adolescent patients for a total of 310 patients and 307 controls, while the remaining included both adolescents and young adults, for a total of 277 patients and 356 controls. Twenty-three studies examined structural imaging. Thirteen studies used structural MRI, 7 used DTI (2 of which provided also structural MRI data) and 3 used MRS. Their description is summarized in Tables 1 and 2. Ten studies examined functional imaging. Six studies performed resting-state fMRI (3 of which performed also structural MRI) and the remaining 4 used SPECT. Their characteristics are presented in Table 3. Risk of bias assessment is presented in Supplemental Table S2a,b.

Table 1. Structural imaging studies—sample characteristics.

Study	Study Design	Subtypes	Males (%)	Mean Age (Years)	Age Range (Years)	Mean BMI (Kg/m²)	Duration of Follow-up (Months)	2nd Imaging Participation	2nd Mean BMI (Kg/m²)	Measure Adapted for 2nd Imaging	Criteria for Diagnosis	Duration of Illness (Months)	Patients under Medication (%)
MRI													
Katzman (1996)	Cross-sectional	AN-R: 13 HC: 8	0	15.2	13.3–17.0	15.6	-	-	-	-	DSM-III-R	11.3	0
Olivo (2018)	Cross-sectional	Atypical AN: 22 HC: 38	0	14.7	13–18	19.3	-	-	-	-	DSM-V	7.9	0
Myrvang (2018)	Cross-sectional	AN-R: 33 HC: 28	0	15.8	12.4–19.2	16.3	-	-	-	-	DSM-V	19.2	23.3
King (2015)	Cross-sectional	AN-R: 36 AN-BP: 4 HC: 40	0	15.9	12–23	14.8	-	-	-	-	DSM-IV	18	Not mentioned
Yue (2018)	Cross-sectional	AN-R: 17 AN-BP: 18 HC: 20	0	19.3	15–23	15.3	-	-	-	-	DSM-IV TR	33.3	0
Fujisawa (2015)	Cross-sectional	AN-R: 20 HC: 14	0	14.2	12–17	14.4	-	-	-	-	DSM-IV TR	23.55	0
Neumärker (2000)	Cross-sectional (longitudinal)	AN-R: 14 AN-BP: 4 HC: 25	0	14.5	13–16	14.9	Not mentioned	100%	17.8	Weight normalization	ICD-10	267.8	Not mentioned
Castro-Fornieles (2009)	Cross-sectional (longitudinal)	AN-R: 9 AN-BP: 3 HC: 9	8.3	14.5	11–17	14.8	6	100%	18.8	Weight normalization.	DSM-IV TR	8.3	8.3
Monzon (2017)	Cross-sectional (longitudinal)	AN: 26 HC: 10	0	16.5	14–19	16.7	2	38%	18.9	Weight gain	DSM-V	Less than 36	Not mentioned
Golden (1996)	Cross-sectional (longitudinal)	AN: 12 HC: 12	0	16.1	11–22	14.3	11	100%	17.9	Weight normalization	DSM-III	Not mentioned	Not mentioned

Table 1. Cont.

Study	Study Design	Subtypes	Males (%)	Mean Age (Years)	Age Range (Years)	Mean BMI (Kg/m^2)	Duration of Follow-up (Months)	2nd Imaging Participation	2nd Mean BMI (Kg/m^2)	Measure Adapted for 2nd Imaging	Criteria for Diagnosis	Duration of Illness (Months)	Patients under Medication (%)
Akgül (2016)	Cross-sectional (longitudinal)	AN: 9 HC: 9	11	15.8	13–21	16.3	14	100%	19.2	Weight normalization	DSM-IV	8.7	0
Bernardoni (2016)	Cross-sectional (longitudinal)	AN-R: 43 AN-BP: 4 HC: 35	0	15.5	12–23	14.8	3	35	18.7	Weight gain	DSM-IV	Not mentioned	0
Katzman (1997)	Cross-sectional (longitudinal)	AN: 6 HC: 6	0	17.0	15–19	15.9	24	100%	23.0	Weight normalization	DSM-III-R	22.5	0
MRS													
Schlemmer (1997)	Cross-sectional	AN-R: 8 AN-BP: 2 HC: 17	0	16.0	14.9–19	14.7	-	-	-	-	DSM-IV	Not mentioned	0
Blasel (2012)	Cross-sectional	AN-R: 19 AN-BP: 2 HC: 29	0	14.4	11–17	14.4	-	-	-	-	DSM-IV	11	0
Castro-Formieles (2007)	Cross-sectional (longitudinal)	AN-R: 9 AN-BP: 3 HC: 12	8.3	14.5	11–17	14.8	7	100%	-	Weight normalization	DSM-IV-TR	Not mentioned	8.3
MRI-DTI													
Pfuhl (2016)	Cross-sectional	AN: 35 HC:62	0	16.1	12–24	14.7	-	-	-	-	DSM-IV	Not mentioned	0
Hu (2017)	Cross-sectional	AN-R: 8 HC:14	0	17.6	15–22	14.3	-	-	-	-	DSM-IV	10.5	Not mentioned
Gaudio (2017)	Cross-sectional	AN-R: 14 HC:15	0	15.7	13–18	16.2	-	-	-	-	DSM-IV-TR	4.9	0
K. E.Travis (2015)	Cross-sectional	AN-R: 15 HC:15	0	16.6	14–18	16	-	-	-	-	DSM-IV	16.3	2

Table 1. Cont.

Study	Study Design	Subtypes	Males (%)	Mean Age (Years)	Age Range (Years)	Mean BMI (Kg/m²)	Duration of Follow-up (Months)	2nd Imaging Partici-Pation	2nd Mean BMI (Kg/m²)	Measure Adapted for 2nd Imaging	Criteria for Diagnosis	Duration of Illness (Months)	Patients under Medication (%)
K. Vogel (2016)	Cross-sectional (longitudinal)	AN-R: 19 AN-BP: 3 HC: 21	0	15.03	10–18	15.36	4.76	41%	17.4	Weight gain	DSM-IV	13.49	1
G. Olivo (2018)	Cross-sectional	AAN: 25 HC:25	0	14.08	13–18	18.6	-	-	-	-	DSM-V	8.4	0
Von Schwanenflug (2018)	Cross-sectional (longitudinal)	AN-R: 53 AN-BP: 3 HC:60	0	15.8	12–27	14.7	3	83%	18.7	Weight gain	DSM-IV	14.5	Not mentioned

Table 2. Structural imaging studies—methods, main findings and clinical interpretations.

Study	Method and Procedure	Data Analysis	Hydration before Imaging for DTI Studies	Presentation of the Main Findings	Clinical Interpretations
MRI					
Katzman (1996)	MRI 1.5T Tested at one time point.	Not mentioned		Significantly larger total CSF volume and reduced total GM and WM volumes. Alterations correlated with BMI and cortisol levels. No correlation with disease duration.	No clinical interpretations. Deficits in GM volume were associated with severity but not disease duration and were related to hypercortisolemia.
Olivo (2018)	MRI 3T Tested at one time point.	Voxel based morphometry (VBM)		Total GM, WM, and CSF volumes were not significantly different between groups.	The preservation of GM volume might indeed differentiate atypical AN from AN. Alternatively, there may be a weight cut-off under which GM alterations become obvious.
Myrvang (2018)	MRI 3T Tested at one time point.	Magnetization Prepared— RApid Gradient Echo (MPRAGE)-sequence		Statistically significant volume reduction in GM, total hippocampal volume and in all hippocampal subfields apart from fissure.	Hippocampal atrophy may be attributed to hypercortisolemia due to high levels of stress.

Table 2. *Cont.*

Study	Method and Procedure	Data Analysis	Hydration before Imaging for DTI Studies	Presentation of the Main Findings	Clinical Interpretations
King (2015)	MRI 3T Tested at one time point.	Source based morphometry (SBM)		Significant GM thickness reduction in a total of 86% of the cortical surface, apart from bilateral temporal pole and entorhinal cortex. Reduced volume of nucleus accumbens, amygdala, cerebellum, hippocampus, putamen and thalamus.	A correlation was found between cortical thickness and "drive for thinness" in a broad region of the right lateral occipitotemporal cortex. The normal neurodevelopmental trajectory of cortical thickness (CT) across adolescence and young adulthood may be interrupted in AN.
Yue (2018)	MRI 3T Tested at one time point.	Not mentioned		Significantly reduced total GM volume and ventricular enlargement. Reduced thalamus volume CT in the left precuneus and a larger ratio of caudate volume.	The relative preservation of caudate volume and reduced CT of the left precuneus may be involved in body image distortion.
Fujisawa (2015)	MRI 3T Tested at one time point.	VBM		Significant volume decreases in total GM as well as in bilateral inferior frontal gyrus (IFG) (19,1% left and 17,6% right). Significant correlations were found between regional reduction of GM in the bilateral IFG and age, BMI and age at disease onset.	Volumetric decreases in the IFG might explain the impulsive behaviors observed in patients with AN.
Neumärker (2000)	MRI 1.5T Tested at three time points: at admission (T1), with 50% weight restoration (T2), with normal weight (T3).	Not mentioned		**T1:** Significant larger lateral ventricles and wider fissures of Sylvius bilaterally. Mesencephalon was also markedly reduced. **T2&T3:** Reduced mesencephalon size persisted.	Volumetric alterations were related to the degree of impairment in arithmetic performance. Intact number processing abilities may be a good predictor for weight restoration.
Castro-Fornieles (2009)	MRI 1.5T Tested at two time points: before treatment (T1) and after weight recovery (T2).	VBM		**T1:** Lower global GM and higher CSF volumes and not statistically significant differences in WM. In regional VBM study, significantly decreased GM was observed in bilateral parietal, right temporal cortex and cingulum. **T2:** Decreased GM volume remained in cingulum, not to the same extent as in the first assessment.	Overall, GM reduction at first assessment correlated with Rey Complex Figure Test copy time, indicating a relationship to slowness in complex mental processing.

Table 2. Cont.

Study	Method and Procedure	Data Analysis	Hydration before Imaging for DTI Studies	Presentation of the Main Findings	Clinical Interpretations
Monzon (2017)	MRI 3T 26 AN(T1) patients evaluated at the beginning, 10 AN(T2) patients re-examined after reaching at least 85% of expected body weight.	VBM		T1: Significantly reduced GM volume in OFC, dlPFC, mPFC, insular cortex and hippocampus, anterior cingulate cortex (ACC), medial cingulate cortex (MCC), posterior cingulate cortex (PCC) and the precuneus bilaterally. Additionally, in bilateral amygdala and thalamus. No significant difference in total brain volume between groups. T2: Significantly reduced GM volume remained in ACC, caudate nucleus and right hippocampus. GM volume increase after weight gain in thalamus was negatively correlated to the presence of eating concern symptoms, while in left OFC was negatively correlated to shape-concern symptoms evaluated by the EDE-Q.	Alterations found in PFC, insular and cingulate cortices, hippocampal region, amygdala and parietal cortex could explain distorted body image, emotional disturbances and cognitive deficits.
Golden (1996)	MRI 1T Tested at two time points: before treatment (T1) and after weight gain (T2).	Not mentioned		T1: Ventricular enlargement, especially of the third ventricle. T2: Significantly decreased total ventricular volume. An inverse relationship was found between ventricular volume and BMI.	Atrophy of the cerebral cortex may occur as a result of decreased protein synthesis caused by malnutrition. Structural changes and cognitive functioning seem to improve with weight gain.
Akgül (2016)	MRI 1.5T-MTI Tested at two time points: T1 at admission, T2 after weight recovery.	Regions of interest (ROIs)		T1: Magnetization Transfer Ratio (MTR) did not differ. MRI identified widening of the cerebral sulci in 7 patients with no other gross abnormalities. (ROIs: Left dlPFC, left cerebellar hemisphere, thalamus, amygdala, pons, corona radiata). T2: MTR did not differ.	No clinical interpretations. Adiposity-related variations in phospholipid composition of brain lipids during adolescence could be related to the reversibility of functional impairment.

Table 2. *Cont.*

Study	Method and Procedure	Data Analysis	Hydration before Imaging for DTI Studies	Presentation of the Main Findings	Clinical Interpretations
Bernardoni (2016)	MRI 3T Tested at two time points: T1 at admission, T2 after weight recovery.	SBM-ROIs		T1: Global cortical thinning. AN(T1) vs. AN(T2): 84% of CT restored. AN(T2) vs. HC: CT normalised apart from left temporal pole and enthorhinal cortex. Subcortical GM volume was increased in all ROIs apart from pallidum where a decrease was observed.	Normalization of CT following partial weight restoration is independent of improvements in psychopathology.
Katzman (1997)	MRI 1.5T Tested at two time points: at low weight (T1) and at normal weight (T2) 2–3 years later.	Not mentioned		T1: GM and WM volume decrease and ventricular enlargement. T2: Findings persisted apart from WM volume decrease. Increase of GM volume correlated with BMI increase.	Hypercortisolemia may lead to neuronal damage and persistent brain abnormalities.
MRS					
Blasel (2012)	MRI 3T and MRS Tested at one time point.	Separate analysis of region1: anterior region rostral of the anterior commissure & region 2: posterior region dorsal of the anterior commissure.		No difference between GM fraction. WM fraction was significantly lower to region 2. Significant differences in metabolite concentrations were determined in GM with higher concentrations of tCho, tCr, tNAA, Glx. No difference was found in WM metabolites. MI concentrations did not differ between patients and controls.	The Glx increase may indicate a psychiatric or neurodegenerative origin of AN rather than the result of nutrition depletion.
Castro-Formieles (2007)	MRI 1.5T and MRS Tested at two time points: T1 before treatment and T2 after weight recovery.	Not mentioned		T1: Significantly lower NAA, Glx and mI. No difference was found in the concentration of Cr and Chol. A positive correlation was reported between NAA & T3 and NAA & Wechsler Intelligence Scale for children (WISC). No difference in metabolites concentration between males and females. T2: A statistically significant increase in NAA and a non-significant increase in Glx in frontal GM.	No clinical interpretations.

Table 2. Cont.

Study	Method and Procedure	Data Analysis	Hydration before Imaging for DTI Studies	Presentation of the Main Findings	Clinical Interpretations
Schlemmer (1997)	MRI 1.5T and MRS Tested at one time point.	Two ROIs: the parieto-occipital WM and the thalamus.		A 25% elevation of Cho/Cr and a 25% depression of NAA/Cho were observed in the parieto-occipital WM. No statistically significant differences were found in thalamus. No correlations were found between the metabolic ratios and age, weight or BMI.	No clinical interpretations. The abnormal phospholipid metabolism of membranes might be responsible for brain atrophy.
MRI-DTI					
Pfuhl (2016)	DTI, MRI Tested at one time point.	Global tractography	Urine specific gravity	No significant volumetric differences or microstructural abnormalities in 18 WM tracts. All four diffusivity indices were evaluated (FA, MD, AD, RD).	The preserved WM microstructure may explain why adolescents often do not show marked impairment in executive functioning.
Hu (2017)	DTI Tested at one time point.	VBM	At least 1 week of supervised meals and hydration.	Decreased FA in the left superior frontal gyrus, medial frontal gyrus, ACC, middle frontal gyrus, IFG, thalamus and bilateral insula. Positive correlations between the FA of the left IFG, insula, thalamus and BMI.	WM alterations in prefrontal cortex, parietal lobe and subcortical regions may be associated with impaired cognitive functions.
Gaudio (2017)	DTI Tested at one time point.	VBM	Not assessed	Decreased FA in the left anterior and superior corona radiata and in the SLF. Decreased AD in the left superior and anterior corona radiata and in the SLF bilaterally, external capsule, posterior limb of the internal capsule and posterior thalamic radiation. No differences in MD, RD. No significant correlations.	WM alterations may be involved in impaired cognitive flexibility and body image distortion.

Table 2. Cont.

Study	Method and Procedure	Data Analysis	Hydration before Imaging for DTI Studies	Presentation of the Main Findings	Clinical Interpretations
Travis (2015)	DTI Tested at one time point.	Tractography, relaxometry	Not assessed	Twenty-six WM tracts were identified, 9 bilateral cerebral and 8 subdivisions of the corpus callosum. FA was found decreased in 4 of 26 tracts (including bilateral fimbria—fornix and right SLF and motor subdivisions of corpus callosum) and increased in 2 (including right anterior thalamic radiation and left SLF). R1 was decreased in 11 of 26 tracts mainly in corticospinal tracts and subdivisions of the corpus callosum—body and splenium. No significant associations between BMI and clinical measures.	WM alterations seem to be related to myelin quality, affecting cognitive, emotional and social functions.
Vogel (2016)	DTI Tested at one time point.	TBSS	Urine specific gravity	T1: Increased FA in bilateral frontal, parietal and temporal areas, including bilateral superior corona radiata, corpus callosum, anterior and posterior thalamic radiation, anterior and posterior limb of internal capsule and left inferior longitudinal fasciculus. FA increase due to reduced RD, not altered AD. Most areas with FA increase exhibited reduced MD. T2: No differences in FA after weight rehabilitation. Higher FA was associated with faster weight loss.	The different pattern of WM microstructural changes in adolescents compared to adults may reflect a different susceptibility and reaction to semi starvation in the still developing brain or a time-dependent pathomechanism differing with extent of chronicity.
Olivo (2018)	DTI Tested at one time point.	TBSS	Patients were instructed to eat before the scanning.	No differences detected in diffusivity indices (FA, MD, RD, AD).	Preserved WM microstructure in patients with atypical AN suggests that alterations observed in full syndrome may constitute state-related consequences of severe weight loss.

Table 2. Cont.

Study	Method and Procedure	Data Analysis	Hydration before Imaging for DTI Studies	Presentation of the Main Findings	Clinical Interpretations
Von Schwanenflug (2019)	DTI Tested at two time points: At baseline (T1) and after partial weight restoration (T2).	TBSS	Urine specific gravity	**T1:** In acAN significantly decreased FA and increased MD, AD, RD in corpus callosum, mainly in the body and increased FA in the right corticospinal tract. Additionally, increased FA in the right SLF. **T2:** After partial weight restoration significantly increased FA and decreased MD, AD, RD in the fornix extending into bilateral optic radiation. No clinical correlations.	The decreased FA in corpus callosum may contribute to the distorted body image.

Table 3. Functional imaging studies—sample characteristics.

Study	Study Design	Sybtype	Males (%)	Mean Age (Years)	Age Range (Years)	Mean BMI (Kg/m^2)	Duration of Follow-up (Months)	2nd Imaging Participation	2nd Mean BMI (Kg/m^2)	Measure Adapted for 2nd Imaging	Criteria for Diagnosis	Duration of Illness (Months)	Patients under Medication (%)
SPECT													
Kojima (2005)	Cross-sectional (longitudinal)	AN-R: 12 HC: 11	0	18.6	15.1–22.1	12.5	3.46	100%	15.6	Weight gain	DSM-IV	Not mentioned	Not mentioned
Takano (2001)	Cross-sectional	AN-R: 8 AN-BP: 6 HC: 8	0	21.2	-	14.0	-	-	-	-	DSM-IV	16.8	0
Matsumoto (2006)	Longitudinal	AN-R: 5 AN-BP: 3 HC: 8	0	18.5	12.3–24	12.9	6	100%	18.8	Weight normalization.	DSM-IV	28	0
Komatsu (2010)	Longitudinal	AN: 10 HC: 10	0	13.2	11.0–14.3	13.1	3	100%	16.6	Weight gain	DSM-IV	Early onset	0

Table 3. *Cont.*

Study	Study Design	Sybtype	Males (%)	Mean Age (Years)	Age Range (Years)	Mean BMI (Kg/m²)	Duration of Follow-up (Months)	2nd Imaging Participation	2nd Mean BMI (Kg/m²)	Measure Adapted for 2nd Imaging	Criteria for Diagnosis	Duration of Illness (Months)	Patients under Medication (%)
fMRI													
S. Gaudio (2015)	Cross-sectional	AN-R: 16 HC:16	0	15.8	13–18	16.2	-	-	-	-	DSM-IV TR	4	0
I. Boehm (2014)	Cross-sectional	AN-R: 33 AN-BP: 2 HC: 35	0	16.1	12–23	14.8	-	-	-	-	DSM-IV	18.9	0
F. Amianto (2013)	Cross-sectional	AN-R: 12 HC:10	0	20.0	16–24	16.3	-	-	-	-	DSM-IV	11.5	0
S. Gaudio (2018)	Cross-sectional	AN-R: 15 HC:15	0	15.7	13–18	16.1	-	-	-	-	DSM-IV TR	4	0
D. Geisler (2015)	Cross-sectional	AN: 35 HC:35	0	16.1	12–23	14.8	-	-	-	-	DSM-IV	18.9	0
S. Ehrlich (2015)	Cross-sectional	AN-R: 33 AN-BP: 2 HC: 35	0	16.1	12–23	14.8	-	-	-	-	DSM-IV	18.9	0

3.2. Results of Individual Studies

3.2.1. Results of Structural Imaging Studies

MRI Studies

Thirteen studies using MRI scan to investigate structural abnormalities in participants with AN were systematically reviewed in the present study. Overall, the studies included 247 individuals with a current diagnosis of AN (148 with the restrictive subtype of the disease, 30 with the binge/purging subtype, 22 with atypical AN and 47 with unspecified AN) and 298 HC, mostly females (2 males only). All of the studies were cross-sectional, while 7 included also a longitudinal follow-up. Eight of the included studies were conducted in a sample of exclusively adolescent patients. Nine patients in total had a co-morbid disorder, either depression or anxious disorder and were under medication. The research groups used different methodological approaches to analyze their data. In detail, four studies used VBM, two used SBM and two were region-of-interest studies (ROIs). Table 2 presents scanning methods, main findings and clinical interpretations.

Overall, the majority of studies reported volumetric differences between AN patients and HC. In detail, total GM seemed to be predominantly affected. Significant global reduction of GM volume was reported in seven studies. Region-specific changes in GM were also identified. Specifically, local decreases in GM volume were detected in the parietal and temporal lobes, bilateral frontal gyrus, dorsolateral and medial prefrontal cortex, insular cortex, cerebellum and mesencephalon [29,42–45]. Apart from GM volume, cortical thickness was found also to be reduced either globally (except for the temporal poles and the entorhinal cortex) or regionally in the left precuneus [44,46]. Along with cortical GM reduction, ten studies *reported* regional volumetric differences in the GM of various subcortical areas and brain structures. In particular, reduced GM volume was reported in the amygdala, hippocampus and cingulate gyrus [29,44,47]. Additionally, one study investigated hippocampal subfields and found all volumes but one to be significantly reduced [47]. Similarly, apart from hippocampus and amygdala, GM volume was found also reduced in other subcortical nuclei, such as thalamus, nucleus accumbens and putamen [44,46,48]. Nonetheless, two articles presented no differences in caudate nucleus [44,46]. In discordance with findings concerning GM, WM volume appeared to be considerably less affected. Only one out of eleven studies identified significant reduction of global WM volume [49]. Regarding total brain volume, only one research group reported a significant reduction [47], while increased CSF volume was found in five studies. In seven studies, participants were re-examined with a second MRI after partial or full weight restoration. Apart from one study which examined patients after 2 years of treatment, the remaining had a relatively short follow up period ranging from 12 to 14 months (mean = 7 months). Significant total GM volume increase and normalization of ventricular enlargement was reported in six studies [42,45,48–52], while in one study enlargement remained [53]. Significant regional volume reduction was reported in ACC, temporal poles and entorhinal cortex, caudate nucleus, mesencephalon and hippocampus [45,48,52]. Along with brain morphology normalization, improvement in disease symptoms was reported as well [52].

MRS Studies

Three cross-sectional studies using MRS were systematically reviewed in the present paper. One included also a longitudinal follow-up. In total, 42 female and one male patient with a current diagnosis of AN were included (36 R-AN and 7 BP-AN) and compared with 58 HC. All patients were adolescents. Only one patient had depression and was under antidepressant therapy. Demographics and neuroimaging findings are shown in Tables 1 and 2 respectively.

The researchers investigated the metabolism of both GM and WM. In detail, in patients with acute AN significantly higher concentrations of tCho, tCr and Glx were found, while low levels of NAA, Glx, and mI were detected in the frontal cortex, with a tendency to normalize after weight restoration [15,54]. Finally, using metabolite ratios in order to evaluate alterations, a significantly higher Cho-Cr ratio and lower NAA-Cho ratio were pointed out in the WM of the parietal-occipital region of patients [55].

DTI Studies

Seven DTI studies in participants with AN were systematically reviewed in the present paper. Overall, the studies included 175 individuals with a current diagnosis of AN (109 with the restrictive subtype of the disease, 6 with the binge/purging subtype, 35 with unspecified AN and 25 with atypical AN) and 209 HC, all females. Table 1 reports the sample characteristics. All studies were cross-sectional while two of them included also a longitudinal follow-up, after partial body weight restoration. Four of the included studies were conducted in a sample of exclusively adolescent patients, while the remaining included both adolescents and young adults. Three patients in total had a co-morbid disorder, either depression or anxiety disorder and were under medication. Two studies provided also volumetric data from structural MRI [56,57]. The research groups used different methodological approaches to analyze their data. In detail, two studies adopted VBM, three studies TBSS and two studies applied tractography. Table 2 presents scanning methods, main findings and clinical interpretations.

Overall, the majority of studies reported widespread alterations in diffusion parameters in several WM tracts. Only two studies did not detect any differences in the microstructure of WM comparing patients with controls [56,58]. Starting with association fibers, three studies reported WM abnormalities in the SLF, although findings were inconsistent [30,57,59]. Specifically, in the right SLF, FA was found decreased by Travis et al. and increased by Von Schwanenflug et al. [57,59]. Similarly, in the left SLF, FA was reported increased by Travis et al. and reduced by Gaudio et al., who additionally found decreased AD in the same WM tract [30,59]. Three studies pointed out WM alterations in the thalamic radiation [57,59,60]. In particular, FA was increased in the acute stage when compared with controls [59,60] but was also increased in patients having partially restored their body weight when compared with the acute stage of the disease [57], while no difference was encountered at baseline. In this patient group, Von Schwanenflug et al. found additionally higher FA in the fornix [57]. One more study reported results regarding the fornix. In particular, Travis et al. found decreased FA in this area [59]. Two studies reported WM alterations in the corona radiata [30,60]. Gaudio et al. showed decreased FA and AD in the left superior and anterior corona radiate [30]. On the other hand, Vogel et al. found increased FA in the bilateral superior corona radiata as well as the anterior and posterior limb of the internal capsule [60]. Following with commissural fibers, three studies highlighted WM alterations in the corpus callosum [57,59,60]. Again, findings were conflicting, with FA value being reported either increased or decreased. Moreover, Travis et al. estimated R1, a myelin index, which was measured decreased mainly in the body and splenium of the corpus callosum [59]. The same index was also reduced in corticospinal tracts. With regard to projection fibers, only one study reported reduced FA in the right corticospinal tract with weight gain, while no difference was detected in the acute stage compared to controls [57]. In contrast with the other research groups, Hu et al. localized their results in GM, reporting decreased FA in several cortical regions, mainly in the frontal lobe, the cingulum, the thalamus and the insula [61]. Finally, as already mentioned two studies did not find any differences between patients and HC, in any of the diffusion indices [56,58].

3.2.2. Results of Functional Imaging Studies

fMRI Studies

Six resting-state fMRI studies in participants with a current diagnosis of AN were systematically reviewed in the present paper. Overall, the studies included 78 individuals with a current diagnosis of AN (76 with the restrictive subtype of the disease and 2 with the binge/purging subtype and 76 HC, all females. Table 3 reports the sample characteristics. All were case-control studies. Two of the included studies were conducted in a sample of exclusively adolescent patients, while the remaining included both adolescents and young adults. Only one patient in total had a co-morbid disorder and was under antidepressant medication. Three studies provided also volumetric data from structural MRI. The research groups used different methodological approaches to analyze their data, either whole brain approaches, or network based. Table 4 presents scanning methods, main findings and clinical interpretations.

Overall, all studies reported disturbed widespread functional connectivity alterations in several brain regions. The variety in the location of findings defies the strict categorization of results by area of interest. In detail, as already mentioned, two studies included only adolescent patients at the earliest stage of the disease. In the first one, Gaudio et al. identified eight widely accepted resting-state networks [62] and found decreased functional connectivity between the ECN and the ACC, which correlated positively with BMI [63]. In the second study in adolescents, Gaudio et al. reported decreased connectivity in a subnetwork involving the ACC, the paracentral lobule, the cerebellum, the insula, the orbitofrontal gyrus and the occipital gyrus (see Table 4 for details) [64]. Neither of the two studies found volumetric differences between patients and HC. Of the remaining four studies, one research group focused as well on resting-state functional networks. In particular, Bohem et al. reported increased functional connectivity between the angular gyrus and other parts of the FPN and also between the anterior insula and the DMN [65]. One study, that of Amianto et al. centered on the intrinsic connectivity of the cerebellum and found increased connectivity within the insula, vermis, temporal poles and PCC and decreased connectivity with the parietal lobes [66]. Cerebellar atrophy was an additional finding. Finally, two research groups pointed out decreased functional connectivity in the thalamo-insular network [67,68]. Furthermore, Geisler et al. highlighted an altered global network architecture [67].

SPECT Studies

Four articles performing SPECT scan in adolescents and young adults with acute AN met the inclusion criteria. A total of 44 patients were included (25 with R-AN, 9 with BP-AN and 10 unspecified) along with 19 HC, all females. Two studies were cross-sectional, one of which re-examined 12 patients after partial weight gain and two were longitudinal studies re-examining their patients ($n = 18$) after partial weight gain or normalization. One study was conducted in a sample of exclusively adolescent patients. None of the patients had any co-morbid disorders. Demographic data and clinical findings are presented in Tables 3 and 4, respectively.

Hypoperfusion was reported in frontal, parietal, temporal, and occipital regions in acutely ill individuals compared to HC [69,70]. Decreased perfusion was positively correlated with BMI [69]. After partial recovery, blood perfusion showed a tendency to increase and reached almost normal levels. Conversely, elevated blood flow was reported in the thalamus, amygdala and hippocampus [69,70].

When examining patients after a BMI elevation by 50%, a significant increase in rCBF was reported in the right dlPFC, the medial parietal cortex including the precuneus and in the PCC. In contrast, a decrease in rCBF was found in the right putamen and a positive correlation was reported between rCBF in the right DLPFC and the interoceptive awareness score in patients before treatment, while after treatment no correlation was found [71]. After an increase in BMI by 25%, significantly increased rCBF was found in bilateral parietal lobes and right posterior cingulate gyrus and a positive correlation was reported between BMI and rCBF in the right thalamus, parietal lobe, and cerebellum [72].

Table 4. Functional imaging studies—methods, main findings and clinical interpretations.

Study	Method and Procedure	Data Analysis	Presentation of the Main Findings	Clinical Interpretations
SPECT				
Kojima (2005)	SPECT Tested at two time points: at baseline (T1) and after weight recovery (T2).	(HMPAO)	**AN (T1) vs. HC**: Decreased rCBF in AN in the bilateral frontal lobes, including the ACC, PCC, bilateral precentral gyri, right insula, and right lingual gyrus. A positive correlation between the rCBF and BMI in the occipital lobe was found. **AN (T2) vs. HC**: Significant increases in the right parietal lobe and the left superior frontal gyrus. Decreases in the left superior temporal gyrus, left putamen, right IFG, right amygdala, and right cerebellum.	Hypoperfusion in the ACC and the parietal lobe may be associated not only with low body weight but also with abnormal brain functions relative to clinical features of AN.
Takano (2001)	SPECT Tested at one time point.	I-123-MIBG SPM approach	**AN vs. HC**: Hypoperfusion in the mPFC and ACC. Hyperperfusion in the thalamus and amygdala-hippocampus complex.	Hypoperfusion of the ACC may reflect depressive symptoms, while hyperactivity of the thalamus may be associated with chronic and refractory AN.
Matsumoto (2006)	SPECT Tested at two time points: at baseline (T1) and before discharge (T2).	123I-IMP	**AN-T1 vs. AN-T2**: Significant increase in rCBF in right dlPFC and medial parietal cortex including the precuneus and in the PCC. At the same lower threshold ($p < 0.002$) rCBF in the ACC and mPFC increased to an almost significant level. Significant decrease of rCBF in the right putamen.	Changes in rCBF may be associated with the improvement of interoceptive awareness following treatment.
Komatsu (2010)	SPECT Tested at two time points: at baseline (T1) and after 3 months (T2).	123I-IMP SPM approach	**AN-T1 vs. AN-T2**: Significant increased rCBF in bilateral parietal lobes and right PCC. No regions of decreased rCBF. A positive correlation between BMI and rCBF in right thalamus, right parietal lobe and right cerebellum.	PCC activation after weight gain might reflect affective changes for eating motivation during the recovery process of early-onset AN.
fMRI				
Gaudio (2015)	fMRI + MRI Tested at one time point.	whole brain ICA analysis	**AN vs. HC**: Eight networks were identified. Statistically significant reduced connectivity between the Executive control network (ECN) and the ACC. The decrease in functional connectivity in the ACC was positively correlated with BMI and negatively correlated with drive for thinness, perfectionism and harm avoidance scores. No significant differences in GM volumes.	The decreased functional connectivity between the ECN and the ACC could explain the cognitive inflexibility in relation to body image.
Boehm (2014)	fMRI Tested at one time point.	ICA network based analysis	**AN vs. HC**: The networks of interest were the Fronto parietal network (FPN), DMN, Salience network (SN), visual and sensory-motor network. Increased functional connectivity between the angular gyrus and the FPN and between the anterior insula and the DMN. Positive correlations for both networks (DMN, FPN) with self-report measures in healthy controls. Functional connectivity in the anterior insula was positively associated with interoceptive difficulties in HC.	Increased functional connectivity within the FPN might be related to excessive cognitive control. The increased functional connectivity of insula with the DMN may mirror difficulties to disengage from thoughts about food and body appearance when not engaged in a task.

Table 4. Cont.

Study	Method and Procedure	Data Analysis	Presentation of the Main Findings	Clinical Interpretations
Amianto (2013)	fMRI, MRI Tested at one time point.	ICA network based analysis	**AN vs. HC:** Within the cerebellar intrinsic connectivity network, a greater connectivity was found with insulae, temporal poles, vermis and paravermis and a lesser connectivity with parietal lobe. Additionally, GM volume reduction in cerebellar hemispheres, cingulate cortex, precuneus and OFC.	The vermian hyper-connection could be linked to some psychopathological core features, such as "drive for thinness" which express the dissatisfaction with body weight. The cerebellar-parietal network dysfunction could be related to the disturbances in the body image perception. A stronger connection between cerebellum and temporal lobes may be related to greater emotional activation elicited by social behaviors in subjects with AN.
Gaudio (2018)	fMRI, MRI Tested at one time point.	Graph analysis whole brain and network based	**AN vs. HC:** Decreased connectivity in the sub-network including the left and right rostral ACC, left paracentral lobule, left cerebellum, left posterior insula, left medial orbito-frontal gyrus and right superior occipital gyrus. No significant differences in GM, WM, and CSF volumes.	The altered sub-network functional connectivity may sustain an altered self-body imge through an impaired integration of somatosensory, visual and interoceptive signals.
Geisler (2015)	fMRI Tested at one time point.	Graph analysis whole brain	**AN vs. HC:** Decreased functional connectivity in the thalamo-insular subnetwork. Longer average routes between nodes and more nodes with a similar connectedness link together. Additionally, altered global network architecture.	The altered network global topology indicates wide-scale disturbance in information flow across brain networks. The local thalamo-insular network disruption may explain the impaired integration of visuospatial and homeostatic signals.
Ehrlich (2015)	fMRI Tested at one time point.	Network based statistics	**AN vs. HC:** Reduced functional connectivity in the thalamo-insular network (in particular in a subnetwork consisting of the thalamus, amygdala, basal ganglia, fusiform gyrus and posterior insula).	The decreased functional connectivity in the thalamo-insular network may explain the striking discrepancy between patient's actual and perceived internal body state.

4. Discussion

4.1. Discussion of Structural Imaging Studies

Starting with MRI, the most frequently used neuroimaging method, total and regional GM volume reduction appears to be the prominent finding, although some heterogeneity arises in terms of severity and localization of findings. This 'pseudo-atrophy' shows the tendency to reverse after weight gain, at least in non-chronic patients. In addition to global GM reduction, particular regions appear to be more susceptible to volume loss, such as the parietal cortex, precuneus, insula, thalamus, as well as limbic structures, such as the PFC, cingulate cortex, hippocampus and amygdala [9,10].

Although several pathophysiological mechanisms have been suggested, the exact etiology of GM atrophy remains unknown. It is widely believed to be the result of extreme malnutrition and not a predisposing factor to the disease. Patients with AN follow a restrictive diet pattern, excluding polyunsaturated fatty acids, proteins and neuroprotective nutrients, such as B-complex vitamins and antioxidants [14]. Polyunsaturated fatty acids are exclusively received through diet and are essential for neuronal membranes integrity and function. Their nutritional deficiency is associated with neuronal apoptosis and interruption of the normal cortex maturation during adolescence, which may explain the greater GM vulnerability during this period [73]. In addition, the decreased protein synthesis due to the extreme nutrient deprivation is thought to result in a reduced number of synaptic connections and delayed synaptogenesis [50]. Other published theories to explain atrophy are brain shrinkage due to dehydration and fluid shifting to extracellular space due to osmotic alterations [74]. However, in almost every included study, MRI imaging was conducted after the initial stabilization of patients and with albumin and electrolytes serum levels within the normal range. Thus, dehydration or osmotic alterations do not seem to adequately explain findings. Considering the hormonal status of the patients, elevated cortisol levels, which is a common finding, are significantly associated mainly with intraparenchymatic GM volume depletion [49]. The underlying mechanism is still unknown, but it is likely that cortisol may be responsible for alterations in protein catabolism [75]. Moreover, secondary insulin growth factor-1 (IGF-1) deficiency due to malnutrition can result in loss of oligodendrocyte proliferation and differentiation, inhibition of myelination and eventually brain volume reduction [76].

An interesting theory that has been proposed to explain the greater GM loss in adolescents, is that the disease seems to modify the normal process of brain maturation (pruning), leading to a more "ergonomic" cortical architecture in order to save energy and maintain an adequate network efficiency despite starvation and malnutrition. This theory may also explain the clinical observation that patients feel actually more alert when starving, at the early stages of the illness [77]. Interestingly, in adolescents with a recent diagnosis of atypical AN, no significant volumetric differences were detected, and no clinical correlations were found. It is worth mentioning though, that patients had a significantly lower BMI than HC and that 40% of them presented with secondary amenorrhea. It is therefore suggested, that a critical BMI limit exists, below which the loss of GM begins to become apparent [78]. This hypothesis is supported by a positive correlation between volumetric alterations and the weight loss rate, emphasizing the importance of early diagnosis and intervention [79]. Overall, the positive correlation between patient's BMI (and not disease duration) and global GM volume depletion in combination with atrophy reversion after partial weight gain, lean towards the concept that atrophy is a temporary effect of semi-starvation and not a consequence of major cell apoptosis, at least in non-chronic patients [50,80].

As already mentioned, specific brain regions appear to be more affected in terms of GM loss, indicating either a higher vulnerability to the disease or a potential involvement in AN pathogenesis. In particular, the parietal lobe is reported by several research groups to be primarily affected [42,46,48]. This finding has been linked to the reported cognitive deficits in verbal memory and to the impairment of visuospatial and concentration ability of patients [9]. Additionally, parietal volume loss may contribute to size overestimation, an important element of disturbed body image. Interestingly, the distortion of self-body image in AN patients is quite similar to the distortion reported after right parietal lobe damage (e.g., stroke), indicating the existence of a cognitive, non-emotional component of body misperception [81]. Another prominent finding is the involvement of limbic structures. The hyperactive adolescent limbic system is believed to have its own special role in the neurobiology of AN [82]. Hippocampus and amygdala in particular, appear to be more susceptible to volume loss. Hippocampal atrophy is reported in several other serious psychiatric disorders, such as major depression [83]. Lower hippocampal volumes in these individuals appear to be a result of longer illness duration or greater number of episodes, instead of a premorbid vulnerability factor [84]. Excessive cortisol levels due to chronic stress have been proposed as the driving mechanism [85]. In AN, hypercortisolemia may serve as a compensatory mechanism, increasing gluconeogenesis and providing vital nutrients [86]. Nonetheless, patients often have co-morbid anxiety disorders, so stress can actually be a confounding factor [87]. This notion is supported by the partial increase in the hippocampal volume following the administration of antidepressants [88]. When comparing studies conducted in teens to those in adults, greater atrophy is shown in adolescent hippocampus [7,47,89]. This exceptional vulnerability to stress during this period may be the result of rapid brain development and increased plasticity, in combination with the existence of numerous stress-hormone receptors in this area [90].

Another limbic structure that seems to have a pivotal involvement in the disease symptomatology and potentially pathophysiology is the amygdala, the brain's "threat detector" [91]. Exaggerated activity of the amygdala is observed in healthy adolescents compared with adults [92]. This hyperactivity is argued to have a central role in AN [93]. Specifically, it has been suggested that a trait amygdala hypersensitivity exists for individuals who will develop AN contributing to the experience of emotion as overwhelming and aversive, and which may become further aggravated during adolescence corresponding with disorder onset [94]. In detail, AN patients, especially those with R-AN, experience food stimuli very aversively, displaying an increased reactivity of the right amygdala [93]. In line with this finding, fMRI studies report hyperactivity of the amygdala when patients are exposed to gustatory [19], or body-related paradigms [95,96], or even disease specific words [97]. These results are suggestive of a multimodal amygdalar reactivity independent of the sensory mode. Likewise, this amygdalar hyperactivity is elicited by disorder-unrelated (emotional) stimuli, reflecting a heightened negative emotional arousal [98]. It could be argued that AN patients are biased towards both emotional (disease-unrelated) and non-emotional (disease-related), a feature that persists following recovery [94,99]. Interestingly, increased activation of the amygdala during anticipation of food is reported also in siblings of AN patients, a finding that supports further the notion of amygdalar hypersensitivity as a premorbid biomarker [100]. Amygdala activation after gustatory stimulation may be the result of intense fear of weight gain [19]. It has been proposed that increased activity in the amygdala may lead to fearful emotional processing concerning body image issues, and in turn influences calorie intake and weight gain [97]. Reduced amygdala volume in AN patients has been associated with less body image uncertainty and reduced phobia scores, possibly contributing to the disease maintenance [101]. It is also worth mentioning that the amygdala, along with the insula and other limbic structures, is part of complex neural circuits related to emotional perception [102]. Thus, in the backdrop of an hyperactive amygdala sending high levels of negative emotional threat information, the insula is unable to integrate basic emotion detection [94]. The pivotal role of the insula in the disease is discussed further along with other functional alterations.

Apart from volumetric changes, alterations in GM metabolism have been studied as well with MRS imaging, although this is not a widely used technique across neuroimaging research of eating disorders. In general, the rarity of MRS data precludes definite conclusions.

MRI imaging has not revealed significant volumetric changes regarding WM. However, changes in the microarchitecture of WM became evident through DTI studies. Overall, multiple WM alterations have been demonstrated, with some degree of overlap across studies but also with a relative inconsistency regarding the location and direction of alterations. With regard to localization of findings, the microarchitecture of WM appears to be affected mainly in thalamo-cortical connections (corona radiata, thalamic radiation), in interhemispheric connections (corpus callosum), in tracts connecting cortical regions as well as in various regions of the limbic system such as the fornix, insula, cingulum and frontal areas [103]. The abovementioned WM tracts and GM areas are involved in somatosensory, emotional and reward processing, in high order cognitive functions and in the formation of body image perception. Therefore, WM alterations may have potential clinical implications related to the symptomatology of the disease.

In detail, the corona radiata is a key WM structure of the DMN, connecting the cerebral cortex to the basal ganglia and the brain stem [104,105]. Disruption of WM could be related to cognitive and emotion regulation deficits in anorectic patients, as has already been demonstrated in individuals with bipolar depression [106]. The posterior thalamic radiation connects thalamus with the parietal and occipital lobe, regions that are anatomically and functionally linked to body image. It could be hypothesized that alterations in WM micro-architecture of thalamic radiation may correlate with distorted body image. However, further research is needed to verify this assumption. The corpus callosum is the principal WM fiber bundle of the brain, involved in motor, perceptual and cognitive functions. Alterations in WM could be related to reduced quantity and speed of information between these areas [33]. Furthermore, corpus callosum atrophy has been correlated with cognitive flexibility, another core feature of the disease [107]. Likewise, the SLF is a major intrahemispheric WM and a major link between the PFC and the parietal lobe concerning the perception of the visual space, providing a means by which the PFC can regulate the focusing on attention in different parts of space [108]. Altered SLF microstructure could give rise to body size misperception, by disrupting information flow across cortical regions implicated in visual attention, spatial perception, and body-specific processing [108–110]. Finally, the fornix is a major limbic structure which is involved in reward processing and feeding regulation [111]. Previous studies have reported consistently reduced FA in the fornix in AN linking this structure with disease symptomatology and potentially pathophysiology [111]. In our review, FA was found either decreased or increased [57,59]. It is worth mentioning that both research groups took into account that FA may be biased by ventricular enlargement which is often encountered in AN patients, due to the partial volume effect (PVE), which occurs when voxels contain heterogenous tissue types, i.e., WM tissue and CSF in the case of the fornix [112]. For that reason, the former estimated ventricular size prior to DTI scanning, while the latter considered ventricular volume as a covariate in their analysis.

As already mentioned, there is a relative discrepancy concerning the localization of findings, which may be attributed to the different methodological approaches utilized for data analysis, (i.e., VBM, TBSS, tractography) leading researchers to focus on different brain regions. Given this variance, it is worth mentioning the study of Pfuhl et al. who found no differences between patients and controls [56]. The researchers applied a global probabilistic tractography, a different analysis that may not detect subtle or more localized alterations [57]. On the other hand, the inconsistency in terms of the direction of the alterations is quite impressive, if not unexpected. In particular, FA was reported either decreased or increased in the same regions of interest by different researchers, a finding that comes in contrast with previous findings in adults who have consistently reported decreased FA [113–115]. Increased FA is a finding encountered principally in adolescents, in line with previous studies [116]. This discrepancy was pointed out in the meta-analysis of Barona et al. as well [31]. It is a fact, that the interpretation of the DTI findings is challenging, as indices of diffusion are open to many biological interpretations. FA in particular, is a highly sensitive but non-specific biomarker of brain WM microstructure [117]. Decreased FA combined with increased MD is typically interpreted as disturbed WM integrity, whereas increased FA is thought to reflect increased myelination [118]. However, increased FA may not always be a desirable finding. For instance, a higher FA value in auditory fibers has been reported in patients with schizophrenia who suffer from hallucinations [119]. In addition, as was pointed out by Jones et al., FA may be affected by several other factors, such as larger axon diameter, lower fiber density, increased membrane permeability and reduced myelination [120]. FA values could additionally be affected by the reduced WM volume, a phenomenon probably attributed to the reduction in the number of supporting glial cells, in the size of neurons and glia cell bodies, or in altered protein synthesis that results in fewer and smaller dendrites and synaptic junctions [8]. A recent study in an animal model of AN identified strongly reduced astrocyte count and astrocyte volumes in the WM of the brain [121]. The reduction in the surrounding tissue could also be a consequence of dehydration [60]. WM with large axons, such as the corpus callosum and the corticospinal tracts have thicker myelin sheets and larger concentrations of myelin. Thus, they may be more vulnerable to the effects of starvation [122]. Another factor that should be taken into consideration for the interpretation of DTI findings is the phenomenon of crossing fibers. A voxel may be composed of fibers with different spatial orientation resulting in an increase in average FA, without reflecting changes in myelin structure [120]. Moreover, most studies focused on FA, which is the most commonly reported variable, and secondarily on MD. However, these may not be enough to characterize DTI changes. AD and RD are considered to be more specific to underlying biological processes, such as myelin and axonal changes [123].

The neuroimaging findings in adolescent patients are of special interest. The detection of site-specific WM alterations in young patients and at the earliest stages of the disease, as described in two studies, supports the hypothesis that these alterations may represent premorbid trait markers [30,59]. On the other hand, Vogel et al. reported widespread alterations, which could be hardly correlated with specific symptoms of the disease and which rapidly normalized with weight restoration [60]. Additionally, the researchers found a positive correlation between FA and the speed of weight loss. Taken together, these findings are against the aforementioned hypothesis. Interestingly, Olivo et al. did not detect any diffusivity abnormalities in adolescents with atypical AN, supporting the notion that undernutrition is the underlying mechanism of FA alterations [58]. This subgroup of patients is characterized by the typical features of AN but with a body weight within the normal limits. In an attempt to interpret the results, it could be speculated that the developing adolescent brain reacts to malnutrition in a different way compared to adults, in a way that even the minimum limitation of food intake could affect the WM development. Alternatively, the increase in FA, which is the prominent finding in adolescents, could reflect a compensatory mechanism to starvation before the long-lasting deprivation of food results in the reduction of FA in adulthood. One way or another, during adolescence, WM maturation is characterized by continual widespread changes of increased FA and increased MD in widespread areas of cerebral and cerebellar WM, prominently in the frontal lobes and association fibers that connect them to other parts of the brain. These changes are driven by reductions in both AD and RD [124]. AD reduces with age, probably as a result of increased numbers of brain fibers or increased axonal caliber and the growth of glial cells. RD also reduces with age as a result of increased myelin development in the majority of brain areas [124]. Thus, normal baseline and age-related RD and AD values should be taken into consideration when investigating pathological conditions in this age group.

Overall, literature indicates that WM is affected in young patients with AN. However, the exact nature of WM alterations is unclear, and no safe conclusions can be drawn whether these alterations bear on disease pathophysiology or not.

4.1.1. Discussion of Functional Imaging Studies

Overall, the researchers reported an altered functional connectivity across various brain regions and large-scale resting-state networks. Despite the discrepancies among studies (in terms of data analysis method and distribution of findings), results indicate functional abnormalities across several areas and networks related to core features of AN such as cognitive inflexibility, disturbed body image and deficits in emotional processing and executive control. In particular, most of the abovementioned areas belong to either the limbic or reward system and additionally are considered to be part of the well identified resting-state networks [24].

One of these areas of special interest is the ACC, a region with multiple functions and several functional connections at rest. The ACC lies in the medial wall of each cerebral hemisphere and is connected to both the "emotional" limbic system and the "cognitive" prefrontal cortex [125]. It is also considered a part of the ECN [63]. It is involved in cognitive and sensorimotor functions as well as in affect-regulation, i.e., the ability to control and manage uncomfortable emotions [126,127]. Stimuli-based fMRI studies in healthy individuals have revealed the role of the ACC in the emotion-regulation process, through a generalized "top-down" control from the prefrontal cortex, which provides the capacity to regulate an over-activated emotional response from the limbic system [125,128]. On the other hand, fMRI studies in patients with psychiatric disorders have reported that both hyper- and hypo-activation of the ACC is involved in impaired emotion regulation characterizing depression, schizophrenia and posttraumatic stress disorder (PTSD) [129–131]. Likewise, altered functional connectivity of the ACC in AN could support the notion that emotion dysregulation is associated with the appearance, maintenance and outcome of the disease [132]. It is finally worth mentioning that functional alterations of the ACC were early recognized by SPECT imaging. Hypoperfusion of this region was a consistent finding, not completely normalizing after weight restoration. However, with the introduction of PET imaging to eating disorders research, further data from SPECT no longer exist.

Another area of interest is the insula. The insular cortex is implicated in an overwhelming variety of functions such as sensorimotor processing, emotional awareness, autonomical control, risk prediction, decision-making and complex social functions like empathy [133,134]. An additional key function of the insula is the integration of interoceptive information, i.e., internal physical sensations including pain, hunger and thirst [87]. The right insula specifically is involved in "self—recognition" [135]. MRI studies have revealed increased volume of the right insula in adolescent and adult patients with AN [116]. This finding has also been correlated with the rumination of being fat while actually being emaciated [136]. Furthermore, the anterior insula is the primary gustatory cortex. Along with the ACC and the OFC, the anterior insula codes the sensory-hedonic response to taste. Moreover, it may play a crucial role in linking sensory-hedonic experiences to the motivational component of reward, which urges an individual to approach food [87]. This potential contribution of the insula to eating behavior has been highlighted in functional neuroimaging. Previous fMRI studies in recovered AN patients have reported a reduced insula response to sweet taste when compared to controls [137,138]. Likewise, a study in participants with acute AN has revealed insula activation in response to drinking chocolate milk in controls but not in patients, in the satiety state [19]. In contrast, a neuroimaging study in healthy individuals pointed out that food deprivation, compared to the satiety state, produces greater insula activation [139]. Adding to these findings, altered functional connectivity at rest between the insula and various regions, as well as within the networks that pass through it, supports the hypothesis that the insula has a central role in the pathophysiology of AN [140]. Interestingly, Bohem et al. found a positive correlation of functional connectivity in the anterior insula with difficulties in interoceptive awareness [65]. These findings come in line with the suggestion that many of the symptoms, such as distorted body image, lack of recognition of the severity of the situation (due to inappropriate response to hunger) and diminished motivation to change could be related to disturbed interoceptive awareness [87].

The prominent finding of altered functional connectivity of the ACC and insula could be interpreted in the context of adolescent brain maturation. It has been suggested that ACC is a key neural substrate of adolescent neurodevelopment [141]. Critically, ACC connectivity undergoes tremendous reorganization during adolescence [142]. In detail, the rostral ACC becomes more strongly connected to the DMN, whereas dorsal ACC shows increasing connectivity with the SN [141]. These developmental changes may contribute to the appearance of AN psychopathology during adolescence, given that most mental disorders are currently considered neurodevelopmental. Likewise, widely accepted theories regarding neurocognitive development in adolescence emphasize the different developmental trajectories of subcortical motivational and cortical control regions [143]. Specifically, limbic regions involved in reward and affective processing mature earlier than PFC regions for the executive control of the behavior, thus creating an imbalance in decision making. The fact that insula serves as a key hub in the interface between emotional processing and executive control [144], brings forward this structure as a central component of adolescent physiological maturation and potentially phychopathology as well. Indeed, research indicates that the fronto-insular connectivity displays the most dramatic developmental effects during puberty [145]. Taken together, this notion opens a new research direction towards the prioritization of the neurodevelopment to understand vulnerability to disease state [146].

Apart from the abovementioned functions, insula appears to be a central hub of some large-scale resting-state networks. A few researchers focused on the study of these networks and highlighted the altered functional connectivity within and between them. In detail, researchers attempted to explore the functional interactions between three core resting state networks (RSNs), the DMN, the ECN and the SN. The DMN is a well-recognized network which encompasses the medial prefrontal cortex, the posterior cingulate cortex, the precuneus, the inferior parietal lobule and the lateral temporal cortex. It has been hypothesized to be active during rest and deactivated when specific goal-directed behavior is needed [147]. In particular, the DMN is the most active brain system when individuals are left to think to themselves undisturbed. It is involved in mental explorations including remembering the past, envisioning the future, considering the thoughts of other people and thinking about one's self [148]. Dysfunction of the DMN has been related to Alzheimer's disease, schizophrenia and autism and virtually to every major psychiatric disorder [149,150]. The ECN covers the dlPFC and the lateral posterior parietal cortex and is responsible for high level cognitive functions such as planning and decision making. ECN disruption is also widespread in most mental disorders [151]. The SN covers the dorsal ACC and the anterior insular cortex and is involved in detecting and filtering internal and external stimuli [151]. Bohem and colleagues attempted to interpret their results in the framework of the triple network model of psychopathology suggested by Menon [65,151]. According to this model, deficits in engagement and disengagement of these three core neurocognitive networks (ECN, DMN, SN) play a significant role in many psychiatric disorders. This model highlights the crucial role of the SN, with the anterior insula as its central hub, in initiating the switch from the DMN to the ECN, for the generation of appropriate behavioral responses to salient stimuli. In detail, the researchers reported increased connectivity between insula and DMN, a finding that is in line with this model representing a difficulty in disengagement from a self-focused state of mind, intensifying the ruminative preoccupation with body image and food. Likewise, in individuals suffering from major depression, increased activation of the DMN has been positively correlated with depressive ruminations [152]. A similar approach was adopted by Uniacke et al. [153]. In their longitudinal study, researchers found reduced SN-ECN connectivity which remained after weight normalization.

Researchers have queried the extent to which this multinetwork model gradually emerges from childhood [146]. Converging evidence suggest the strengthening of intra- and inter- network connectivity in adults compared to children, implying that significant subnetwork reorganization takes place during adolescence [38,39,145]. Network maturation follows a hierarchical modularity, with those networks serving the most basic functions of the organism maturing the earliest [146]. This asynchrony in the timing of network developmental trajectories might result in greater vulnerability to mental disorders during adolescence [146], among those AN as well. This theory has been previously proposed for the greater vulnerability of adolescents to addictive behaviors [146]. Nonetheless, the complex and highly sophisticated methodology of these studies results in sparse data, especially in adolescent populations. Further research is needed therefore, to clarify the potential role of the triple network connectivity in the pathophysiology of the disease and to further investigate the complex inter-network relationships.

Another brain area with a potentially pivotal role in the disease is the OFC. This subregion of the prefrontal cortex has a major role in regulating when to stop eating a particular food, by activating the phenomenon of *sensory specific satiety*, a decline in pleasantness of a food as it is eaten [154,155]. The median OFC has further been associated with food avoidance. Altered functional connectivity in this area comes in accordance with the previously reported reduced grey GM matter volume in adolescents and adults with AN, a finding which has been correlated with disturbed satiety regulation, a possible driving mechanism for restriction of food in anoretic patients [116].

The interpretation of findings raises again the question whether functional connectivity could be affected by undernutrition. For example, Amianto et al. reported GM volume reduction in the same regions where abnormal connectivity was detected [66]. On the other hand, functional alterations in adolescent cohorts were not related to volumetric differences, although a positive correlation between ACC connectivity and BMI was highlighted [63]. Thus, no definite conclusion can be drawn. An additional, open to interpretation, aspect of functional connectivity is the direction of the effect. Although it could be obviously hypothesized that increased connectivity is desirable, its clinical implication is difficult to be assessed. Finally, it is worth mentioning that only two studies reported correlations between functional alterations and core symptoms of the disease [63,65]. Relating encountered differences between groups to relevant clinical variables increases the reproducibility of the results and thus, is an advisable approach for every study [156].

4.1.2. Overall, Synthesis and Limitations

This systematic review attempted a global approach to structural and functional alterations in the brain of youth patients with AN. Young adults were also included in this effort, as they share more common features with the teen population than with older adults, due to the ongoing brain neurodevelopment during the first years of adulthood.

Our findings are consistent with the current literature indicating widespread and regional GM volume reduction, WM microstructure disturbances and resting-state functional alterations. The heterogeneity of findings across all neuroimaging methods may be attributed to the different methodological approaches and the non-uniformity of cohorts regarding multiple clinical variables such as disease duration and severity. Alternatively, it may merely reflect the complexity of the disease. In fact, specific brain regions such as the insula, PFC, parietal cortex, as well as WM tracts and functional networks related to them appear to be consistently affected in young patients, suggesting their potential role in the disease pathophysiology. Typical findings in adult patients such as cerebellar atrophy are not consistently encountered in young individuals, suggesting associations with longer disease duration [12,157,158]. A prominence of limbic structures is also indicative of emotional and reward processing deficits being at the root of the disease. Of course, in the human brain, it is not always possible to ascribe a symptom to a single region. On the other hand, both structural and functional alterations are highly reversible after short weight restoration and long before the psychological recovery, pointing out malnutrition as the underlying causative mechanism, although data from longitudinal studies are limited.

A principal limitation of our review is the exclusion of stimuli or task-based fMRI studies, due to space limitations and in order to limit heterogeneity related to study design oriented to specific tasks. However, this exclusion precluded us from addressing disturbances in neural circuitries involved in reward-processing, which may have a central role in AN according to current neurobiological models of the disease [87,159]. Additionally, the application of stringent criteria in an effort to eliminate potential confounders such as psychiatric comorbidity and medications may have led us to exclude studies with significant results and has resulted in a limited number of resting-state fMRI and DTI studies. Another noticeable limitation of our review is the exclusion of recovered patients. It is a common practice for researchers to enroll recovered individuals in order to avoid the confounding effect of malnutrition and to detect permanent "scars" of the disease [160]. Our rationale behind this exclusion lies on the fact that recovery in AN is open to many clinical interpretations in the existing literature [161]. According to the DSM-V, full remission is achieved when none of the diagnostic criteria are fulfilled for a substantial period of time, without specifying the exact duration of being free of symptoms and without differentiating between adolescents and adults. For adolescents and youth in particular, recovery requires full weight restoration and normalization of eating pattern, pubertal progression and linear growth, if expected, as well as age-appropriate interpersonal, psychosocial, and occupational functioning [5]. Most studies that include recovered patients define recovery as weight restoration and maintenance for at least one year, thus providing comparability between their results. Nonetheless, given the fact that adolescents continue to grow and develop throughout puberty and into young adulthood, a "maintenance weight" restoration is far from characterizing a teen patient recovered [5]. A topic of significant questioning across AN neuroimaging is the potential confounding effect of co-morbid disorders, such as depression, stress disorder and OCD. This notion is further supported by the reported overlapping neuroimaging findings. As already mentioned, hippocampal atrophy is a common finding between AN patients and those with major depressive disorder. Similarly, depressive patients display changes in FA concerning mainly the genu and body of the corpus callosum and the corona radiata [84]. Likewise, adolescents with OCD are characterized by lower GM volume and CT of the parietal lobes [162]. Not only structural but also functional overlaps are apparent between AN and other psychiatric disorders. For instance, the hyperactivation of the PFC and the amygdala which are commonly reported in AN, are also features of the generalized stress disorder [163]. In addition, as mentioned before, altered functional connectivity between and within core RSNs characterizes many other psychiatric disorders, including OCD [162]. It is therefore quite difficult, if not impossible, to overcome the potential biases from co-morbid disorders, since these are the rule rather than the exception in AN patients.

The interpretation of findings needs to be considered in the light of several limitations characterizing all types of neuroimaging techniques. First of all, cohorts are consistently small and thus, with limited ability to control for potential confounding factors and to allow the generalization of the results. As highlighted by Thirion and colleagues, at least 20 subjects or more should be included in functional neuroimaging studies in order to have sufficient reliability [164], which can be quite difficult due to the high cost of the imaging procedures. Difficulty in enrolling patients usually results in heterogeneous samples in terms of demographic data and several clinical variables. Heterogeneity may exist even in samples including exclusively adolescents, due to the different neurodevelopmental stage of the participants. Even more profound is the sparsity of male patients. Interestingly, gender differences exist concerning cortical activation to taste in both the fasting state and satiety [139]. Thus, the neurobiological basis of the disease may differ considerably in males. Likewise, none of the included studies differentiated between the subtypes of the disease. However, it could be hypothesized that binge/purging behaviors may be related to different neurobiological paths from restrictive eating patterns. Another important factor that should be taken into consideration when studying adolescents pertains to the hormonal effects on the developing brain. For instance, research has shown that regional subcortical volumes are related to pubertal development, as measured by Tanner stage [165]. Additionally, a positive association has been reported between circulating estrogen levels and regional GM volumes [166]. Thus, given that pubertal development is partially dissociable from chronological age, matching study groups according to Tanner stage could be a reasonable approach [165]. Future systematic reviews could comparatively assess the present neuroimaging findings on AN versus other forms of malnutrition. Moreover, this systematic review subgrouped studies on the basis of imaging modalities; alternative subgrouping, as for instance according to methods of examining brain volumes, could have been performed but would not have allowed a clear link with the advantages and limitations of each modality.

Finally, as it has been already discussed, the interpretation of DTI findings is subject to additional limitations. First, differences in DTI parameters can emerge due to head motion during the scanning [167]. Only three studies have performed rigorous correction for head motion beyond the simple algorithm that is part of edgy current correction [56,59,60]. Second, dehydration could potentially affect diffusivity values, although the effects of dehydration on brain structure and function in eating disorders is an area of debate [168]. Studies used various methods to assess hydration status and some did not assess it at all (See Table 2). Urine specific gravity has been commonly used as a marker of hydration, however it may not be sufficient to diagnose hydration status and should be combined with other indices such as plasma and urine osmolarity [169]. Concluding, as discussed earlier, diffusion parameters could be affected by partial volume effect, at least in the fornix. Likewise, it could be hypothesized that WM tracts bordering the ventricular system, such as the corpus callosum and thalamic radiation could be affected as well. Consequently, the finding of reduced FA could be biased when ventricular volume has not been considered as a covariable.

Summarizing, our recommendations for future research are:

Since no standardized protocols are available, researchers are encouraged to follow proposed guidelines in order to increase validity, reliability and comparability of their results [168].

Enrolling adolescent patients at the earliest stage of the disease is the key to detect early biomarkers, before the confounding effects of malnutrition become apparent, albeit always considering developmental trajectories and puberty-related structural and functional deviations from normality.

Multi-center, longitudinal studies after long-term, physical and psychological recovery are proposed to conclusively disambiguate between trait-based variations and long-lasting effects of starvation.

Likewise, studying populations at risk before the onset of the disease is essential to differentiate between premorbid trait markers and permanent scars of the disease.

Finally, multimodal neuroimaging techniques combining different methodological approaches for data analysis could offer a more comprehensive view of disease impact on brain. Following the same logic, researchers could ideally utilize both structural and functional imaging to address regions of interest.

5. Conclusions

This systematic review demonstrated potential associations between structural and functional alterations detected in young, anorectic patients and core features of the disease. Of course, the complexity of both the human brain and the disease does not allow the definite attribution of a symptom to a specific area dysfunction. Moreover, further research is needed in order to clarify whether these alterations are state-dependent or pre-morbid markers and therefore, potential targets for early detection and intervention.

Supplementary Materials: The following are available online at https://www.mdpi.com/2227-9067/8/2/137/s1, Table S1: Studies excluded, with their reason for exclusion. Table S2a: Evaluation of the eligible studies with Newcastle-Ottawa scale- Case-Control studies. Table S2b: Evalusation of the eligible studies with Newcastle-Ottawa scale- Cohort studies.

Author Contributions: Conceptualization, G.M., M.T., F.B., T.N.S. and A.T.; methodology, K.K., M.N., A.K., E.P., E.V and T.N.S.; investigation, K.K., M.N., A.K., E.P. and E.V.; writing—original draft preparation, K.K., M.N., A.K., E.P., G.M. and F.G.; writing—review and editing S.M, F.G., F.B., M.T., T.P., T.N.S. and A.T.; visualization E.V., S.M., T.P., F.B. and F.G.; supervision, T.P., S.M., G.M., M.T., A.T. and T.N.S. All authors have read and agreed to the published version of the manuscript.

Funding: This research received no external funding.

Institutional Review Board Statement: The study did not require ethical approval/Not applicable.

Informed Consent Statement: The study did not require ethical approval/Not applicable.

Data Availability Statement: Data is contained within the article.

Conflicts of Interest: The authors declare no conflict of interest.

Abbreviations

ACC: Anterior Cingulate cortex; AD: Axial Diffusivity; AN: Anorexia Nervosa; AN-BP: Anorexia nervosa-Binge Purge type; AN-R: Anorexia Nervosa-Restricting type; BMI: Body Mass Index; Cho: Choline; CSF: Cerebrospinal Fluid; Cr: Creatine; CT: Cortical Thickness; dlPFC: Dorsolateral Prefrontal Cortex; DMN: Default Mode Network; DSM: Diagnostic and Statistical Manual of Mental Disorders; Dstr: Dorsal striatum; DTI: Diffusion Tensor Imaging; ECN: Executive Control Network; FA: Fractional Anisotropy; fMRI: Functional Magnetic Resonance Imaging; FPN: Fronto-Parietal Network; Glutamate/Glutamine: Glx; GM: Grey Matter; HC: Healthy Control participants; ICA: Independent component analysis; IFG: Inferior Frontal Gyrus; MCC: Medial Cingulate Cortex; MD: Mean Diffusivity; mI: myo-Inositol; MFG: Middle Frontal Gyrus; mPFC: Medial Prefrontal Cortex; MRI: Magnetic Resonance Imaging; MRS: Magnetic Resonance Spectroscopy; MTR: Magnetization Transfer Ratio; NAA: N-acetyl-aspartate; OCD: Obsessive Compulsive Disorder; OFC: Orbitofrontal Cortex; PCC: Posterior Cingulate Cortex; PFC: Prefrontal Cortex; PRISMA: Preferred Reporting Items for Systematic Reviews and Meta-Analyses; PTSD: Posttraumatic Stress Disorder; PVE: Partial Volume Effect; RD: Radial Diffusivity; rCBF: Regional Cerebral Blood Flow; ROIs: Regions Of Interest; RSFC: Resting State Functional Connectivity; RSN: Resting State Network; SBM: Surface Based Morphometry; SLF: Superior Longitudinal Fasciculus; SMA: Supplementary Motor Area; SN: Salience Network; SPECT: Single- Photon Emission Computed Tomography; SPM:s Statistical Parametric Mapping; TBSS:tract-based spatial statistics; tCho: total Choline; tCr: total Creatine; VBM: Voxel Based Morphometry; WISC: Wechsler Intelligence Scale for Children; WM: White Matter.

References

1. Gonzalez, A.; Kohn, M.R.; Clarke, S.D. Eating disorders in adolescents. *Aust. Fam. Physician* **2007**, *36*, 614–619.
2. Nicholls, D.; Viner, R.M. Eating disorders and weight problems. *BMJ* **2005**, *330*, 950–953. [CrossRef] [PubMed]
3. American Psychiatric Association (Ed.). *Diagnostic and Statistical Manual of Mental Disorders: DSM-5*, 5th ed.; American Psychiatric Association: Washington, DC, USA, 2013; p. 947.
4. Mitchell, J.E.; Peterson, C.B. Anorexia Nervosa. *N. Engl. J. Med.* **2020**, *382*, 1343–1351. [CrossRef]
5. Campbell, K.; Peebles, R. Eating Disorders in Children and Adolescents: State of the Art Review. *Pediatrics* **2014**, *134*, 582–592. [CrossRef]
6. Van den Eynde, F.; Suda, M.; Broadbent, H.; Guillaume, S.; Van den Eynde, M.; Steiger, H.; Schmidt, U. Structural magnetic resonance imaging in eating disorders: A systematic review of voxel-based morphometry studies. *Eur. Eat. Disord. Rev.* **2012**, *20*, 94–105. [CrossRef]
7. Seitz, J.; Herpertz-Dahlmann, B.; Konrad, K. Brain morphological changes in adolescent and adult patients with anorexia nervosa. *J. Neural Transm.* **2016**, *123*, 949–959. [CrossRef]
8. Seitz, J.; Bühren, K.; Von Polier, G.G.; Heussen, N.; Herpertz-Dahlmann, B.; Konrad, K. Morphological Changes in the Brain of Acutely Ill and Weight-Recovered Patients with Anorexia Nervosa. *Zeitschrift für Kinder und Jugendpsychiatrie Psychotherapie* **2014**, *42*, 7–18. [CrossRef] [PubMed]
9. Titova, O.E.; Hjorth, O.C.; Schiöth, H.B.; Brooks, S.J. Anorexia nervosa is linked to reduced brain structure in reward and so-matosensory regions: A meta-analysis of VBM studies. *BMC Psychiatry* **2013**, *13*, 110. [CrossRef]
10. Seitz, J.; Konrad, K.; Herpertz-Dahlmann, B. Extend, Pathomechanism and Clinical Consequences of Brain Volume Changes in Anorexia Nervosa. *Curr. Neuropharmacol.* **2018**, *16*, 1164–1173. [CrossRef]
11. Zhang, S.; Wang, W.; Su, X.; Kemp, G.J.; Yang, X.; Su, J.; Tan, Q.; Zhao, Y.; Sun, H.; Yue, Q. Psychoradiological investigations of gray matter alterations in patients with anorexia nervosa. *Transl. Psychiatry* **2018**, *8*, 277. [CrossRef] [PubMed]
12. Brooks, S.J.; Barker, G.J.; O'Daly, O.; Brammer, M.; Williams, S.C.; Benedict, C.; Schiöth, H.B.; Treasure, J.; Campbell, I.C. Restraint of appetite and reduced regional brain volumes in anorexia nervosa: A voxel-based morphometric study. *BMC Psychiatry* **2011**, *11*, 179. [CrossRef]
13. Frank, G.K.W.; Shott, M.E.; Hagman, J.; Yang, T.T. Localized brain volume and white matter integrity alterations in adolescent anorexia nervosa. *J. Am. Acad. Child. Adolesc. Psychiatry* **2013**, *52*, 1066–1075.e5. [CrossRef] [PubMed]
14. Lavagnino, L.; Mwangi, B.; Cao, B.; Shott, M.E.; Soares, J.C.; Frank, G.K.W. Cortical thickness patterns as state biomarker of anorexia nervosa. *Int. J. Eat. Disord.* **2018**, *51*, 241–249. [CrossRef] [PubMed]

15. Blasel, S.; Pilatus, U.; Magerkurth, J.; von Stauffenberg, M.; Vronski, D.; Mueller, M.; Hattingen, E. Metabolic gray matter changes of ad-olescents with anorexia nervosa in combined MR proton and phosphorus spectroscopy. *Neuroradiology* **2012**, *54*, 753–764. [CrossRef]
16. Roser, W.; Bubl, R.; Buergin, D.; Seelig, J.; Radue, E.W.; Rost, B. Metabolic changes in the brain of patients with anorexia and bu-limia nervosa as detected by proton magnetic resonance spectroscopy. *Int. J. Eat. Disord.* **1999**, *26*, 119–136. [CrossRef]
17. Simon, J.J.; Stopyra, M.A.; Friederich, H. Neural Processing of Disorder-Related Stimuli in Patients with Anorexia Nervosa: A Narrative Review of Brain Imaging Studies. *J. Clin. Med.* **2019**, *8*, 1047. [CrossRef] [PubMed]
18. Monteleone, A.M.; Monteleone, P.; Esposito, F.; Prinster, A.; Volpe, U.; Cantone, E.; Pellegrino, F.; Canna, A.; Milano, W.; Aiello, M.; et al. Altered processing of rewarding and aversive basic taste stimuli in symptomatic women with anorexia nervosa and bulimia nervosa: An fMRI study. *J. Psychiatr. Res.* **2017**, *90*, 94–101. [CrossRef]
19. Vocks, S.; Herpertz, S.; Rosenberger, C.; Senf, W.; Gizewski, E. Effects of gustatory stimulation on brain activity during hunger and satiety in females with restricting-type anorexia nervosa: An fMRI study. *J. Psychiatr. Res.* **2011**, *45*, 395–403. [CrossRef]
20. Gaudio, S.; Quattrocchi, C.C. Neural basis of a multidimensional model of body image distortion in anorexia nervosa. *Neurosci. Biobehav. Rev.* **2012**, *36*, 1839–1847. [CrossRef]
21. Olivo, G.; Gaudio, S.; Schiöth, H.B. Brain and Cognitive Development in Adolescents with Anorexia Nervosa: A Systematic Review of fMRI Studies. *Nutrients* **2019**, *11*, 1907. [CrossRef]
22. Kühn, S.; Vanderhasselt, M.-A.; De Raedt, R.; Gallinat, J. The neural basis of unwanted thoughts during resting state. *Soc. Cogn. Affect. Neurosci.* **2013**, *9*, 1320–1324. [CrossRef] [PubMed]
23. Cowdrey, F.A.; Filippini, N.; Park, R.J.; Smith, S.M.; McCabe, C. Increased resting state functional connectivity in the default mode network in recovered anorexia nervosa. *Hum. Brain Mapp.* **2014**, *35*, 483–491. [CrossRef] [PubMed]
24. Gaudio, S.; Wiemerslage, L.; Brooks, S.J.; Schiöth, H.B. A systematic review of resting-state functional-MRI studies in anorexia nervosa: Evidence for functional connectivity impairment in cognitive control and visuospatial and body-signal integration. *Neurosci. Biobehav. Rev.* **2016**, *71*, 578–589. [CrossRef] [PubMed]
25. Alfano, V.; Mele, G.; Cotugno, A.; Longarzo, M. Multimodal neuroimaging in anorexia nervosa. *J. Neurosci. Res.* **2020**. [CrossRef] [PubMed]
26. Phillipou, A.; Rossell, S.L.; Castle, D.J. The neurobiology of anorexia nervosa: A systematic review. *Aust. New Zealand J. Psychiatry* **2014**, *48*, 128–152. [CrossRef]
27. Brewerton, T.D. Antipsychotic Agents in the Treatment of Anorexia Nervosa: Neuropsychopharmacologic Rationale and Evidence from Controlled Trials. *Curr. Psychiatry Rep.* **2012**, *14*, 398–405. [CrossRef] [PubMed]
28. Fredrikson, M.; Faria, V. Neuroimaging in Anxiety Disorders. In *Modern Trends in Pharmacopsychiatry*; Baldwin, D.S., Leonard, B.E., Eds.; KARGER AG: Basel, Switzerland, 2013; pp. 47–66.
29. Martin Monzon, B.; Hay, P.; Foroughi, N.; Touyz, S. White matter alterations in anorexia nervosa: A systematic review of diffusion tensor imaging studies. *World J. Psychiatry* **2016**, *6*, 177–186. [CrossRef]
30. Gaudio, S.; Quattrocchi, C.C.; Piervincenzi, C.; Zobel, B.B.; Montecchi, F.R.; Dakanalis, A.; Riva, G.; Carducci, F. White matter abnormalities in treatment-naive adolescents at the earliest stages of Anorexia Nervosa: A diffusion tensor imaging study. *Psychiatry Res. Neuroimaging* **2017**, *266*, 138–145. [CrossRef]
31. Barona, M.; Brown, M.; Clark, C.; Frangou, S.; White, T.; Micali, N. White matter alterations in anorexia nervosa: Evidence from a voxel-based meta-analysis. *Neurosci. Biobehav. Rev.* **2019**, *100*, 285–295. [CrossRef]
32. Meneguzzo, P.; Collantoni, E.; Solmi, M.; Tenconi, E.; Favaro, A. Anorexia nervosa and diffusion weighted imaging: An open methodological question raised by a systematic review and a fractional anisotropy anatomical likelihood estimation me-ta-analysis. *Int. J. Eat. Disord.* **2019**, *52*, 1237–1250. [CrossRef]
33. Zhang, S.; Wang, W.; Su, X.; Li, L.; Yang, X.; Su, J.; Tan, Q.; Zhao, Y.; Sun, H.; Kemp, G.J.; et al. White Matter Abnormalities in Anorexia Nervosa: Psychoradiologic Evidence From Meta-Analysis of Diffusion Tensor Imaging Studies Using Tract Based Spatial Statistics. *Front. Neurosci.* **2020**, *14*, 159. [CrossRef]
34. Spear, L.P. Adolescent neurodevelopment. *J. Adolesc. Health* **2013**, *52* (Suppl. 2), S7–S13. [CrossRef]
35. Lu, L.H.; Dapretto, M.; O'Hare, E.D.; Kan, E.; McCourt, S.T.; Thompson, P.M.; Toga, A.W.; Bookheimer, S.Y.; Sowell, E.R. Relationships between Brain Activation and Brain Structure in Normally Developing Children. *Cereb. Cortex* **2009**, *19*, 2595–2604. [CrossRef]
36. Sharma, S.; Arain, M.; Mathur, P.; Rais, A.; Nel, W.; Sandhu, R.; Haque, M.; Johal, L. Maturation of the adolescent brain. *Neuropsychiatr. Dis. Treat.* **2013**, *9*, 449–461. [CrossRef]
37. Peper, J.S.; Heuvel, M.P.V.D.; Mandl, R.C.; Pol, H.E.H.; Van Honk, J. Sex steroids and connectivity in the human brain: A review of neuroimaging studies. *Psychoneuroendocrinology* **2011**, *36*, 1101–1113. [CrossRef]
38. Supekar, K.; Musen, M.; Menon, V. Development of large-scale functional brain networks in children. *PLoS Biol.* **2009**, *7*, e1000157. [CrossRef] [PubMed]
39. Fair, D.A.; Cohen, A.L.; Power, J.D.; Dosenbach, N.U.F.; Church, J.A.; Miezin, F.M.; Schlaggar, B.L.; Petersen, S.E. Functional brain networks develop from a "local to distributed" organization. *PLoS Comput. Biol.* **2009**, *5*, e1000381. [CrossRef] [PubMed]
40. Stevens, M.C.; Pearlson, G.D.; Calhoun, V.D. Changes in the interaction of resting-state neural networks from adolescence to adulthood. *Hum. Brain Mapp.* **2009**, *30*, 2356–2366. [CrossRef]

41. Liberati, A.; Altman, D.G.; Tetzlaff, J.; Mulrow, C.; Gøtzsche, P.C.; Ioannidis, J.P.A.; Clarke, M.; Devereaux, P.J.; Kleijnen, J.; Moher, D. The PRISMA statement for reporting systematic reviews and meta-analyses of studies that evaluate health care interventions: Explanation and elaboration. *PLoS Med.* **2009**, *6*, e1000100. [CrossRef] [PubMed]
42. Castro-Fornieles, J.; Bargalló, N.; Lázaro, L.; Andrés, S.; Falcon, C.; Plana, M.T.; Junqué, C. A cross-sectional and follow-up voxel-based morphometric MRI study in adolescent anorexia nervosa. *J. Psychiatr. Res.* **2009**, *43*, 331–340. [CrossRef]
43. Fujisawa, T.X.; Yatsuga, C.; Mabe, H.; Yamada, E.; Masuda, M.; Tomoda, A. Anorexia Nervosa during Adolescence Is Associated with Decreased Gray Matter Volume in the Inferior Frontal Gyrus. *PLoS ONE* **2015**, *10*, e0128548. [CrossRef]
44. King, J.A.; Geisler, D.; Ritschel, F.; Boehm, I.; Seidel, M.; Roschinski, B.; Soltwedel, L.; Zwipp, J.; Pfuhl, G.; Marxen, M.; et al. Global Cortical Thinning in Acute Anorexia Nervosa Normalizes Following Long-Term Weight Restoration. *Biol. Psychiatry* **2015**, *77*, 624–632. [CrossRef]
45. Neumärker, K.J.; Bzufka, W.M.; Dudeck, U.; Hein, J.; Neumärker, U. Are there specific disabilities of number processing in adolescent patients with Anorexia nervosa? Evidence from clinical and neuropsychological data when compared to mor-phometric measures from magnetic resonance imaging. *Eur. Child. Adolesc. Psychiatry.* **2000**, *9*, S111–S121. [CrossRef] [PubMed]
46. Yue, L.; Wang, Y.; Kaye, W.H.; Kang, Q.; Huang, J.-B.; Cheung, E.F.; Xiao, S.-F.; Wang, Z.; Chen, J.; Chan, R.C.K. Structural alterations in the caudate nucleus and precuneus in un-medicated anorexia nervosa patients. *Psychiatry Res. Neuroimaging* **2018**, *281*, 12–18. [CrossRef]
47. Myrvang, A.D.; Vangberg, T.R.; Stedal, K.; Rø, Ø.; Endestad, T.; Rosenvinge, J.H.; Aslaksen, P.M. Hippocampal subfields in adolescent ano-rexia nervosa. *Psychiatry Res. Neuroimaging* **2018**, *282*, 24–30. [CrossRef] [PubMed]
48. Martin Monzon, B.; Henderson, L.A.; Madden, S.; Macefield, V.G.; Touyz, S.; Kohn, M.R.; Clarke, S.; Foroughi, N.; Hay, P. Grey matter volume in adolescents with anorexia nervosa and associated eating disorder symptoms. *Eur. J. Neurosci.* **2017**, *46*, 2297–2307. [CrossRef]
49. Katzman, D.K.; Lambe, E.K.; Mikulis, D.J.; Ridgley, J.N.; Goldbloom, D.S.; Zipursky, R.B. Cerebral gray matter and white matter volume deficits in adolescent girls with anorexia nervosa. *J. Pediatr.* **1996**, *129*, 794–803. [CrossRef]
50. Golden, N.H.; Ashtari, M.; Kohn, M.R.; Patel, M.; Jacobson, M.S.; Fletcher, A.; Shenker, I. Reversibility of cerebral ventricular enlargement in anorexia nervosa, demonstrated by quantitative magnetic resonance imaging. *J. Pediatr.* **1996**, *128*, 296–301. [CrossRef]
51. Akgül, S.; Öz, A.; Karlı-Oğuz, K.; Kanbur, N.; Derman, O. Is white matter affected in adolescents with anorexia nervosa? a study using magnetization transfer imaging. *Turk. J. Pediatr.* **2016**, *58*, 282. [CrossRef]
52. Bernardoni, F.; King, J.A.; Geisler, D.; Stein, E.; Jaite, C.; Nätsch, D.; Tam, F.I.; Boehm, I.; Seidel, M.; Roessner, V.; et al. Weight restoration therapy rapidly reverses cortical thinning in anorexia nervosa: A longitudinal study. *NeuroImage* **2016**, *130*, 214–222. [CrossRef]
53. Katzman, D.K.; Zipursky, R.B.; Lambe, E.K.; Mikulis, D.J. A longitudinal magnetic resonance imaging study of brain changes in adolescents with anorexia nervosa. *Arch. Pediatr. Adolesc. Med.* **1997**, *151*, 793–797. [CrossRef]
54. Castro-Fornieles, J.; Bargalló, N.; Lázaro, L.; Andrés, S.; Falcon, C.; Plana, M.T.; Junqué, C. Adolescent anorexia nervosa: Cross-sectional and follow-up frontal gray matter disturbances detected with proton magnetic resonance spectroscopy. *J. Psychiatric Res.* **2007**, *41*, 952–958. [CrossRef] [PubMed]
55. Schlemmer, H.-P.; Möckel, R.; Marcus, A.; Hentschel, F.; Göpel, C.; Becker, G.; Köpke, J.; Gückel, F.; Schmidt, M.H.; Georgi, M. Proton magnetic resonance spectroscopy in acute, juvenile anorexia nervosa. *Psychiatry Res. Neuroimaging* **1998**, *82*, 171–179. [CrossRef]
56. Pfuhl, G.; King, J.A.; Geisler, D.; Roschinski, B.; Ritschel, F.; Seidel, M.; Bernardoni, F.; Müller, D.K.; White, T.; Roessner, V.; et al. Preserved white matter microstructure in young patients with anorexia nervosa? *Hum. Brain Mapp.* **2016**, *37*, 4069–4083. [CrossRef]
57. von Schwanenflug, N.; Müller, D.K.; King, J.A.; Ritschel, F.; Bernardoni, F.; Mohammadi, S.; Geisler, D.; Roessner, V.; Biemann, R.; Marxen, M.; et al. Dynamic changes in white matter microstructure in anorexia nervosa: Findings from a longitudinal study. *Psychol. Med.* **2019**, *49*, 1555–1564. [CrossRef]
58. Olivo, G.; Swenne, I.; Zhukovsky, C.; Tuunainen, A.-K.; Saaid, A.; Salonen-Ros, H.; Larsson, E.-M.; Brooks, S.J.; Schiöth, H.B. Preserved white matter microstructure in adolescent patients with atypical anorexia nervosa. *Int. J. Eat. Disord.* **2019**, *52*, 166–174. [CrossRef] [PubMed]
59. Travis, K.E.; Golden, N.H.; Feldman, H.M.; Solomon, M.; Nguyen, J.; Mezer, A.; Yeatman, J.D.; Dougherty, R.F. Abnormal white matter properties in ado-lescent girls with anorexia nervosa. *Neuroimage Clin.* **2015**, *9*, 648–659. [CrossRef] [PubMed]
60. Vogel, K.; Timmers, I.; Kumar, V.; Nickl-Jockschat, T.; Bastiani, M.; Roebroek, A.; Herpertz-Dahlmann, B.; Konrad, K.; Goebel, R.; Seitz, J. White matter microstructural changes in adolescent anorexia nervosa including an exploratory longitudinal study. *NeuroImage: Clin.* **2016**, *11*, 614–621. [CrossRef]
61. Hu, S.-H.; Feng, H.; Xu, T.-T.; Zhang, H.-R.; Zhao, Z.-Y.; Lai, J.-B.; Xu, D.; Xu, Y. Altered microstructure of brain white matter in females with anorexia nervosa: A diffusion tensor imaging study. *Neuropsychiatr. Dis. Treat.* **2017**, *13*, 2829–2836. [CrossRef]
62. Smith, S.M.; Fox, P.M.; Miller, K.L.; Glahn, D.C.; Mackay, C.E.; Filippini, N.; Watkins, K.E.; Toro, R.; Laird, A.R.; Beckmann, C.F. Correspondence of the brain's functional architecture during activation and rest. *Proc. Natl. Acad. Sci. USA* **2009**, *106*, 13040–13045. [CrossRef]

63. Gaudio, S.; Piervincenzi, C.; Zobel, B.B.; Montecchi, F.R.; Riva, G.; Carducci, F.; Quattrocchi, C.C. Altered resting state functional connectivity of anterior cingulate cortex in drug naïve adolescents at the earliest stages of anorexia nervosa. *Sci. Rep.* **2015**, *5*, 10818. [CrossRef]
64. Gaudio, S.; Olivo, G.; Zobel, B.B.; Schiöth, H.B. Altered cerebellar–insular–parietal–cingular subnetwork in adolescents in the earliest stages of anorexia nervosa: A network–based statistic analysis. *Transl. Psychiatry* **2018**, *8*, 1–10. [CrossRef]
65. Boehm, I.; Geisler, D.; King, J.A.; Ritschel, F.; Seidel, M.; Araujo, Y.D.; Petermann, J.; Lohmeier, H.; Weiss, J.; Walter, M.; et al. Increased resting state functional connectivity in the fronto-parietal and default mode network in anorexia nervosa. *Front. Behav. Neurosci.* **2014**, *8*. [CrossRef]
66. Amianto, F.; D'Agata, F.; Lavagnino, L.; Caroppo, P.; Abbate-Daga, G.; Righi, D.; Scarone, S.; Bergui, M.; Mortara, P.; Fassino, S. Intrinsic Connectivity Networks Within Cerebellum and Beyond in Eating Disorders. *Cerebellum* **2013**, *12*, 623–631. [CrossRef] [PubMed]
67. Geisler, D.; Borchardt-Lohölter, V.; Lord, A.; Boehm, I.; Ritschel, F.; Zwipp, J.; Clas, S.; King, J.A.; Wolff-Stephan, S.; Roessner, V.; et al. Abnormal functional global and local brain connectivity in female patients with anorexia nervosa. *J. Psychiatry Neurosci.* **2016**, *41*, 6–15. [CrossRef] [PubMed]
68. Ehrlich, S.; Lord, A.R.; Geisler, D.; Borchardt, V.; Boehm, I.; Seidel, M.; Ritschel, F.; Schulze, A.; King, J.A.; Weidner, K.; et al. Reduced functional connectivity in the thalamo-insular subnetwork in patients with acute anorexia nervosa. *Hum. Brain Mapp.* **2015**, *36*, 1772–1781. [CrossRef] [PubMed]
69. Kojima, S.; Nagai, N.; Nakabeppu, Y.; Muranaga, T.; Deguchi, D.; Nakajo, M.; Masuda, A.; Nozoe, S.-I.; Naruo, T. Comparison of regional cerebral blood flow in patients with anorexia nervosa before and after weight gain. *Psychiatry Res. Neuroimaging* **2005**, *140*, 251–258. [CrossRef] [PubMed]
70. Takano, A.; Shiga, T.; Kitagawa, N.; Koyama, T.; Katoh, C.; Tsukamoto, E.; Tamaki, N. Abnormal neuronal network in anorexia nervosa studied with I-123-IMP SPECT. *Psychiatry Res. Neuroimaging* **2001**, *107*, 45–50. [CrossRef]
71. Matsumoto, R.; Kitabayashi, Y.; Narumoto, J.; Wada, Y.; Okamoto, A.; Ushijima, Y.; Yokoyama, C.; Yamashita, T.; Takahashi, H.; Yasuno, F.; et al. Regional cerebral blood flow changes associated with interoceptive awareness in the recovery process of anorexia nervosa. *Prog. Neuro Psychopharmacology Biol. Psychiatry* **2006**, *30*, 1265–1270. [CrossRef]
72. Komatsu, H.; Nagamitsu, S.; Ozono, S.; Yamashita, Y.; Ishibashi, M.; Matsuishi, T. Regional cerebral blood flow changes in early-onset anorexia nervosa before and after weight gain. *Brain Dev.* **2010**, *32*, 625–630. [CrossRef]
73. Schwartz, D.H.; Dickie, E.W.; Pangelinan, M.M.; Leonard, G.; Perron, M.; Pike, G.B.; Richer, L.; Veillette, S.; Pausova, Z.; Paus, T. Adiposity is associated with structural properties of the adolescent brain. *NeuroImage* **2014**, *103*, 192–201. [CrossRef]
74. Hoffman, G.W.; Ellinwood, E.; Rockwell, W.; Herfkens, R.J.; Nishita, J.; Guthrie, L.F. Cerebral atrophy in anorexia nervosa: A pilot study. *Biol. Psychiatry* **1989**, *26*, 321–324. [CrossRef]
75. Andela, C.D.; Van Haalen, F.M.; Ragnarsson, O.; Papakokkinou, E.; Johannsson, G.; Santos, A.; Webb, S.M.; Biermasz, N.R.; Van Der Wee, N.J.; Pereira, A.M. Mechanisms in endocrinology: Cushing's syndrome causes irreversible effects on the human brain: A systematic review of structural and functional magnetic resonance imaging studies. *Eur. J. Endocrinol.* **2015**, *173*, R1–R14. [CrossRef] [PubMed]
76. Schorr, M.; Miller, K.K. The endocrine manifestations of anorexia nervosa: Mechanisms and management. *Nat. Rev. Endocrinol.* **2017**, *13*, 174–186. [CrossRef] [PubMed]
77. Collantoni, E.; Meneguzzo, P.; Tenconi, E.; Manara, R.; Favaro, A. Small-world properties of brain morphological characteristics in Anorexia Nervosa. *PLoS ONE* **2019**, *14*, e0216154. [CrossRef]
78. Olivo, G.; Dahlberg, L.S.; Wiemerslage, L.; Swenne, I.; Zhukovsky, C.; Salonen-Ros, H.; Larsson, E.-M.; Gaudio, S.; Brooks, S.J.; Schiöth, H.B. Atypical anorexia nervosa is not related to brain structural changes in newly diagnosed adolescent patients. *Int. J. Eat. Disord.* **2017**, *51*, 39–45. [CrossRef]
79. Bomba, M.; Riva, A.; Veggo, F.; Grimaldi, M.; Villa, R.; Neri, F.; Nacinovich, R. Impact of speed and magnitude of weight loss on the development of brain trophic changes in adolescents with anorexia nervosa: A case control study. *Ital. J. Pediatr.* **2013**, *39*, 14. [CrossRef]
80. Lavagnino, L.; Amianto, F.; Mwangi, B.; D'Agata, F.; Spalatro, A.; Soares, G.B.Z.; Daga, G.A.; Mortara, P.; Fassino, S.; Soares, J.C. The relationship between cortical thickness and body mass index differs between women with anorexia nervosa and healthy controls. *Psychiatry Res. Neuroimaging* **2016**, *248*, 105–109. [CrossRef] [PubMed]
81. Nico, D.; Daprati, E.; Nighoghossian, N.; Carrier, E.; Duhamel, J.-R.; Sirigu, A. The role of the right parietal lobe in anorexia nervosa. *Psychol. Med.* **2009**, *40*, 1531–1539. [CrossRef]
82. Lipsman, N.; Woodside, D.B.; Lozano, A.M. Neurocircuitry of limbic dysfunction in anorexia nervosa. *Cortex* **2015**, *62*, 109–118. [CrossRef]
83. Treadway, M.T.; Waskom, M.L.; Dillon, D.G.; Holmes, A.J.; Park, M.T.M.; Chakravarty, M.M.; Dutra, S.J.; Polli, F.E.; Iosifescu, D.V.; Fava, M.; et al. Illness Progression, Recent Stress, and Morphometry of Hippocampal Subfields and Medial Prefrontal Cortex in Major Depression. *Biol. Psychiatry* **2015**, *77*, 285–294. [CrossRef]
84. Schmaal, L.; Veltman, D.J.; Van Erp, T.; Sämann, P.; Frodl, T.; Jahanshad, N.; Loehrer, E.; Tiemeier, H.; Hofman, A. Subcortical brain alterations in major depressive disorder: Findings from the ENIGMA Major Depressive Disorder working group. *Mol. Psychiatry* **2016**, *21*, 806–812. [CrossRef]

85. Mainz, V.; Schulte-Rüther, M.; Fink, G.R.; Herpertz-Dahlmann, B.; Konrad, K. Structural Brain Abnormalities in Adolescent Anorexia Nervosa Before and After Weight Recovery and Associated Hormonal Changes. *Psychosom. Med.* **2012**, *74*, 574–582. [CrossRef]
86. Gibson, D.; Workman, C.; Mehler, P.S. Medical Complications of Anorexia Nervosa and Bulimia Nervosa. *Psychiatr. Clin. North. Am.* **2019**, *42*, 263–274. [CrossRef] [PubMed]
87. Kaye, W.H.; Wierenga, C.E.; Bailer, U.F.; Simmons, A.N.; Bischoff-Grethe, A. Nothing tastes as good as skinny feels: The neurobiology of anorexia nervosa. *Trends Neurosci.* **2013**, *36*, 110–120. [CrossRef] [PubMed]
88. Jun, H.; Hussaini, S.M.Q.; Rigby, M.J.; Jang, M.-H. Functional Role of Adult Hippocampal Neurogenesis as a Therapeutic Strategy for Mental Disorders. *Neural Plast.* **2012**, *2012*, 854285. [CrossRef] [PubMed]
89. Burkert, N.T.; Koschutnig, K.; Ebner, F.; Freidl, W. Structural hippocampal alterations, perceived stress, and coping deficiencies in patients with anorexia nervosa: Hippocampus, stress, and coping in Anorexia nervosa. *Int J. Eat. Disord.* **2015**, *48*, 670–676. [CrossRef]
90. Tottenham, N.; Galván, A. Stress and the adolescent brain: Amygdala-prefrontal cortex circuitry and ventral striatum as developmental targets. *Neurosci. Biobehav. Rev.* **2016**, *70*, 217–227. [CrossRef] [PubMed]
91. Fossati, P. Neural correlates of emotion processing: From emotional to social brain. *Eur. Neuropsychopharmacol.* **2012**, *22*, S487–S491. [CrossRef]
92. Hare, T.A.; Tottenham, N.; Galvan, A.; Voss, H.U.; Glover, G.H.; Casey, B. Biological Substrates of Emotional Reactivity and Regulation in Adolescence During an Emotional Go-Nogo Task. *Biol. Psychiatry* **2008**, *63*, 927–934. [CrossRef]
93. Joos, A.; Saum, B.; Van Elst, L.T.; Perlov, E.; Glauche, V.; Hartmann, A.; Freyer, T.; Tüscher, O.; Zeeck, A. Amygdala hyperreactivity in restrictive anorexia nervosa. *Psychiatry Res. Neuroimaging* **2011**, *191*, 189–195. [CrossRef]
94. Oldershaw, A.; Startup, H.; Lavender, T. Anorexia Nervosa and a Lost Emotional Self: A Psychological Formulation of the Development, Maintenance, and Treatment of Anorexia Nervosa. *Front. Psychol.* **2019**, *10*, 219. [CrossRef]
95. Vocks, S.; Busch, M.; Grönemeyer, D.; Schulte, D.; Herpertz, S.; Suchan, B. Neural correlates of viewing photographs of one's own body and another woman's body in anorexia and bulimia nervosa: An fMRI study. *J Psychiatry Neurosci.* **2010**, *35*, 163–176. [CrossRef]
96. Miyake, Y.; Okamoto, Y.; Onoda, K.; Kurosaki, M.; Shirao, N.; Okamoto, Y.; Yamawaki, S. Brain activation during the perception of distorted body images in eating disorders. *Psychiatry Res. Neuroimaging* **2010**, *181*, 183–192. [CrossRef] [PubMed]
97. Miyake, Y.; Okamoto, Y.; Onoda, K.; Shirao, N.; Okamoto, Y.; Otagaki, Y.; Yamawaki, S. Neural processing of negative word stimuli concerning body image in patients with eating disorders: An fMRI study. *NeuroImage* **2010**, *50*, 1333–1339. [CrossRef] [PubMed]
98. Seidel, M.; King, J.A.; Ritschel, F.; Boehm, I.; Geisler, D.; Bernardoni, F.; Beck, M.; Pauligk, S.; Biemann, R.; Strobel, A.; et al. Processing and regulation of negative emotions in anorexia nervosa: An fMRI study. *NeuroImage: Clin.* **2018**, *18*, 1–8. [CrossRef] [PubMed]
99. Oldershaw, A.; Hambrook, D.; Stahl, D.; Tchanturia, K.; Treasure, J.; Schmidt, U. The socio-emotional processing stream in Anorexia Nervosa. *Neurosci. Biobehav. Rev.* **2011**, *35*, 970–988. [CrossRef]
100. Horndasch, S.; O'Keefe, S.; Lamond, A.; Brown, K.; McCabe, C. Increased anticipatory but decreased consummatory brain responses to food in sisters of anorexia nervosa patients. *BJPsych Open* **2016**, *2*, 255–261. [CrossRef]
101. Burkert, N.T.; Koschutnig, K.; Ebner, F.; Freidl, W. Body image disturbances, fear and associations with the amygdala in anorexia nervosa. *Wien. Klin. Wochenschr.* **2019**, *131*, 61–67. [CrossRef]
102. Phillips, M.L.; Drevets, W.C.; Rauch, S.L.; Lane, R. Neurobiology of emotion perception I: The neural basis of normal emotion perception. *Biol. Psychiatry* **2003**, *54*, 504–514. [CrossRef]
103. Gaudio, S.; Carducci, F.; Piervincenzi, C.; Olivo, G.; Schiöth, H.B. Altered thalamo–cortical and occipital–parietal– temporal–frontal white matter connections in patients with anorexia and bulimia nervosa: A systematic review of diffusion tensor imaging studies. *J. Psychiatry Neurosci.* **2019**, *44*, 324–339. [CrossRef]
104. Stave, E.A.; De Bellis, M.D.; Hooper, S.R.; Woolley, D.P.; Chang, S.K.; Chen, S.D. Dimensions of Attention Associated with the Microstructure of Corona Radiata White Matter. *J. Child Neurol.* **2017**, *32*, 458–466. [CrossRef] [PubMed]
105. Phillipou, A.; Castle, D.J.; Rossell, S.L. Response: Commentary on Phillipou et al. (2018) anorexia nervosa: Eating disorder or body image disorder? *Aust. New Zealand J. Psychiatry* **2018**, *52*, 288–289. [CrossRef]
106. Karababa, I.F.; Bayazıt, H.; Kılıçaslan, N.; Çelik, M.; Cece, H.; Karakas, E.; Selek, S. Microstructural Changes of Anterior Corona Radiata in Bipolar Depression. *Psychiatry Investig.* **2015**, *12*, 367–371. [CrossRef]
107. Papathanasiou, A.; Messinis, L.; Zampakis, P.; Papathanasopoulos, P. Corpus callosum atrophy as a marker of clinically meaningful cognitive decline in secondary progressive multiple sclerosis. Impact on employment status. *J. Clin. Neurosci.* **2017**, *43*, 170–175. [CrossRef] [PubMed]
108. Makris, N.; Kennedy, D.N.; McInerney, S.; Sorensen, A.G.; Wang, R.; Caviness, V.S.; Pandya, D.N. Segmentation of Subcomponents within the Superior Longitudinal Fascicle in Humans: A Quantitative, In Vivo, DT-MRI Study. *Cereb. Cortex* **2005**, *15*, 854–869. [CrossRef]
109. Catani, M.; de Schotten, M.T. *Atlas of Human Brain Connections*; Oxford University Press: Oxford, UK, 2012.
110. Emori, S.; Oishi, K.; Jiang, H.; Jiang, L.; Li, X.; Akhter, K.; Hua, K.; Faria, A.V.; Mahmood, A.; Woods, R.P.; et al. Stereotaxic white matter atlas based on diffusion tensor imaging in an ICBM template. *NeuroImage* **2008**, *40*, 570–582. [CrossRef]

111. Frank, G.K. Advances from neuroimaging studies in eating disorders. *CNS Spectrums* **2015**, *20*, 391–400. [CrossRef]
112. Kaufmann, L.-K.; Baur, V.; Hänggi, J.; Jäncke, L.; Piccirelli, M.; Kollias, S.; Schnyder, U.; Pasternak, O.; Martin-Soelch, C.; Milos, G. Fornix Under Water? Ventricular Enlargement Biases Forniceal Diffusion Magnetic Resonance Imaging Indices in Anorexia Nervosa. *Biol. Psychiatry Cogn. Neurosci. Neuroimaging* **2017**, *2*, 430–437. [CrossRef] [PubMed]
113. Kazlouski, D.; Rollin, M.D.; Tregellas, J.; Shott, M.E.; Jappe, L.M.; Hagman, J.O.; Pryor, T.; Yang, T.T.; Frank, G.K.W. Altered fimbria-fornix white matter integrity in anorexia nervosa predicts harm avoidance. *Psychiatry Res. Neuroimaging* **2011**, *192*, 109–116. [CrossRef]
114. Via, E.; Zalesky, A.; Sánchez, I.; Forcano, L.; Harrison, B.J.; Pujol, J.; Fernández-Aranda, F.; Menchón, J.M.; Soriano-Mas, C.; Cardoner, N.C.; et al. Disruption of brain white matter microstructure in women with anorexia nervosa. *J. Psychiatry Neurosci.* **2014**, *39*, 367–375. [CrossRef] [PubMed]
115. Frieling, H.; Fischer, J.; Wilhelm, J.; Engelhorn, T.; Bleich, S.; Hillemacher, T.; Dörfler, A.; Kornhuber, J.; De Zwaan, M.; Peschel, T. Microstructural abnormalities of the posterior thalamic radiation and the mediodorsal thalamic nuclei in females with anorexia nervosa—A voxel based diffusion tensor imaging (DTI) study. *J. Psychiatr. Res.* **2012**, *46*, 1237–1242. [CrossRef] [PubMed]
116. Frank, G.K.W. Altered brain reward circuits in eating disorders: Chicken or egg? *Curr. Psychiatry. Rep.* **2013**, *15*, 396. [CrossRef] [PubMed]
117. Alexander, A.L.; Lee, J.E.; Lazar, M.; Field, A.S. Diffusion tensor imaging of the brain. *Neurotherapeutics* **2007**, *4*, 316–329. [CrossRef]
118. Basser, P.J.; Pierpaoli, C. Microstructural and physiological features of tissues elucidated by quantitative-diffusion-tensor MRI. *J. Magn. Reson.* **2011**, *213*, 560–570. [CrossRef]
119. Kubicki, M.; McCarley, R.; Westin, C.-F.; Park, H.-J.; Maier, S.; Kikinis, R.; Jolesz, F.A.; Shenton, M.E. A review of diffusion tensor imaging studies in schizophrenia. *J. Psychiatr. Res.* **2007**, *41*, 15–30. [CrossRef] [PubMed]
120. Jones, D.K.; Knösche, T.R.; Turner, R. White matter integrity, fiber count, and other fallacies: The do's and don'ts of diffusion MRI. *Neuroimage* **2013**, *73*, 239–254. [CrossRef]
121. Frintrop, L.; Liesbrock, J.; Paulukat, L.; Johann, S.; Kas, M.J.; Tolba, R.H.; Heussen, N.; Neulen, J.; Konrad, K.; Herpertz-Dahlmann, B.; et al. Reduced astrocyte density underlying brain volume reduction in activity-based anorexia rats. *World J. Biol. Psychiatry* **2017**, *19*, 225–235. [CrossRef]
122. Paus, T. Growth of white matter in the adolescent brain: Myelin or axon? *Brain Cogn.* **2010**, *72*, 26–35. [CrossRef]
123. Song, S.-K.; Sun, S.-W.; Ramsbottom, M.J.; Chang, C.; Russell, J.; Cross, A.H. Dysmyelination revealed through MRI as increased radial (but unchanged axial) diffusion of water. *Neuroimage* **2002**, *17*, 1429–1436. [CrossRef]
124. Qiu, D.; Tan, L.-H.; Zhou, K.; Khong, P.-L. Diffusion tensor imaging of normal white matter maturation from late childhood to young adulthood: Voxel-wise evaluation of mean diffusivity, fractional anisotropy, radial and axial diffusivities, and correlation with reading development. *NeuroImage* **2008**, *41*, 223–232. [CrossRef] [PubMed]
125. Stevens, F.L.; Hurley, R.A.; Taber, K.H. Anterior cingulate cortex: Unique role in cognition and emotion. *J. Neuropsychiatry Clin. Neurosci.* **2011**, *23*, 121–125. [CrossRef]
126. Kelly, A.C.; Di Martino, A.; Uddin, L.Q.; Shehzad, Z.; Gee, D.G.; Reiss, P.T.; Margulies, D.S.; Castellanos, F.X.; Milham, M.P. Development of Anterior Cingulate Functional Connectivity from Late Childhood to Early Adulthood. *Cereb. Cortex* **2008**, *19*, 640–657. [CrossRef] [PubMed]
127. Margulies, D.S.; Kelly, A.M.C.; Uddin, L.Q.; Biswal, B.B.; Castellanos, F.X.; Milham, M.P. Mapping the functional connectivity of anterior cingulate cortex. *NeuroImage* **2007**, *37*, 579–588. [CrossRef]
128. Blair, K.S.; Smith, B.W.; Mitchell, D.G.; Morton, J.; Vythilingam, M.; Pessoa, L.; Fridberg, D.; Zametkin, A.; Sturman, D.; Nelson, E.E.; et al. Modulation of emotion by cognition and cognition by emotion. *NeuroImage* **2007**, *35*, 430–440. [CrossRef]
129. Fitzgerald, P.B.; Laird, A.R.; Maller, J.; Daskalakis, Z.J. A meta-analytic study of changes in brain activation in depression. *Hum Brain Mapp.* **2008**, *29*, 683–695. [CrossRef] [PubMed]
130. Minzenberg, M.J.; Laird, A.R.; Thelen, S.; Carter, C.S.; Glahn, D.C. Meta-analysis of 41 Functional Neuroimaging Studies of Executive Function in Schizophrenia. *Arch. Gen. Psychiatry* **2009**, *66*, 811–822. [CrossRef]
131. Etkin, A.; Wager, T.D. Functional Neuroimaging of Anxiety: A Meta-Analysis of Emotional Processing in PTSD, Social Anxiety Disorder, and Specific Phobia. *Am. J. Psychiatry* **2007**, *164*, 1476–1488. [CrossRef]
132. Rowsell, M.; Macdonald, D.E.; Carter, J.C. Emotion regulation difficulties in anorexia nervosa: Associations with improvements in eating psychopathology. *J. Eat. Disord.* **2016**, *4*, 17. [CrossRef] [PubMed]
133. Uddin, L.Q.; Nomi, J.S.; Hébert-Seropian, B.; Ghaziri, J.; Boucher, O. Structure and Function of the Human Insula. *J. Clin. Neurophysiol.* **2017**, *34*, 300–306. [CrossRef]
134. Gogolla, N. The insular cortex. *Curr. Biol.* **2017**, *27*, R580–R586. [CrossRef]
135. Devue, C.; Collette, F.; Balteau, E.; Degueldre, C.; Luxen, A.; Maquet, P.; Brédart, S. Here I am: The cortical correlates of visual self-recognition. *Brain Res.* **2007**, *1143*, 169–182. [CrossRef]
136. Konstantakopoulos, G.; Varsou, E.; Dikeos, D.; Ioannidi, N.; Gonidakis, F.; Papadimitriou, G.; Oulis, P. Delusionality of body image beliefs in eating disorders. *Psychiatry Res.* **2012**, *200*, 482–488. [CrossRef]
137. Wagner, A.; Aizenstein, H.J.; Mazurkewicz, L.; Fudge, J.L.; Frank, G.K.W.; Putnam, K.; Bailer, U.F.; Fischer, L.; Kaye, W.H. Altered Insula Response to Taste Stimuli in Individuals Recovered from Restricting-Type Anorexia Nervosa. *Neuropsychopharmacology* **2008**, *33*, 513–523. [CrossRef]

138. Oberndorfer, T.A.; Frank, G.K.; Simmons, A.N.; Wagner, A.; McCurdy, D.; Fudge, J.L.; Yang, T.T.; Paulus, M.P.; Kaye, W.H. Altered Insula Response to Sweet Taste Processing After Recovery From Anorexia and Bulimia Nervosa. *Am. J. Psychiatry* **2013**, *170*, 1143–1151. [CrossRef]
139. Haase, L.; Green, E.; Murphy, C. Males and females show differential brain activation to taste when hungry and sated in gustatory and reward areas. *Appetite* **2011**, *57*, 421–434. [CrossRef]
140. Nunn, K.; Frampton, I.; Fuglset, T.S.; Törzsök-Sonnevend, M.; Lask, B. Anorexia nervosa and the insula. *Med. Hypotheses* **2011**, *76*, 353–357. [CrossRef] [PubMed]
141. Lichenstein, S.D.; Verstynen, T.; Forbes, E.E. Adolescent brain development and depression: A case for the importance of connectivity of the anterior cingulate cortex. *Neurosci. Biobehav. Rev.* **2016**, *70*, 271–287. [CrossRef] [PubMed]
142. Fair, D.A.; Dosenbach, N.U.F.; Church, J.A.; Cohen, A.L.; Brahmbhatt, S.; Miezin, F.M.; Barch, D.M.; Raichle, M.E.; Petersen, S.E.; Schlaggar, B.L. Development of distinct control networks through segregation and integration. *Proc. Natl. Acad. Sci. USA* **2007**, *104*, 13507–13512. [CrossRef] [PubMed]
143. Casey, B.J.; Jones, R.M.; Somerville, L.H. Braking and Accelerating of the Adolescent Brain. *J. Res. Adolesc.* **2011**, *21*, 21–33. [CrossRef]
144. Craig, A.D.B. How do you feel—now? The anterior insula and human awareness. *Nat. Rev. Neurosci.* **2009**, *10*, 59–70. [CrossRef]
145. Uddin, L.Q.; Supekar, K.S.; Ryali, S.; Menon, V. Dynamic Reconfiguration of Structural and Functional Connectivity Across Core Neurocognitive Brain Networks with Development. *J. Neurosci.* **2011**, *31*, 18578–18589. [CrossRef] [PubMed]
146. Ernst, M.; Torrisi, S.; Balderston, N.L.; Grillon, C.; Hale, E.A. fMRI Functional Connectivity Applied to Adolescent Neurodevelopment. *Annu. Rev. Clin. Psychol.* **2015**, *11*, 361–377. [CrossRef] [PubMed]
147. Damoiseaux, J.S.; Rombouts, S.A.R.B.; Barkhof, F.; Scheltens, P.; Stam, C.J.; Smith, S.M.; Beckmann, C.F. Consistent resting-state networks across healthy subjects. *Proc. Natl. Acad. Sci. USA* **2006**, *103*, 13848–13853. [CrossRef]
148. Buckner, R.L.; Andrews-Hanna, J.R.; Schacter, D.L. The brain's default network: Anatomy, function, and relevance to disease. *Ann. N. Y. Acad. Sci.* **2008**, *1124*, 1–38. [CrossRef]
149. Raichle, M.E. The brain's default mode network. *Annu. Rev. Neurosci.* **2015**, *38*, 433–447. [CrossRef]
150. Broyd, S.J.; Demanuele, C.; Debener, S.; Helps, S.K.; James, C.J.; Sonuga-Barke, E.J. Default-mode brain dysfunction in mental disorders: A systematic review. *Neurosci. Biobehav. Rev.* **2009**, *33*, 279–296. [CrossRef] [PubMed]
151. Menon, V. Large-scale brain networks and psychopathology: A unifying triple network model. *Trends Cogn. Sci.* **2011**, *15*, 483–506. [CrossRef]
152. Hamilton, J.P.; Farmer, M.; Fogelman, P.; Gotlib, I.H. Depressive Rumination, the Default-Mode Network, and the Dark Matter of Clinical Neuroscience. *Biol. Psychiatry* **2015**, *78*, 224–230. [CrossRef]
153. Uniacke, B.; Wang, Y.; Biezonski, D.; Sussman, T.; Lee, S.; Posner, J.; Steinglass, J. Resting-state connectivity within and across neural circuits in anorexia nervosa. *Brain Behav.* **2019**, *9*, e01205. [CrossRef] [PubMed]
154. Shott, M.E.; Cornier, M.-A.; Mittal, V.A.; Pryor, T.L.; Orr, J.M.; Brown, M.S.; Frank, G.K. Orbitofrontal cortex volume and brain reward response in obesity. *Int. J. Obes.* **2015**, *39*, 214–221. [CrossRef]
155. Wilkinson, L.L.; Brunstrom, J.M. Sensory specific satiety: More than "just" habituation? *Appetite* **2016**, *103*, 221–228. [CrossRef]
156. Fox, M.D.; Greicius, M. Clinical applications of resting state functional connectivity. *Front Syst. Neurosci.* **2010**, *4*, 19. [CrossRef] [PubMed]
157. Boghi, A.; Sterpone, S.; Sales, S.; D'Agata, F.; Bradac, G.B.; Zullo, G.; Munno, D. In vivo evidence of global and focal brain alterations in anorexia nervosa. *Psychiatry Res. Neuroimaging* **2011**, *192*, 154–159. [CrossRef]
158. Amianto, F.; Caroppo, P.; D'Agata, F.; Spalatro, A.; Lavagnino, L.; Caglio, M.; Righi, D.; Bergui, M.; Abbate-Daga, G.; Rigardetto, R.; et al. Brain volumetric abnormalities in patients with anorexia and bulimia nervosa: A Voxel-based morphometry study. *Psychiatry Res. Neuroimaging* **2013**, *213*, 210–216. [CrossRef]
159. Frank, G.K.; DeGuzman, M.C.; Shott, M.E. Motivation to eat and not to eat—The psycho-biological conflict in anorexia nervosa. *Physiol. Behav.* **2019**, *206*, 185–190. [CrossRef]
160. Wagner, A.; Bs, N.C.B.; Frank, G.K.W.; Bailer, U.F.; Wonderlich, S.A.; Crosby, R.D.; Bs, S.E.H.; Bs, V.V.; Plotnicov, K.; McConaha, C.; et al. Personality traits after recovery from eating disorders: Do subtypes differ? *Int. J. Eat. Disord.* **2006**, *39*, 276–284. [CrossRef] [PubMed]
161. Khalsa, S.S.; Portnoff, L.C.; McCurdy-McKinnon, D.; Feusner, J.D. What happens after treatment? A systematic review of relapse, remission, and recovery in anorexia nervosa. *J. Eat. Disord.* **2017**, *5*, 1–12. [CrossRef] [PubMed]
162. Boedhoe, P.S.; Schmaal, L.; Abe, Y.; Alonso, P.; Ameis, S.H.; Anticevic, A.; Arnold, P.; Batistuzzo, M.C.; Benedetti, F.; Beucke, J.C.; et al. Cortical Abnormalities Associated With Pediatric and Adult Obsessive-Compulsive Disorder: Findings From the ENIGMA Obsessive-Compulsive Disorder Working Group. *Am. J. Psychiatry* **2018**, *175*, 453–462. [CrossRef] [PubMed]
163. Madonna, D.; DelVecchio, G.; Soares, J.C.; Brambilla, P. Structural and functional neuroimaging studies in generalized anxiety disorder: A systematic review. *Rev. Bras. Psiquiatr.* **2019**, *41*, 336–362. [CrossRef] [PubMed]
164. Thirion, B.; Pinel, P.; Mériaux, S.; Roche, A.; Dehaene, S.; Poline, J.-B. Analysis of a large fMRI cohort: Statistical and methodological issues for group analyses. *NeuroImage* **2007**, *35*, 105–120. [CrossRef] [PubMed]
165. Goddings, A.-L.; Mills, K.L.; Clasen, L.S.; Giedd, J.N.; Viner, R.M.; Blakemore, S.-J. The influence of puberty on subcortical brain development. *NeuroImage* **2014**, *88*, 242–251. [CrossRef]

166. Neufang, S.; Specht, K.; Hausmann, M.; Güntürkün, O.; Herpertz-Dahlmann, B.; Fink, G.R.; Konrad, K. Sex Differences and the Impact of Steroid Hormones on the Developing Human Brain. *Cereb. Cortex* **2008**, *19*, 464–473. [CrossRef] [PubMed]
167. Yendiki, A.; Koldewyn, K.; Kakunoori, S.; Kanwisher, N.; Fischl, B. Spurious group differences due to head motion in a diffusion MRI study. *NeuroImage* **2014**, *88*, 79–90. [CrossRef] [PubMed]
168. Frank, G.K.W.; Favaro, A.; Marsh, R.; Ehrlich, S.; Lawson, E.A. Toward valid and reliable brain imaging results in eating disorders. *Int. J. Eat. Disord.* **2018**, *51*, 250–261. [CrossRef]
169. Armstrong, L.E.; Maughan, R.J.; Senay, L.C.; Shirreffs, S.M. Limitations to the use of plasma osmolality as a hydration biomarker. *Am. J. Clin. Nutr.* **2013**, *98*, 503–504. [CrossRef] [PubMed]

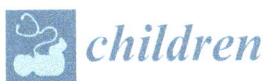

Review

Nutritional Status of Pediatric Cancer Patients at Diagnosis and Correlations with Treatment, Clinical Outcome and the Long-Term Growth and Health of Survivors

Vassiliki Diakatou [1,2] and Tonia Vassilakou [2,*]

1. Children's & Adolescents' Oncology Radiotherapy Department, Athens General Children's Hospital "Pan. & Aglaia Kyriakou", GR-11527 Athens, Greece; vdiakatou@hotmail.com
2. Department of Public Health Policy, School of Public Health, University of West Attica, Athens University Campus, 196 Alexandras Avenue, GR-11521 Athens, Greece
* Correspondence: tvasilakou@uniwa.gr; Tel.: +30-213-2010-283

Received: 1 October 2020; Accepted: 5 November 2020; Published: 7 November 2020

Abstract: Malnutrition is caused either by cancer itself or by its treatment, and affects the clinical outcome, the quality of life (QOL), and the overall survival (OS) of the patient. However, malnutrition in children with cancer should not be accepted or tolerated as an inevitable procedure at any stage of the disease. A review of the international literature from 2014 to 2019 was performed. Despite the difficulty of accurately assessing the prevalence of malnutrition, poor nutritional status has adverse effects from diagnosis to subsequent survival. Nutritional status (NS) at diagnosis relates to undernutrition, while correlations with clinical outcome are still unclear. Malnutrition adversely affects health-related quality of life (HRQOL) in children with cancer and collective evidence constantly shows poor nutritional quality in childhood cancer survivors (CCSs). Nutritional assessment and early intervention in pediatric cancer patients could minimize the side effects of treatment, improve their survival, and reduce the risk of nutritional morbidity with a positive impact on QOL, in view of the potentially manageable nature of this risk factor.

Keywords: childhood cancer; pediatric oncology; nutritional status; malnutrition

1. Introduction

The importance of nutrition in children with cancer is indisputable [1]. Nutrition influences most cancer control parameters in pediatric oncology, including prevention, epidemiology, biology, treatment, supportive care, recuperation, and survival [2]. It is widely recognized that the nutritional status (NS) of children diagnosed with and treated for cancer will be probably affected during the course of the disease.

NS of pediatric cancer patients has been researched for a lengthy time and nutritional problems have long-been recognized [3–8]. Indeed, publications on childhood cancer related undernutrition have appeared since the 1970s [9], however its management remains variable [1,4,10], with many undernourished children not timely recognized and therefore not treated [11].

The importance of NS in childhood cancer patients concerns its potential impact on disease progression and survival [1]. The NS at the time of diagnosis can affect outcomes in terms of morbidity and mortality [12]. Additionally, nutrition related problems can affect the quality of life (QOL) of survivors, as well as predispose them to other chronic diseases [2]. This fact highlights the need for scientific management and nutritional support for this population.

At the same time, the available data regarding the prevalence of poor nutritional status are derived at different phases of the disease and are highly variable among diagnostic groups, as well as between developed and developing countries [1,13–15]. The heterogeneity of diagnoses, the different stages of treatment and the followed treatment protocols complicate any straightforward comparison among studies. Moreover, the variety of definitions for malnutrition, the methodology used to assess the NS—in terms of anthropometric measurements—as well as criteria and cut-off points, make an accurate estimation of the prevalence of cancer related malnutrition very difficult.

This review aims to identify NS alterations that occur during the management of childhood cancer. The purpose of the study is to investigate how neoplastic diseases affect the NS of children and adolescents, as well as how the nutritional profile affects treatment response, clinical outcome and long-term growth and health of survivors. By investigating the multifactorial components of nutrition in childhood cancer morbidity, this work aims to be the trigger to recognize the importance of nutrition in order to become an integral part of cancer treatment in children and adolescents in Greece.

2. Materials and Methods

An electronic search of the international literature was performed, using the Cochrane Library, MEDLINE, SCOPUS, and PUBMED to identify systematic reviews, meta-analyses, randomized controlled trials and observational studies published during the period 2014–2019. The search strategy identified the following keywords and medical subject heading searches (MeSH): "childhood cancer", "pediatric oncology", "nutritional status", and "malnutrition". The reference list of all relevant articles was also examined, and possibly relevant corresponding articles were hand-searched. Particular attention has been paid to most recent articles, meta-analyses and systematic reviews conducted in countries with different socioeconomic status in order to identify possible influence. Studies involving adult patients were excluded.

3. Results

3.1. Nutritional Status at Diagnosis

Many former and recent studies have investigated the issue of weight changes in children diagnosed with cancer. Pediatric cancer includes a heterogeneous group of diagnoses, while the repercussions, prognosis and the therapeutic planning differ according to tumor location, histological type, nature as well as biological behavior and age of incidence [16]. Such differences also influence the NS, in a way that some patients present with weight loss at diagnosis, thus being at higher risk for suboptimal NS during the anticancer treatment [17,18]. NS at the time of the diagnosis is an important factor which influences the response to the treatment as well as the possibility of recovery [1].

In the cross-sectional observational study of Maia Lemos et al. [16], the authors assessed the NS of 1154 children and adolescents with malignant neoplasms in Brazil at the time of diagnosis. At that time point, 67.63% of patients presented adequate body mass index (BMI). The overall prevalence of undernutrition was 10.8%, 27.3%, 24.5% and 13.6%, based on BMI, triceps skinfold thickness (TSFT), mid-upper arm circumference (MUAC), and arm muscle circumference (AMC), respectively [16].

Villanueva et al. [19] studied the NS of 1060 patients diagnosed with cancer in Guatemala. NS was evaluated by MUAC, TSFT, and serum albumin (ALB) levels. Children were nutritionally classified as adequately nourished, moderately depleted, and severely depleted. With regard to diagnoses, leukemia accounted for 51% of all diagnoses, followed by solid tumors (33%), lymphomas (11%), and brain tumors (BT) (5%). At diagnosis, 47% ($n = 495$) of patients were severely nutritionally depleted, 19% ($n = 207$) were moderately depleted, and 34% ($n = 358$) were adequately nourished.

In total, 74 pediatric oncology patients newly diagnosed with hematological malignancies ($n = 56$) or solid tumors ($n = 18$), were included in a prospective observational cohort study conducted in Istanbul [20]. Anthropometric measurements included body weight, height, BMI, BMI for age percentile, MUAC, TSFT as well as z-scores for weight for age (WFA), height for age (HFA), BMI for age, weight for height for age, MUAC for age, and TSFT for age. At diagnosis, undernutrition (BMI for age z<−2 standard deviation (SD)) was evident in nine (12.3%) of 74 patients, including six (10.9%) patients with hematological malignancies and three (16.7%) patients with solid tumors, whereas undernutrition (BMI<5th age percentile) was evident in 10 (13.7%) of 74 patients, including six (10.9%) patients with hematological malignancies and four (22.2%) patients with solid tumors. In addition, increased body weight (BMI for age z > 2 SD) was evident in five (6.8%) patients.

Pribnow et al. [21] conducted a retrospective review of newly diagnosed patients with acute lymphoblastic leukemia (ALL), acute myeloid leukemia (AML), Wilms tumor, Hodgkin lymphoma (HL), or Burkitt lymphoma (BL) in Nicaragua. A total of 473 patients were assessed and 282 patients were recruited in the study. At diagnosis weight, height or length measurements were recorded and NS assessment included BMI, MUAC, TSFT, and levels of serum albumin. At diagnosis, on the basis of NS categories, 67% of patients were undernourished, 19.1% suffered from moderate undernutrition and 47.9% were severely undernourished. Undernutrition rates were higher in patients with Wilms tumor (85.7%) and BL (75%) and lower in those with HL (58.3%). Patients with high-risk malignancies were inclined to have inferior NS regardless diagnosis, when comparing adequately nourished (37.3% of patients with high-risk disease) to severely undernourished (62.7% of those with high-risk disease) groups ($p = 0.08$). Similar trends are also observed in high-income countries (HICs) and can be attributed to disease burden.

In the same country, a cohort of 104 patients was screened for NS at diagnosis [22]. The NS assessment was based on weight, height or length and the anthropometric measures of MUAC and TSFT. Thirty-four patients were affected by ALL, five by AML, 13 by lymphomas and 52 by solid tumors, including BT ($n = 20$), retinoblastoma ($n = 3$), bone and soft-tissue sarcoma ($n = 15$), Wilms' tumor ($n = 7$) and others ($n = 7$). Yet, diseases were clustered in two groups—leukemia/lymphomas and solid tumors—for further analyses. According to their anthropometric measurements, patients were overall classified as 65.4% severely depleted, 13.5% moderately depleted, and 21.1% borderline/adequately nourished, that is considered at risk of developing undernutrition during treatment.

In the largest study so far from India, a total of 1693 new patients were enrolled, of whom 1187 had all anthropometric measurements performed [23]. The prevalence of undernutrition—defined by World Health Organization (WHO) criteria—at the time of diagnosis was very high ranging from 40–80% depending on the method used for assessment, being higher with MUAC and lowest with BMI. Specifically, the prevalence of undernutrition was 38%, 57%, 76%, 69%, and 81% on the basis of BMI, TSFT, MUAC, AMC, and arm TSFT + MUAC, respectively. Addition of BMI and serum albumin to arm anthropometry increased the proportion classified as severely nutritionally depleted by a mere 2% and 1.5% respectively. Among disease groups, no considerable differences were found in undernutrition rates, consistent with findings of a similar large study published at that time [24]. On the other extreme, only 14 (0.8%) of children in this study were obese among the whole group, much lower than the 14% rate of obesity in a recent large study from the United States of America (USA), reflecting the socio-economic influence on NS [25].

Another study conducted in India, analyzed retrospectively weight records collected at diagnosis for patients with ALL, AML, solid tumors, and lymphomas [26]. A total of 295 pediatric patients were enrolled in the analysis. Patients' weight was plotted on WFA growth charts of Center for Disease Control and Prevention (CDC) [27]. At diagnosis, 153 out of 295 (52%) of patients had WFA between 3rd and 97th centile and were therefore considered to be well-nourished, 130 out of 295 (44%) patients were undernourished and 12/295 (4%) patients were obese. The prevalence of undernutrition at admission among males and females was 44% and 42%, respectively. As regards the diagnosis, there was no significant difference in NS at diagnosis between hematological malignancies and solid tumors ($p = 0.8$).

NS at the time of cancer diagnosis is dependent on a cancer type, its localization and clinical stage of the disease [1]. In addition, prevalence rates of malnutrition depend not only on methods and criteria used to assess NS, timing of assessment and composition of the study population—in terms of types of malignancies—, but also on socio-economic status [3]. Studies carried out in countries with better socio-economic conditions showed different results from the above mentioned. Moreover, other factors such as poverty, lack of adequate education and health support can aggravate nutritional risk especially in developing countries [16]. In general, undernutrition rates have been found much higher in low- or low-middle-income countries (LMICs) (40–90%) in comparison to countries with high or medium income (0–30%) [4,24,28–30].

In the USA, a cohort of 2,008 children treated for high-risk ALL enrolled in Children's Oncology Group study CCG–1961 (Children's Cancer Group) [25]. Weight status by z-score and percentile was determined as per guidelines from the CDC using BMI for children age 2–20 years and Weight for Length (WFL) for those age <2 years [31,32]. Of the 2.008 evaluable children, 279 (14%) were obese and 117 (6%) 17 were underweight at diagnosis.

In Italy, 126 newly diagnosed pediatric cancer patients were included in the study of Triarico et al. [33]. For each patient, nutritional risk has been assessed with STRONGKids—a quick, reliable, and practical screening tool—to identify patients with risk of undernutrition [34,35]. Subsequently, anthropometric measurements—such as weight, height, BMI z-scores—were evaluated. The analysis showed a 100% rate of patients at risk of undernutrition at diagnosis. Respectively at diagnosis 90 patients (71.4%) presented a moderate risk of undernutrition (STRONGkids 2 or 3), whereas the other 36 (28.6%) were at high risk of undernutrition (STRONGkids 4 or 5). Sixteen patients (12.7%) presented mild undernutrition (BMI z-score from (−1)–(−1.9)), two patients (1.6%) presented moderate undernutrition (BMI z-score from (−2)–(−2.9)) and four patients (3.1%) showed severe undernutrition (BMI z-score ≤ −3).

In Poland, the authors of [36] studied the frequency of undernutrition and obesity at diagnosis. A study group of 734 patients with various diagnoses was enrolled. Patients were divided into groups depending on the type of neoplasms: ALL, acute non-lymphoblastic leukemia (ANLL), HL, non-Hodgkin lymphoma (NHL), neuroblastoma (NB), Wilms' tumor, and mesenchymal malignant tumor (MMT). Body weight and height were measured, and BMI was calculated at the time of diagnosis. At cancer diagnosis moment, 21.5% (158) of patients were undernourished, 64.7% (475) weighed properly and 13.8% (101) were overweight. Height deficiency was observed in 8% (57) of the patients, of whom 10% (34) were boys and 9% (23) were girls. Both underweight and short stature were found in 2% (15) of the patients. Among diagnoses, there were no notable difference considering height deficiencies. Patients in the ALL group were overweight more often than the rest of the study group (Risk Ratio (RR) = 1.82, Confidence Interval (CI) 95% 1.26–2.63, p = 0.002)—18.6% of them were overweight. However, children with MMT were less susceptible to overweight than the rest of the patients (RR = 0.36, CI 95% 0.15–0.87, p = 0.021)—only 5.4% of them were overweight. Girls with ALL were undernourished more often than other patients (RR = 1.72, CI 95% 1.08–2.75, p = 0.03). There were no significant differences in the undernutrition/obesity frequency in other neoplasms groups.

In Australia, Small et al. [37] retrospectively reviewed the growth and NS—assessed by BMI—of children diagnosed with NB. One hundred fifty-four children were diagnosed with NB, while only 129 of them had length/height and weight measurements recorded at diagnosis. At that moment, almost a quarter—31 children—(24.0%) were classified as underweight indicating a high incidence of undernutrition, while the percentage of overweight patients was 11.6% (n = 15). There was no noteworthy difference in gender, age, or disease stage at diagnosis across children who were classified as underweight, normoweight or overweight.

It is therefore understood that weight and height are important measurements for assessing a child's NS. According to Brinksma et al. [38], the evaluation of weight and height at the time of diagnosis in comparison with the measurements prior to diagnosis is particularly important in children who have recently been diagnosed with cancer. However, children who suffer from severe weight loss or lack of linear growth, but have what is considered appropriate weight and height parameters—between −2 and +2 standard deviation scores (SDS)—, may also be poorly nourished [38]. The authors studied a group of 95 patients, 45 (47%) of which were females. Children were diagnosed with hematological malignancies (57%), solid (26%) and brain (17%) tumors. At diagnosis, weight and height measurements were recorded and compared with the child's own growth potential—authors used data collected in Primary Health Care Corporation (PHCC). Undernutrition was observed in 2% (2 out of 95), 4% (4 out of 95), and 7% (7 out of 95) of the children according to zWFA<-2 SDS, zHFA<-2 SDS, and z-scores for weight for height (WFH) <-2 SDS, respectively. However, when compared to their growth curves another 20–24% of children lost more than 0.5 SDS in WFA, HFA, and WFH z-score. In conclusion comparison of weight and height at diagnosis with data from growth curves indicated that—on average—children's z-scores of weight and height at diagnosis were lower than predicted from their growth curves. Actually, more children were poorly nourished than weight and height at diagnosis indicated [38].

In the same country, Loeffen et al. [39] studied—amongst others—malnutrition at diagnosis within a heterogeneous childhood cancer population. The study sample consisted of 269 children with cancer, receiving treatment for various malignancies. BMI z-scores were used as indicator of NS. At the time of diagnosis, 14 children (5.2%) were classified as undernourished (BMI z-score < −2), 229 children (56.9%) were adequately nourished while 19 (7.1%) were over-nourished (BMI z-score > 2). Undernourished children showed poorer survival versus adequately nourished (hazard ratio (HR) = 3.63, 95% confidence interval (CI) = 1.52–8.70, $p = 0.004$).

According to published studies, the majority of data on NS of children with cancer at the time of diagnosis relates to undernutrition. Numerous studies include diverse measures and assessment methods, leading to a highly variable prevalence of undernutrition at diagnosis [1]. Table 1 summarizes the characteristics of eligible studies that assess nutritional status at the time of diagnosis.

The reported differences between studies are due to the fact that nutrition related problems—particularly the prevalence of undernutrition—depend on factors such as the timing of nutritional assessment. Nutritional assessment at diagnosis is often postponed in the context of many other procedures that may have a higher priority, some of which may even affect it [40]. In addition, there is no clinical "gold standard" to assess the NS [1]. The methods used make the criteria of malnutrition heterogeneous, as the process depends on the sensitivity and specificity of the parameters [8]. Furthermore, the time of cancer development is not the same for all diagnoses. If cancer develops more rapidly—e.g., hematological malignancies against solid tumors—the shortage of weight is lower, as there is not enough time to develop severe nutrition deficiencies [36]. Moreover, the reported differences as regards the prevalence of undernutrition are due to the composition of each study population regarding the types of malignancies. In the majority of studies, patients are categorized into hematologic, solid, and brain malignancies [3].

Nutritional assessment at the time of diagnosis, is probably the most appropriate time to prevent the deterioration of NS. Undernutrition worsens as the disease progresses, meaning that the longer the diagnosis is delayed, the higher the risk of undernutrition [41]. Therefore, the early diagnosis of undernutrition and early intervention should be a priority in all interdisciplinary oncological teams in an effort to solve at least part of the problem [24].

Table 1. Characteristics of listed studies that assess NS at diagnosis.

Author, Year (Location)	Study Design	Patients (N)	Diagnosis	Assessment Method	Nutritional Related Problems
Maia Lemos et al., 2016 [16] (Brazil)	Cross-sectional observational study	1154	Various diagnoses	BMI [1], TSFT [2], MUAC [3], AMC [4]	Undernutrition
Villanueva et al., 2019 [19] (Guatemala)	Retrospective cohort study	1060	Hematological Malignancies Solid tumors Brain tumors	TSFT, MUAC, ALB [5] levels	Undernutrition
Yoruk et al., 2018 [20] (Istanbul)	Prospective observational cohort study	74	Hematological malignancies Solid tumors	BMI, TSFT, MUAC, WFA [6], HFA [7]	Malnutrition
Pribnow et al., 2017 [21] (Nicaragua)	Retrospective study	282	ALL [8], AML [9], HL [10], BL [11], Wilms tumors	BMI, TSFT, MUAC, ALB levels	Undernutrition
Peccatori et al., 2018 [22] (Nicaragua)	Intervention study	104	Hematological malignancies Solid tumors	TSFT, MUAC, Height, Weight	Undernutrition
Shah et al., 2014 [23] (India)	Retrospective observational study	1693	Various diagnoses	BMI, TSFT, MUAC, ALB levels	Malnutrition
Radhakrishnan et al., 2015 [26] (India)	Retrospective study	295	Various diagnoses	WFA	Malnutrition
Orgel et al., 2014 [25] (USA)	Retrospective cohort study	2008	High-risk ALL	BMI	Malnutrition
Triarico et al., 2019 [33] (Italy)	Retrospective study	126	Hematological malignancies Solid tumors CNS [12] tumors,	STRONGkids score	Undernutrition
Połubok et al., 2017 [36] (Poland)	Retrospective cohort study	734	ALL, ANLL [13], HL, NHL [14], NB [15], MMT [16], Wilms tumors	BMI	Malnutrition
Small et al., 2015 [37] (Australia)	Retrospective review	154	NB	Height, Weight, BMI	Malnutrition
Brinksma et al., 2015 [38] (The Netherlands)	Retrospective study	95	Hematological Malignancies Solid tumors Brain tumors	Height, Weight	Growth alterations
Loeffen et al., 2015 [39] (The Netherlands)	Retrospective study	269	Hematological Malignancies Solid tumors Brain tumors	BMI	Malnutrition

[1] Body Mass Index (BMI), [2] Triceps Skinfold Thickness (TSFT), [3] Mid–Upper Arm Circumference (MUAC), [4] Arm Muscle Circumference (AMC), [5] Serum albumin (ALB), [6] Weight for Age (WFA), [7] Height for Age (HFA), [8] Acute Lymphoblastic Leukemia (ALL), [9] Acute Myeloid Leukemia (AML), [10] Hodgkin Lymphoma (HL), [11] Burkitt Lymphoma (BL), [12] Central Nervous System (CNS), [13] Acute Non-Lymphoblastic Leukemia (ANLL), [14] Non-Hodgkin Lymphoma (NHL), [15] Neuroblastoma (NB), [16] Mesenchymal Malignant Tumor (MMT).

3.2. Nutritional Status during Treatment

NS at the time of diagnosis is an important factor which influences the response to the treatment, as well as the possibility of recovery [1]. However, malnutrition in pediatric patients with cancer is dynamic and development of impaired NS is commonly seen during subsequent treatment [42]. The adverse effects of nutritional problems during treatment, such as reduced tolerance of chemotherapy, alterations in drug metabolism, reduced immunity, increased risk of infection, and compromised QOL, have been established, however the quality of the evidence supporting each of these effects is variable [43].

Previous reports addressing the impact of weight on treatment-related toxicity (TRT) and event-free survival (EFS) in acute leukemia were limited by taking into account patient's weight only at diagnosis [44–46]. As weight varies significantly during the treatment course of pediatric ALL [47], Orgel et al. [25] evaluated the effect of weight alterations on EFS and development of TRT, all along the treatment period in contrast to weight at diagnosis. A multitudinous group of children diagnosed with and treated for high-risk ALL was enrolled in the analysis. Orgel et al. [25] observed that only those children with constant underweight or obese status across intensive phases of treatment for high-risk ALL were at substantially higher risk for TRT occurrence, relapse, or death. Furthermore, for patients whose NS status-either obesity or underweight-was constant for > half of pre-maintenance therapy, the risk for future relapse or death was up to double compared with patients who remained normoweight during the treatment course. Contrarily, the risk of patients who began treatment obese or underweight and subsequently ended up normoweight/overweight, decreased to become comparable to being normoweight throughout. In addition, obese or underweight children were facing greater risk for specific toxicity profiles, an essential independent issue in efforts to decrease morbidity resulting from effective but toxic treatment protocols.

Paciarotti et al. [48] performed a prospective cohort study, aiming to determine both the prevalence of undernutrition and over-nutrition—overweight and obesity—and to detect critical changes in NS with reference to tumor type, treatments, and nutritional interventions. NS assessment combined several parameters—dietary intake, BMI centile, TSFT and MUAC—and was performed at diagnosis and at three months after treatment initiation. In terms of diagnosis, cohort was grouped in children with leukemia and in children with other types of cancer. Undernutrition prevalence—determined by BMI centiles—was highest among the "other cancers" group at diagnosis. The low BMI centiles were correlated with a higher prevalence rate of undernourished children in comparison to the anticipated undernutrition rate for the UK population [28]. On the other hand, the "leukemia" group, demonstrated excess BMI centiles at both time points and the prevalence of obesity was greater than the expected for the UK population. The BMI alterations, as time went on, followed the anthropometric variations. The "leukemia" patients had excess fat reserves during treatment course—measured by Upper Arm Fat Area (UAFA)—being 130% of standard at three-month time. The "other cancers" group had depleted fat stores, with UAFA values getting lower from 78% at diagnosis to 70% of standard at three months of treatment, suggesting a negative energy status existing prior to diagnosis. Consequently, both undernutrition and obesity are frequent disorders during the first phase of treatment for pediatric cancer with clear differences among cancer diagnoses.

There are several studies that present data on malnutrition in children with cancer, however little is known about the timing of under- and over-nutrition onset, as well as their respective causes. Brinksma et al. [49] intended to determine in which treatment phase NS deterioration occurred, and which factors lead to these alterations. A prospective cohort study of 133 newly diagnosed cancer patients with hematological malignancies, solid and brain tumors was performed. Anthropometric measurements and related date were recorded at admission and at three, six and 12 months after diagnosis. Despite initial weight loss at the beginning of treatment in patients with hematological and solid malignancies, BMI, and fat mass (FM) increased within three months by 0.13 SDS ($p < 0.001$) and 0.05 SDS ($p = 0.021$) respectively. Increase continued during the following months and resulted in a doubling of the number of over-nourished patients. Fat-free mass (FFM)—which was already low at diagnosis—remained low. During the entire study period about 17% of the patients were undernourished on the basis of low FFM. The most important changes took place within three months after diagnosis. Particularly WFA and BMI decreased at first, in patients with hematological malignancies and solid tumors, while tended to increase in patients with brain tumors. In a three–month period both WFA and BMI increased in all diagnoses, compared to the time of diagnosis. Furthermore, HFA decreased in all diagnostic groups, whereas MUAC increased. TSFT, % FM, and FM were higher, especially for patients with BT. FFM was constant and values were lower in patients with brain tumors in comparison to children with hematological malignancies and solid tumors. Furthermore, stagnation of growth in terms of height contributed to increase in BMI. Consequently, it is imperative for clinicians to comprehend that in order to prevent increase in BMI during treatment, weight should remain stable until growth in height continues.

Iniesta et al. [50] performed a prospective cohort study to examine the prevalence of malnutrition, NS alterations and factors contributing to nutritional disorders in Scottish pediatric cancer patients aged < 18 years. Clinical and nutritional data, as well as anthropometric measurements—MUAC and TSFT—were recorded at specific periods up until 36 months after diagnosis. The study population was grouped conforming to the wider definition of solid and brain tumors, hematologic malignancies, and other associated diagnoses. The prevalence of malnutrition—undernutrition, overweight and obesity—differed at various time points and among the anthropometric measurements. Overall, undernutrition was higher at diagnosis than at any other time whereas no patient was undernourished at the end, i.e., 30 and 36 months. In contrast, overnutrition increased over time. Particularly overweight was highest at 36 months and obesity was most prevalent at 30 months. As to diagnoses, patients with brain tumors and other associated diagnoses had the highest prevalence of overweight and obesity, even at the start of treatment. Contrarily, children diagnosed with solid tumors had the highest prevalence of undernutrition, followed by brain tumors and hematological malignancies during the first stages of treatment. In conclusion, the study highlights that children diagnosed with and treated for cancer are at high risk of undernutrition—notably during the first three months of treatment—and of over-nutrition at later stages. The most significant component contributing to undernutrition during the first three months of treatment was high treatment risk.

With regard to solid tumors, NB is one of the most common solid tumors in children [51]. Small et al. [37] wanted to examine retrospectively the BMI status of children treated for NB. One hundred and twenty-nine children diagnosed with NB were recruited in the study. Anthropometric measurements were collected at diagnosis as well as at various time points, up until five years after diagnosis. At diagnosis 24% of children were classified as undernourished and 11.6% were overweight. At six months after diagnosis, children in almost all disease stages showed a significant decrease in age and sex adjusted BMI. Subsequently, weight z-scores began to increase so that at 12 months' time higher BMI z-scores were observed in children in all disease stages. Over the following four years, BMI z-scores either gradually changed or stabilized depending on the stage of the disease. Almost five years after diagnosis, the proportion of underweight children decreased to 8.7% while the proportion of children who were classified as overweight doubled to 28%. Even though low BMI values are common in children with NB—particularly at diagnosis and during treatment—the authors did not find any association between BMI and survival rates. Yet, the high proportion of overweight children at follow-up underscores the importance of nutritional interventions [37].

In India, Radhakrishnan et al. [26] conducted a study to look at the prevalence of malnutrition and to assess the impact of treatment on NS of pediatric cancer patients. A total of 295 pediatric patients were enrolled in the analysis. They were provided all meals and nutritional supplements by the hospital during their treatment duration. Data on WFA were available for 295 patients at diagnosis, 282 patients at midway through treatment, and 152 patients at the end of treatment. At diagnosis, undernutrition was seen in 44% patients, which increased to 46% midway during treatment, and decreased to 27% at the end of treatment ($p = 0.0005$). Even though undernutrition is a common problem in patients in resource-poor countries such as India, this study highlights that active nutritional intervention and education were able to significantly reduce the prevalence of undernutrition in patients at the end of treatment.

Nutritional support aims to reverse undernutrition seen at diagnosis, prevent undernutrition associated with treatment and promote weight and growth. There is no doubt that a poor nutritional state is a clear prognostic factor for treatment response and has an effect on the outcome of children with cancer [42].

3.3. Nutritional Status and Clinical Outcome

The presence of undernutrition correlates with a greater number of complications and relapses, as well as with decreased level of recovery [1,52]. Undernutrition can adversely affect the overall survival (OS), because it may reduce the tolerance to chemotherapy, increasing treatment-related morbidity (TRM) and decreasing EFS [21,39,53].

According to Barr et al. [43], two landmark retrospective studies were performed in the (CCG). Lange [54] conducted a study which included 768 children and adolescents with AML. Eighty-four patients (10.9%) of the study population underwent weight loss and 114 (14.8%) were overweight or obese, defined by BMI (≤10th percentile and ≥95th percentile respectively). Children with abnormal weight had remarkably worse survival than normoweight because of higher TRM rates.

Butturini et al. conducted the subsequent report, regarding >4000 children and adolescents with ALL. The CCG researchers focused on the effect of obesity, again as defined by BMI. The five-year EFS was poorer and the relapse rate higher in obese ($n = 343,8\%$) compared to non-obese patients, but only in those aged 10 years and older. After these two landmark studies in pediatric leukemia, multiple analyses from international research centers have since described inconsistent associations between obesity and leukemia survival [25,45,55–58], raising uncertainty as to whether such a relation exists and, if so, to what extent.

Amankwah et al. [59] performed a meta-analysis which further complicated data interpretation through inclusion of a wide variety of leukemia types, therapeutic modalities, and differences in baseline survival rates between high- and low-income countries (LICs) [60,61]. The authors aimed to evaluate the association between BMI at diagnosis and pediatric acute leukemia mortality and relapse. An increased risk of mortality with a high BMI at diagnosis was observed (OS: HR = 1.30, 95% CI = 1.16–1.46 and EFS: HR = 1.46, 95% CI = 1.29–1.64). Sub-group analysis for ALL, the most prevalent form of pediatric acute leukemia, revealed a stronger association for both OS (HR = 2.25, 95% CI = 1.33–3.82, $p = 0.002$) and EFS (HR = 1.49, 95% CI = 1.30–1.71, $p < 0.001$). Overall a high BMI at diagnosis was associated with poor OS and EFS among pediatric acute leukemia patients [59].

In contrast to the previous review [59], Orgel et al. [62] included in their analysis a relatively uniform population from HICs in order to determine whether a higher BMI at diagnosis of pediatric ALL or AML is associated with worse EFS, OS, and cumulative incidence of relapse (CIR). As regards ALL, the authors observed poorer EFS in children with a higher BMI (RR = 1.35, 95% CI = 1.20–1.51) than in those with a lower BMI. A higher BMI was associated with significantly increased mortality (RR = 1.31, 95% CI = 1.09–1.58) and a statistically nonsignificant trend toward greater risk of relapse (RR = 1.17, 95% CI = 0.99–1.38) compared with a lower BMI. In AML, a higher BMI was significantly associated with poorer EFS and OS (RR = 1.36, 95% CI = 1.16–1.60 and RR = 1.56, 95% CI = 1.32–1.86, respectively) than was a lower BMI. However, other studies have reported different outcomes.

In the recent retrospective analysis, Saenz et al. [63] evaluated the association between overweight/obesity (BMI ≥ 85th percentile) at pediatric leukemia diagnosis and relapse or mortality. The study included 181 pediatric patients diagnosed with ALL, AML, and chronic myeloid leukemia (CML). The authors observed a statistically significant association between mortality and obesity status in unadjusted models that disappeared in both age- and sex-adjusted and multivariable-adjusted analysis. Analysis limited to ALL patients—the most common type of leukemia—showed no association between relapse or mortality and obesity status. As expected, analysis based on the small number of AML cases only, did not show any statistically significant association for relapse (HR = 3.93,

95% CI = 0.71–21.82, p = 0.12) or mortality (HR = 1.39, 95% CI = 0.31–6.27, p = 0.67) either. A meta–analysis combining these findings with those of previous studies was also performed. Concerning ALL overweight/obese patients, the meta-analysis revealed an increased mortality and relapse risk (HR = 1.79, 95% CI = 1.03–3.10) and (HR = 1.28, 95% CI = 1.04–1.57) respectively. Similarly, an association between obesity and increased risk of mortality was observed for AML patients (HR = 1.64, 95% CI = 1.32–2.04) [63].

Aldhafiri et al. [55] conducted a study in the UK, on a cohort of 1,033 patients. The authors found no evidence to support the association between overweight/obesity at diagnosis and childhood leukemia relapse [55]. These findings are consistent with previous studies as well. In the UK, Weir et al. [64] examined the effects of BMI at diagnosis on leukemia relapse in children (n = 1,025) and found no statistically significant association between obesity and relapse. Two more studies in the US [57,65] also failed to detect an association between obesity at diagnosis and risk of relapse in children with ALL. In Turkey, Karakurt et al. [66] did not observe any difference between mean BMI at diagnosis and relapsed or non-relapsed patients. The authors of [67] did not find any association between BMI at diagnosis and prognosis for children aged 2–9 years, but they observed a trend for improved outcome in overweight patients aged 10–17 years.

So far, data have been related to hematological malignancies, while studies evaluating the role of NS in pediatric solid tumors are lacking. Joffe et al. [68] conducted a study aiming to summarize data reporting on the association of NS and treatment-related outcomes—TRT, EFS, CIR and OS—in children and adolescents diagnosed with a solid tumor. Finally, 10 reports met the criteria and were included in the review. Up to 62% of patients were over- or undernourished at diagnosis [69]. Four out of 10 included studies identify abnormal BMI as a poor prognostic indicator in this group of patients [70–73]. Abnormal BMI was associated with worse OS in Ewing sarcoma (HR = 3.46, p = 0.022), osteosarcoma (HR = 1.6, p < 0.005), and there was a trend toward poorer OS in rhabdomyosarcoma (HR = 1.70, p = 0.0596). High BMI in osteosarcoma was associated with increased nephrotoxicity and postoperative complications. Regarding other included disease categories, NS was not a significant predictor of outcomes.

Iniesta et al. [74] aimed to evaluate the primary research on the prevalence of malnutrition in children with cancer and determine whether there are correlations between malnutrition and clinical outcomes. According to the authors [74], correlations between undernutrition and clinical outcomes remain unclear, with some researchers arguing that undernutrition is associated with worse outcomes [8,75–77] and others claiming that there are no such associations [64,78]. Undernutrition may be associated with higher mortality [8,77]. Yet, both studies referred to developing countries, so findings may have been affected by other factors regarding mortality. As regards undernutrition and relapse, two large studies [8,64] found no associations. Obesity in children with ALL was not associated with a decrease in EFS, when obese children were compared with normoweight children [65]. On the contrary, Butturini et al. [44] found that obesity at diagnosis independently predicted the likelihood of relapse in pre-teenagers and adolescents with ALL.

Moreover, the majority of research studies regarding the effect of malnutrition on infections and mortality have been conducted in homogenous populations including patients with one diagnosis. Loeffen et al. [39] investigated whether malnutrition is a prognostic factor for infection rates and survival, within a heterogeneous childhood cancer population. The authors of [39] showed the strong association between rapid weight reduction within the first three months of treatment and increased rate of Febrile Neutropenia (FN) episodes. A group 269 children diagnosed with and treated for cancer were enrolled in the analysis. During the first year after diagnosis, 332 admissions for FN were recorded. As regards the incidence of these episodes, there were no statistically remarkable difference between patients who were adequately nourished at diagnosis and patients who were under- or over-nourished. Nevertheless, BMI z-score decrease >1.0 (n = 13) and weight loss >5% of the initial body weight within the first three months after diagnosis, were strongly associated with FN episodes occurrence—(p = 0.010) and (p = 0.004) respectively. Regarding NS, survival was notably worse ($p = 0.01$) for undernourished children at diagnosis ($n = 14$) than for those who were adequately and over-nourished ($n = 248$).

Pribnow et al. [21] examined the correlations between NS and cancer type, TRM and EFS. A total of 282 patients diagnosed with Wilms tumor, ALL, AML, HL or BL were included in the study. Children diagnosed with Wilms tumor had the highest prevalence of undernutrition (85.7%), followed by children with BL (75%) and AML (74.3%). As regards TRM, 92.2% of patients experienced morbidity during the first three months of treatment whereas 84% of patients experienced severe morbidity. TRM in pediatric patients with cancer was associated with NS, as morbidity was greater in children with severe undernutrition than in those with adequate nutrition ($p = 0.023$). Another crucial finding in this study was the association between NS and severe infection, as infection is a major cause of mortality and was the second leading cause of death during the study period (22.9%). Particularly undernutrition was associated with severe infection ($p = 0.033$). In addition, undernourished patients had inferior median EFS ($p = 0.049$) and abandoned therapy more frequently ($p = 0.015$).

With regard to the increased risk of infections and their incidence, Triarico et al. [33] recently confirmed their association with nutrition related problems. In their retrospective study 126 newly diagnosed children 3–18 years old were included. Overall, 298 admissions for FN occurred during the first year after diagnosis. On average, children had two admissions for FN while 54 patients (42.9%) had ≥3 admissions for FN during the first year after diagnosis. A number of hospitalization for FN ≥3 was found in children moderately to severely undernourished at three and six months after diagnosis, in patients with weight loss ≥5% at three months, in the case of a weight loss ≥10% at six months and finally in patients with a BMI z-score decrease ≥1 at six months. Analyses of weight loss and BMI z-score decrease demonstrate that in a period of three and six months from diagnosis there was a three-fold increase of the rate of at least moderate undernutrition, from 4.7% to 14.3% and 13.5% respectively. Indeed, at three months 58 children (46%) underwent weight loss ≥5%. At six months, they were 63 (50%), while 28 of them (22.2%) had lost ≥10% of their body weight. Furthermore, weight loss ≥5% at three months and weight loss ≥10% at six months after diagnosis were remarkably associated with higher mortality. Mortality risk increased by 294% in patients who lost ≥5% of weight in a three-month period after diagnosis and by 110% in patients who reported weight loss ≥10% at six-month time.

Given the high prevalence of nutrition related problems during childhood cancer treatment and their impact on clinical outcomes, nutritional assessment should be mandatory from diagnosis and during treatment, in view of the possible manageable nature of this risk factor. Early adaptation of the NS screening for pediatric cancer patients could not only improve their survival, but also their QOL [33].

3.4. Nutritional Status and Health-Related Quality of Life

Malnutrition during treatment for childhood cancer has not only substantial clinical implications, but may also adversely affect a child's QOL [79]. Until recently, QOL in children with cancer was unexplored [80]. In recent decades, cancer survival rates have increased thus emphasizing the importance of children's personal needs. As a result, health-related quality of life (HRQOL) in childhood cancer patients has become a crucial issue in clinical practice [79]. HRQOL of children and adolescents is complex as children grow and develop. On the other hand, multimodal therapy that combines intensive chemotherapeutic protocols, surgery and radiotherapy induces many side effects which adversely affect children's HRQOL [81].

Tsiros et al. [82] conducted a literature review on HRQOL in healthy, though obese children and adolescents. Findings support that being overweight/obese has an unfavorable impact on social and emotional functioning. In addition, other previous studies [83–86] have found that children diagnosed with and treated for malignancies had the lowest HRQOL, in comparison to healthy peers or children with other diseases. Broadly, it is considered that HRQOL in undernourished patients is lower when compared with adequately nourished patients [87] and that NS amelioration will lead to better HRQOL.

However, the correlation between NS and HRQOL in childhood cancer patients had not been examined until 2015.

Brinksma et al. are the first to examine the association between NS and HRQOL across childhood cancer patients. Notably, they studied the association of undernutrition, over-nutrition, weight loss, weight gain with HRQOL in a heterogeneous group of children with cancer one year after diagnosis. In total, 104 patients (aged 2–18 years) diagnosed with hematological (43%), solid (33%), or brain malignancies (24%) participated in the study. Weight, height, and BMI were assessed and expressed as SDS. Furthermore, FFM and FM were calculated based on bioelectrical impedance analysis (BIA). The child- and parent-report versions of the PedsQL 4.0 Generic scale [86,88] and the PedsQL 3.0 Cancer Module [89] were used in order to measure generic and cancer-specific HRQOL. According to Brinksma et al. [79] nutrition related problems adversely affect HRQOL in childhood cancer patients. Undernourished as well as over-nourished children experienced poorer QOL than children who were well-nourished. Similarly, both noteworthy weight loss and weight gain led to worse HRQOL. Actually, impaired physical functioning prevailed in undernourished patients and in patients with weight loss. It is widely known that undernutrition and weight loss are associated with muscle mass deficit and muscle deficiency, resulting in fatigue [90]. Therefore, undernourished children did not have the vitality and muscle strength needed to involve themselves in physical activities. Furthermore, undernutrition adversely affected children's social functioning. This finding can be justified by the pain, nausea, and tiredness these children encounter, which impair their ability to sufficiently participate in physical and social activities with their peers. As regards the psychosocial field, both over-nourished children and children with weight gain showed impaired functioning—when compared to adequately nourished patients—particularly in the emotional and cognitive sphere. They were more susceptible to feelings of fear, sorrow, and anger. Hence, they experienced more difficulties in interacting with others and they struggled to perform cognitive tasks—compared to adequately nourished patients with cancer.

These results have implications in clinical practice as they indicate the significance of adequate NS in children with cancer. Although the study could not demonstrate a causal relationship between nutrition related problems and HRQOL, undernourished and over-nourished patients experienced the lowest HRQOL across all cancer patients.

3.5. Nutritional Status during Survivorship

Advances in treatment have resulted in considerable improvements in survival rates of pediatric cancer. This success translates into a growing population of long-term survivors [91]. However, almost two-third of childhood cancer survivors (CCSs) will encounter at least one late effect while 40% of them are vulnerable to experience a disabling or potentially fatal condition even 30 years after diagnosis [92]. Even though late effects and chronic health conditions may be largely attributed to cancer and its treatment [93], the effects of NS that extend into survivorship put survivors at risk for numerous nutrition-related morbidities considering the pre-existing risk factors CCSs are facing [94]. There is a significant body of literature on NS among cancer survivors in childhood and adolescence after completion of treatment in HICs [43]. Special attention has been paid to ALL diagnosis, given its dominant prevalence in this age group worldwide [95] (Table 2).

Zhang et al. [96] performed a meta-analysis on the prevalence of obesity in pediatric ALL survivors in order to evaluate whether survivors are more likely to be obese than a reference population. Forty-seven studies met the inclusion criteria reporting on 9223 pediatric ALL survivors. Even though there was significant heterogeneity among studies, pediatric ALL survivors had considerably higher BMI than the reference population. There was a consistently high prevalence of overweight/obesity in both recent and long-term survivors regardless of patient- and treatment-related characteristics.

Table 2. Characteristics of listed studies that assess NS in CCSs.

Author, Year (Location)	Study Design	Survivors, N/(Control)	Diagnosis	Assessment Criteria	Nutritional Related Problems
Zhang et al., 2014 [96] (USA)	Systematic Review and Meta-analysis	9223	ALL	BMI	Overweight/obesity
Zhang et al., 2014 [97] (USA)	Retrospective cohort study	83	ALL	BMI	Overweight/obesity
Zhang et al., 2015 [98] (USA)	Systematic Review and Meta-analysis	1791	ALL	BMI	Overweight/obesity
Collins et al., 2017 [99] (Canada)	Cross-sectional cohort study	75	ALL	Arm anthropometry BMI	Malnutrition
Karlage et al., 2015 [100] (USA)	Longitudinal cohort study	1361	Various diagnoses	DXA [1] Anthropometry LBM [2] FM [3]	Overweight/obesity Sarcopenic obesity
Marriott et al., 2018 [101] (Canada)	Cross-sectional study	75	ALL	Whole-body BMC [4] Bone densitometry	Overweight/obesity BMD [5]
Molinari et al., 2017 [102] (Brazil)	Cross-sectional study	101	ALL	Anthropometry BMI	Overweight/obesity
Wang et al., 2018 [103] (Canada)	Systematic Review and Meta-analysis	2032	BT [6]	FM	
Warner et al., 2014 [104] (USA)	Population-based study	1060/(5410)	Various diagnoses	BMI	Malnutrition
Prasad et al., 2015 [105] (India)	Retrospective cohort study	648	Various diagnoses	BMI	Malnutrition MS [7]

[1] Dual-energy X-ray Absorptiometry (DXA), [2] Lean Body Mass (LBM), [3] Fat Mass, [4] Bone Mineral Content (BMC), [5] Bone Mineral Density (BMD), [6] Brain Tumors, [7] Metabolic Syndrome (MS).

Although many studies have focused on obesity and the consequences of being overweight, it was unclear at which time period survivors experienced excessive weight gain. Zhang et al. [97] performed a retrospective cohort study of 83 children with ALL. BMI status was examined at various time points during and after treatment, as well as annually up to five years after treatment. The percentage of patients who were overweight or obese (BMI ≥ 85th percentile) doubled from 20% at diagnosis to about 40% after treatment completion [97]. Particularly, 26.7% of normoweight children became overweight/obese at the end of treatment and 36.1% were overweight/obese five years post-treatment. Among those who were overweight/obese at diagnosis, 81.3% and 66.7% remained overweight/obese at the end of treatment and five years post-treatment, respectively. The overall increase in BMI z-score from diagnosis to the end of treatment was associated with a more than threefold increased risk of being overweight/obese five years after treatment. The study reveals that patients with pediatric ALL were at risk of becoming overweight or obese early during treatment, while these changes in weight status remained throughout treatment and after treatment completion.

Zhang et al. [98] conducted a subsequent meta-analysis and come to similar conclusions. Findings demonstrated significant increase in mean BMI z-score and weight during treatment that persisted beyond treatment completion. Actually, unsound weight gain was prevalent in pediatric ALL patients regardless of receipt of cranial irradiation therapy (CRT), sex, and weight status [98].

Collins et al. [99] performed arm anthropometry to assess the NS in long-term survivors of ALL in childhood and adolescence, as BMI does not distinguish muscle from adipose tissue [106]. Seventy-five patients diagnosed with ALL at least before a decade, were enrolled in the study. According to BMI values only six survivors were undernourished and none of them severely. Twenty-five survivors were overweight/obese, while only six (8%) were actually obese. However, 15 (20%) survivors were obese—assessed by TSFT—and only 3% suffered from sarcopenia according to MUAC. As it results, malnutrition rates varied according to assessment methods performed.

Karlage et al. [100] reported similar inconsistencies regarding BMI and anthropometric measurements of body composition. Obesity rates varied between 40% determined by BMI, 62% by three site skinfolds and 85% by Dual-energy X-ray Absorptiometry (DXA). Even though skinfolds undervalued the percent body fat of CCSs when compared with DXA, they indicated higher sensitivity than BMI when used to assort survivors as obese or not obese. Particularly nearly 47% of males and 53% of females of the study population were misclassified as non-obese when assessed by BMI, which may result in CCSs not receiving appropriate nutritional support and guidance.

As regards to body composition, Marriott et al. [101] conducted a study focusing on skeletal muscle mass (SMM) alterations. The study included 75 long-term survivors—37 male and 38 female—diagnosed with ALL at least before a decade. Whole-body DXA scans were obtained, as well as measures of lean body mass (LBM), FM, and whole-body bone mineral content (BMC). According to fat mass index (FMI), the majority of females and two-thirds of males were overweight/obese—12% and 18% were obese respectively. On the basis of BMI, the percentages of overweight/obese became 35.3% for females and 31.3% for males—5.9% and 9.8% were obese respectively. The analysis of appendicular lean mass (ALM) showed that 50% of survivors ≤18 years old suffered from SMM deficit. Thirty-two survivors (43%) were identified with positive z-scores for FMI and negative scores for appendicular lean mass index (ALMI). Consequently, sarcopenic obesity prevails in long-term survivors of ALL, which puts them at risk of both excess body fat and insufficient SMM.

Apart from body composition alterations, changes in bone metabolism constitute extensive adverse late effects of cancer treatment. They represent a major cause of morbidity in the CCSs population through pain, fractures, decrease of BMD and chronic deterioration of bone function [107,108]. Molinari et al. [102] evaluated BMD and body composition in 101 patients treated for ALL, using bone densitometry and anthropometric data. As regards to NS, 22.8% of survivors were overweight and 15.8% were obese. As to body composition the LBM levels and BMC were higher in males, while FM levels and fat percentages were higher in females. The more time had passed from treatment completion until the time of the study, the higher the values of LBM, FM, percentage of fat and BMC. Among children and adolescents <20 years old (*n* = 79), three survivors (2.9%) had low BMD and 16 (15.8%) were classified as at risk for low BMD. Among survivors aged >20 years old, eight (7.9%) had osteopenia and none of them had osteoporosis. In comparison to the reference population most of the survivors had normal BMD values. However, the risk group—considered by the literature as with normal BMD—actually presented significantly lower bone mass values. Eventually, ALL survivors can regain lost bone mass during the post-treatment period. Yet, some of them will never achieve their higher BMD acquisition potential, presenting considerable bone deficit [109].

So far, most publications on the NS of CCSs focus on ALL. Wang et al. [103] systematically reviewed the prevalence of overweight and obesity of CCSs diagnosed with BT. As it emerges, evidence for weight gain and obesity among survivors of childhood brain tumors (SCBT) varies. Some studies report an increase [110,111], whereas others have shown no significant differences compared to healthy controls [112,113]. Among participants, survivors diagnosed with brain tumors other than craniopharyngioma and craniopharyngioma survivors were analyzed in separate groups in order not to overrate the prevalence of obesity in overall SCBT population, as patients diagnosed with craniopharyngioma are known to be at high risk of developing obesity [114,115]. According to BMI measures, overweight and obesity rates were similar for SCBT and general population—rate of combined overweight and obesity 42.6% and 40.4%, respectively. Yet, survivors had higher adiposity. As regards to craniopharyngioma, the participants had higher prevalence of obesity and combined overweight and obesity than SCBT and healthy controls. Specifically, overweight and obesity affected almost two-thirds of patients with craniopharyngioma.

Warner et al. [104] conducted a population-based study in order to evaluate the prevalence of undernutrition and overweight/obesity among 1060 adult CCSs of various diagnoses. The most prevalent diagnoses among female survivors were epithelial cancer (26.1%) and lymphoma (17.4%), while for males were lymphoma (23.8%) and central nervous system (CNS) tumors (16.3%). Considering all diagnoses, there were no differences between female or male survivors versus the age- and sex-matched comparison population, regarding the risk of being underweight or overweight/obese. However, according to BMI values 36% of females and 61% of male survivors were classified as overweight/obese. When further analyzed by cancer diagnosis, female epithelial survivors were less likely to be overweight or obese than the comparison population and only male CNS survivors had a slightly higher risk of being overweight or obese than the reference cohort.

Even though overweight, obesity, and MS have been broadly reported in the Western literature, data from developing countries are lacking. Prasad et al. [105] conducted a retrospective study and NS was assessed in a cohort of 648 Indian CCSs. At the time of the study 471 survivors were <18 years—child and adolescent survivors (CASs)—and 177 were 18 years or older. The prevalence of obesity, overweight, normal NS and undernutrition was 2.6%, 10.8%, 62.7%, and 28.8% for CASs while 0%, 8.5%, 62.7% and 28.8% for adult survivors, respectively. Regarding adult survivors, those >30 years old had higher prevalence of overweight compared to those <30 years old (22.2% vs. 6.9%, $p = 0.004$). None of them fit the strict criteria of MS, though 17 (9.6%) fit the lenient criteria which included overweight survivors as well as obese. As to CASs none participant fit the strict criteria for MS. However, 11 (2.4%) survivors had features of MS when the weight criteria were lenient. There was a higher prevalence of overweight/obesity between those diagnosed with ALL or BT (16.5% and 20.7%, respectively, $p = 0.07$) and the rest of survivors (13.6%). Overall the prevalence of obesity/overweight was lower in this cohort when compared to western literature. Yet, it is unclear whether these rates reflect the underlying undernutrition in developing countries such as India or the CCSs population of this study differ from their western counterparts. Despite the lower prevalence of overweight/obesity and MS in this cohort of survivors, CCSs remain at high risk for cardiometabolic complications.

Some of the risk factors for overweight, obesity and MS are modifiable and in the hands of CCSs themselves. There are guidelines for promoting health in cancer survivors, including encouraging healthy nutrition, physical exercise and avoiding high-risk behaviors [116,117]. Yet, dietary guidelines developed for cancer survivors—such as those developed by the American Cancer Society [118] and the World Cancer Research Fund/the American Institute for Cancer Research (WCRF/AICR) [119]—do not elaborate on CCSs. Furthermore, the long-term follow-up guidelines for CCS developed by the Children's Oncology Group (COG) do not include cancer- and treatment-specific guidelines on nutrition [120].

Nevertheless, according to Brinkman et al. [121] healthy diet and physical exercise can moderate several late effects of cancer treatment, including obesity, hyperlipidemia, diabetes mellitus, cardiovascular disease, hypertension, and osteoporosis. Unfortunately, many CCSs do not meet the recommended dietary guidelines, with 54% of them exceeding their daily caloric requirements [122]. According to Zhang et al. [123], only 4%, 19%, 24%, and 29% of survivors follow the guidelines for vitamin D, sodium, calcium, and saturated fat intake, respectively. Nevertheless, nutritional intake in CCS has not been adequately studied [123]. Even though there are a few existing studies providing evidence that current dietary guidelines are not met [124–127], data are mainly derived from small groups of survivors or focus on specific cancer diagnoses—such as pediatric lymphoblastic leukemia. Zhang et al. [128] aimed to evaluate diet quality and dietary intake in a large cohort of 2570 adult CCSs. As regards diagnoses, leukemia was the most prevalent followed by lymphoma, embryonal tumor, sarcoma, and CNS tumor. The overall evidence emerges poor diet quality in CCSs, while older survivors had better diet quality than younger survivors did.

Unhealthy dietary behaviors have been associated with increased risk for health threatening conditions [94]. In addition, according to preliminary studies among CCSs, better quality diets may conduce to improved long-term health outcomes. There is developing evidence indicating that healthy dietary behaviors may reduce the risk of nutrition-related chronic conditions [94], thus it becomes essential to incorporate nutrition interventions and particularly dietary counseling into the clinical framework of survivorship care.

4. Discussion

Childhood cancer is an illness related to severe morbidity and mortality. The malignancy itself remains the main cause of death among childhood cancer patients [129,130]. Concurrently nutrition is a fundamental part of the pediatric cancer patients' care. Adequate and appropriate nutrition is required to maintain optimal growth and development. Furthermore, adequate nutrition is likely to enhance survival outcome, reduce toxicity and improve QOL [53].

It has been widely recognized in literature that the NS of children diagnosed with and treated for cancer is likely to be affected at some point during the disease trajectory. Actually, for many childhood cancer patients, the early progression of the disease and the commencement of antineoplastic therapies can affect the NS, leading to malnutrition with many adverse consequences [8,74,131].

One of the most important findings of this review—that focuses on NS alterations that occur during the management of childhood cancer—is that the reported prevalence of malnutrition—undernutrition, overweight and obesity—varies between different types of cancer, different stages of the disease, type of treatment, as well as among studies, highlighting the complexity and diversity of this population. Children diagnosed with specific cancer types develop nutrition related problems more often than others. For instance, at diagnosis prevalence of undernutrition is higher in patients with solid tumors—especially Wilms tumor or neuroblastoma—and much lower in children with ALL and HL [4,11,14,21]. At the same time patients with brain tumors demonstrate high prevalence of overweight and obesity [50]. During treatment, children with solid tumors are more frequently nutritionally depleted, followed by brain tumors and hematological malignancies [49,74]. The detected differences in malnutrition among various diagnoses are inconsistent in LMICs, as delays in diagnosis and limited access to healthcare may lead to higher undernutrition rates, regardless of cancer type [21]. In addition, undernutrition is more often observed in high-risk diseases across all cancer types [21].

The majority of data that focus on NS of children with cancer at the time of diagnosis relates to undernutrition, the prevalence of which ranges from 10.8% [16] to 76% [23]. These reported differences between studies are due both to the stage of the disease at diagnosis and the parameters used to assess NS [8]. To date, there is a lack of consensus on the definition of malnutrition [1,28]. In addition, the criteria for NS assessment are heterogeneous [1,8,28]. Nutritional assessment is a process that depends on the sensitivity and specificity of the parameters performed [8]. Unfortunately, this procedure is often postponed in the context of many other procedures that may have a higher priority, some of which may even affect it [40]. Most studies refer to BMI as, it is widely used in clinical practice. Yet, it is not the most appropriate method for NS assessment because it does not measure body fat directly. Even though every method for clinical assessment of NS has restrictions, indicators such as MUAC, TSFT, and BIA provide more information regarding body composition changes that occur in paediatric cancer patients. Nonetheless, the diversity among different indicators of NS does not allow any straightforward comparisons among them. The prevalence of nutrition related problems depends not only on the methods and criteria used to assess the NS [8], the timing of the assessment [40] and the composition of the study population [3]—in terms of types of malignancies—but also on the socio-economic status. In general, undernutrition rates were much higher in LICs than in HICs [3,23,25].

Clearly, the NS at the time of diagnosis is an important prognostic factor that affects treatment response as well as the possibility of recovery [1]. However, nutrition related problems in pediatric cancer patients are dynamic and their development is usually observed during subsequent treatment.

Currently, the most relevant research is retrospective or cross-sectional. The few prospectively designed studies that have been published principally concern children diagnosed with hematological malignancies while most of them do not refer to the NS at all stages of treatment [74]. In addition, research has focused on the study of undernutrition during cancer treatment, while excessive energy intake or poor diet quality is being overlooked [74]. The adverse effects of undernutrition during treatment have been established [43]. Among others these include reduced tolerance to chemotherapy, changes in the metabolism of medicinal products, reduced immunity, increased risk of infections and degraded QOL [43]. However, the quality of data supporting each of these results varies.

Studies that investigate the association between NS at diagnosis and clinical outcome suggest that NS may affect cancer prognosis in children with cancer. Particularly, observed inferior survival was generally stable among studies [59]. The presence of undernutrition was associated with a large number of complications and relapses, as well as a reduced level of recovery [1,52,68]. On the other hand, excess weight gain and obesity negatively affected the response to treatment and led to reduced cure rates [1,4,52,53]. Yet, the correlations between nutrition related problems and clinical outcomes remain unclear, with some researchers claiming that they are associated to worse outcomes and others claiming that there are no such associations [53,74].

The NS status of children with cancer has not only significant clinical implications, but also can adversely affect the long–term development and health of survivors, including children's QOL which as shown by the review remains underestimated [79]. There is a significant body of research on the NS of childhood and adolescent cancer survivors. Most studies focus on children with hematological malignancies—mainly in HICs—taking into account their predominant prevalence [43]. Furthermore, many reports confirm the impact of low or excessive body weight on survival, while collective evidence consistently shows poor diet quality in CCSs [128].

The lack of standard protocols and algorithms for assessment and treatment of nutritional problems, as well as limited in time dietary interventions are important factors that contribute to significant rates of malnutrition according to the literature. Meanwhile there is a lack of international specific dietary guidelines for children with cancer. Future scientific research should emphasize on proposing certain criteria that could assist the establishment of dietary instructions, such as cancer type, NS at diagnosis, treatment protocol, as well as children's gender and age.

Nutritional assessment should be mandatory from diagnosis and during treatment, in view of the possible manageable nature of this risk factor [33]. Therefore, early assessment of NS and timely intervention should be a priority in all interdisciplinary oncology teams, in order to integrate nutritional counseling into the clinical framework of care in an effort to address at least part of the problem [24].

5. Conclusions

NS of pediatric cancer patients plays a crucial role during the disease trajectory. The malignancy itself and the progression of the disease cause NS alterations, leading to malnutrition. In addition, the commencement of antineoplastic therapies affects energy balance with many negative consequences.

Malnutrition—undernutrition, overweight, and obesity—is linked to adverse outcomes from diagnosis to long-term survivorship. NS at the time of diagnosis is an important prognostic factor that affects treatment response and the possibility of recovery. The impact of impaired NS on clinical outcome and cancer prognosis is related to treatment intolerance due to nutrient deficiency and immune incompetence. Increased risk of infection and alterations in drug metabolism lead to delays and treatment cessation that result in higher relapse rates and lower survival rates. In addition, undernutrition during treatment correlates to a greater number of complications, increasing TRM and decreasing EFS. Yet, correlations between NS alterations and clinical outcomes remain unclear. Nutrition related problems can also adversely affect the long-term health of survivors, including children's HRQOL. The effects of NS that extend into survivorship put survivors at risk for numerous nutrition-related morbidities.

Given the high prevalence of malnutrition during childhood cancer and as NS represents a modifiable risk factor, nutritional assessment should be mandatory from diagnosis, during treatment and subsequently. There are several methods for the clinical assessment of NS and each one of them has limitations and constraints. Among those performed in clinical practice MUAC, TSFT and BIA provide more information concerning body composition changes than BMI does. Nonetheless, the diversity among different indicators of NS prevents us from extracting safe results regarding the most suitable one. Ideally, the most appropriate indicator is the one that would not allow a malnourished child to remain underdiagnosed.

As regards pediatric oncology, advances in treatment and follow-up care are significant. However, there is still a lack of international specific dietary guidelines for children with cancer. Hopefully, future scientific research should emphasize establishing cancer- and treatment-specific guidelines for nutrition. Early monitoring and adaptation of pediatric cancer patients' NS as well as timely nutritional intervention could improve their treatment response, their clinical outcome, their survival, but also their QOL.

Author Contributions: Conceptualization, V.D. and T.V.; methodology, V.D. and T.V.; investigation, V.D.; writing–original draft preparation, V.D.; writing–review and editing, V.D. and T.V.; visualization, V.D.; supervision, T.V. All authors have read and agreed to the published version of the manuscript.

Funding: This research received no external funding.

Acknowledgments: The authors wish to thank Elena Vlastou, medical physicist, for her constructive advice and general support.

Conflicts of Interest: The authors declare no conflict of interest.

References

1. Sala, A.; Pencharz, P.; Barr, R.D. Children, Cancer, and Nutrition—A Dynamic Triangle in Review. *Cancer* **2004**, *100*, 677–687. [CrossRef]
2. Rogers, P.C. Importance of Nutrition in Pediatric Oncology. *Indian J. Cancer* **2015**, *52*, 176. [CrossRef]
3. Antillon, F.; Rossi, E.; Molina, A.L.; Sala, A.; Pencharz, P.; Valsecchi, M.G.; Barr, R. Nutritional Status of Children during Treatment for Acute Lymphoblastic Leukemia in Guatemala. *Pediatr. Blood Cancer* **2013**, *60*, 911–915. [CrossRef] [PubMed]
4. Brinksma, A.; Huizinga, G.; Sulkers, E.; Kamps, W.; Roodbol, P.; Tissing, W. Malnutrition in Childhood Cancer Patients: A Review on Its Prevalence and Possible Causes. *Crit. Rev. Oncol. Hematol.* **2012**, *83*, 249–275. [CrossRef] [PubMed]

5. Jaime-Pérez, J.C.; González-Llano, O.; Herrera-Garza, J.L.; Gutiérrez-Aguirre, H.; Vázquez-Garza, E.; Gómez-Almaguer, D. Assessment of Nutritional Status in Children with Acute Lymphoblastic Leukemia in Northern México: A 5-Year Experience. *Pediatr. Blood Cancer* **2008**, *50*, 506–508. [CrossRef] [PubMed]
6. Odame, I.; Reilly, J.J.; Gibson, B.E.S.; Donaldson, M.D.C. Patterns of Obesity in Boys and Girls after Treatment for Acute Lymphoblastic Leukaemia. *Arch. Dis. Child.* **1994**, *71*, 147–149. [CrossRef] [PubMed]
7. Reilly, J.J. Obesity during and after Treatment for Childhood Cancer. *Endocr. Dev.* **2009**, *15*, 40–58.
8. Sala, A.; Rossi, E.; Antillon, F.; Molina, A.L.; de Maselli, T.; Bonilla, M.; Hernandez, A.; Ortiz, R.; Pacheco, C.; Nieves, R.; et al. Nutritional Status at Diagnosis Is Related to Clinical Outcomes in Children and Adolescents with Cancer: A Perspective from Central America. *Eur. J. Cancer* **2012**, *48*, 243–252. [CrossRef]
9. Van Eys, J. Malnutrition in Children with Cancer: Incidence and Consequence. *Cancer* **1979**, *43*, 2030–2035.
10. Reilly, J.J.; Dorosty, A.R.; Emmett, P.M. Prevalence of Overweight and Obesity in British Children: Cohort Study. *BMJ* **1999**, *319*, 1039. [CrossRef]
11. Antillon, F.; de Maselli, T.; Garcia, T.; Rossi, E.; Sala, A. Nutritional Status of Children during Treatment for Acute Lymphoblastic Leukemia in the Central American Pediatric Hematology Oncology Association (AHOPCA): Preliminary Data from Guatemala. *Pediatr. Blood Cancer* **2008**, *50*, 502–505. [CrossRef] [PubMed]
12. Barr, R.D. Nutritional Status in Children with Cancer: Before, during and after Therapy. *Indian J. Cancer* **2015**, *52*, 173. [CrossRef] [PubMed]
13. Barr, R.; Atkinson, S.; Pencharz, P.; Arguelles, G.R. Nutrition and Cancer in Children. *Pediatr. Blood Cancer* **2008**, *50*, 437. [CrossRef]
14. Sala, A.; Rossi, E.; Antillon, F. Nutritional Status at Diagnosis in Children and Adolescents with Cancer in the Asociacion de Hemato-Oncologia Pediatrica de Centro America (AHOPCA) Countries: Preliminary Results from Guatemala. *Pediatr. Blood Cancer* **2008**, *50*, 499–501. [CrossRef]
15. Sala, A.; Antillon, F.; Pencharz, P.; Barr, R.; AHOPCA Consortium. Nutritional Status in Children with Cancer: A Report from the AHOPCA Workshop Held in Guatemala City, August 31-September 5, 2004. *Pediatr. Blood Cancer* **2005**, *45*, 230–236. [CrossRef] [PubMed]
16. Dos Maia Lemos, P.S.; Ceragioli Oliveira, F.L.; Monteiro-Caran, E.M. Nutritional Status at Diagnosis in Children with Cancer in Brazil. *Pediatr. Ther.* **2016**, *6*. [CrossRef]
17. Ladas, E.J.; Sacks, N.; Brophy, P.; Rogers, P.C. Standards of Nutritional Care in Pediatric Oncology: Results from a Nationwide Survey on the Standards of Practice in Pediatric Oncology. A Children's Oncology Group Study. *Pediatr. Blood Cancer* **2006**, *46*, 339–344. [CrossRef]
18. Rogers, P.C.; Melnick, S.J.; Ladas, E.J.; Halton, J.; Baillargeon, J.; Sacks, N. Children's Oncology Group (COG) Nutrition Committee. *Pediatr. Blood Cancer* **2008**, *50*, 447–450. [CrossRef]
19. Villanueva, G.; Blanco, J.; Rivas, S.; Molina, A.L.; Lopez, N.; Fuentes, A.L.; Muller, L.; Caceres, A.; Antillon, F.; Ladas, E.; et al. Nutritional Status at Diagnosis of Cancer in Children and Adolescents in Guatemala and Its Relationship to Socioeconomic Disadvantage: A Retrospective Cohort Study. *Pediatr. Blood Cancer* **2019**, *66*, e27647. [CrossRef]
20. Yoruk, M.A.; Durakbasa, C.U.; Timur, C.; Sahin, S.S.; Taskin, E.C. Assessment of Nutritional Status and Malnutrition Risk at Diagnosis and Over a 6-Month Treatment Period in Pediatric Oncology Patients with Hematologic Malignancies and Solid Tumors. *J. Pediatr. Hematol. Oncol.* **2018**, *41*, e308–e321. [CrossRef]
21. Pribnow, A.K.; Ortiz, R.; Báez, L.F.; Mendieta, L.; Luna-Fineman, S. Effects of Malnutrition on Treatment-Related Morbidity and Survival of Children with Cancer in Nicaragua. *Pediatr. Blood Cancer* **2017**, *64*, e26590. [CrossRef]
22. Peccatori, N.; Ortiz, R.; Rossi, E.; Calderon, P.; Conter, V.; Garcia, Y.; Biondi, A.; Espinoza, D.; Ceppi, F.; Mendieta, L.; et al. Oral/Enteral Nutritional Supplementation In Children Treated For Cancer In Low-Middle-Income Countries Is Feasible And Effective: The Experience Of The Children's Hospital Manuel De Jesus Rivera "La Mascota" In Nicaragua. *Mediterr. J. Hematol. Infect. Dis.* **2018**, *10*, e2018038. [CrossRef] [PubMed]
23. Shah, P.; Jhaveri, U.; Idhate, T.B.; Dhingra, S.; Arolkar, P.; Arora, B. Nutritional Status at Presentation, Comparison of Assessment Tools, and Importance of Arm Anthropometry in Children with Cancer in India. *Indian J. Cancer* **2015**, *52*, 210–215.
24. Dos Lemos, P.S.M.; de Oliveira, F.L.C.; Caran, E.M.M. Nutritional Status of Children and Adolescents at Diagnosis of Hematological and Solid Malignancies. *Rev. Bras. Hematol. E Hemoter.* **2014**, *36*, 420–423. [CrossRef]

25. Orgel, E.; Sposto, R.; Malvar, J.; Seibel, N.L.; Ladas, E.; Gaynon, P.S.; Freyer, D.R. Impact on Survival and Toxicity by Duration of Weight Extremes During Treatment for Pediatric Acute Lymphoblastic Leukemia: A Report From the Children's Oncology Group. *J. Clin. Oncol.* **2014**, *32*, 1331–1337. [CrossRef]
26. Radhakrishnan, V.; Ganesan, P.; Rajendranath, R.; Ganesan, T.S.; Sagar, T.G. Nutritional Profile of Pediatric Cancer Patients at Cancer Institute, Chennai. *Indian J. Cancer* **2015**, *52*, 207. [CrossRef]
27. CDC Growth Charts. Available online: http://www.cdc.gov/growthcharts/ (accessed on 4 August 2020).
28. Garófolo, A.; Lopez, F.A.; Petrilli, A.S. High Prevalence of Malnutrition among Patients with Solid Non-Hematological Tumors as Found by Using Skinfold and Circumference Measurements. *Sao Paulo Med. J.* **2005**, *123*, 277–281. [CrossRef]
29. Smith, D.E.; Stevens, M.C.G.; Booth, I.W. Malnutrition at Diagnosis of Malignancy in Childhood: Common but Mostly Missed. *Eur. J. Pediatr.* **1991**, *150*, 318–322. [CrossRef]
30. Tazi, I.; Hidane, Z.; Zafad, S.; Harif, M.; Benchekroun, S.; Ribeiro, R. Nutritional Status at Diagnosis of Children with Malignancies in Casablanca. *Pediatr. Blood Cancer* **2008**, *51*, 495–498. [CrossRef]
31. Kuczmarski, R.J.; Ogden, C.L.; Grummer-Strawn, L.M.; Flegal, K.M.; Guo, S.S.; Wei, R.; Mei, Z.; Curtin, L.R.; Roche, A.F.; Johnson, C.L. CDC Growth Charts: United States. *Adv. Data* **2000**, *314*, 1–27.
32. Mei, Z.; Grummer-Strawn, L.M.; Pietrobelli, A.; Goulding, A.; Goran, M.I.; Dietz, W.H. Validity of Body Mass Index Compared with Other Body-Composition Screening Indexes for the Assessment of Body Fatness in Children and Adolescents. *Am. J. Clin. Nutr.* **2002**, *75*, 978–985. [CrossRef] [PubMed]
33. Triarico, S.; Rinninella, E.; Cintoni, M.; Capozza, M.A.; Mastrangelo, S.; Mele, M.C.; Ruggiero, A. Impact of Malnutrition on Survival and Infections among Pediatric Patients with Cancer: A Retrospective Study. *Eur. Rev. Med. Pharmacol. Sci.* **2019**, *23*, 1165–1175. [PubMed]
34. Huysentruyt, K.; Alliet, P.; Muyshont, L.; Rossignol, R.; Devreker, T.; Bontems, P.; Dejonckheere, J.; Vandenplas, Y.; De Schepper, J. The STRONG(Kids) Nutritional Screening Tool in Hospitalized Children: A Validation Study. *Nutr.* **2013**, *29*, 1356–1361. [CrossRef]
35. Joosten, K.F.M.; Hulst, J.M. Nutritional Screening Tools for Hospitalized Children: Methodological Considerations. *Clin. Nutr.* **2014**, *33*, 1–5. [CrossRef]
36. Połubok, J.; Malczewska, A.; Rąpała, M.; Szymocha, J.; Kozicka, M.; Dubieńska, K.; Duczek, M.; Kazanowska, B.; Barg, E. Nutritional Status at the Moment of Diagnosis in Childhood Cancer Patients. *Pediatr. Endocrinol. Diabetes Metab.* **2017**, *23*, 77–82. [CrossRef]
37. Small, A.G.; Thwe, L.M.; Byrne, J.A.; Lau, L.; Chan, A.; Craig, M.E.; Cowell, C.T.; Garnett, S.P. Neuroblastoma, Body Mass Index, and Survival: A Retrospective Analysis. *Medicine.* **2015**, *94*, e713. [CrossRef] [PubMed]
38. Brinksma, A.; Roodbol, P.F.; Sulkers, E.; Hooimeijer, H.L.; Sauer, P.J.J.; van Sonderen, E.; de Bont, E.S.J.M.; Tissing, W.J.E. Weight and Height in Children Newly Diagnosed with Cancer: Weight and Height in Children With Cancer. *Pediatr. Blood Cancer* **2015**, *62*, 269–273. [CrossRef]
39. Loeffen, E.A.H.; Brinksma, A.; Miedema, K.G.E.; de Bock, G.H.; Tissing, W.J.E. Clinical Implications of Malnutrition in Childhood Cancer Patients—Infections and Mortality. *Support. Care Cancer* **2015**, *23*, 143–150. [CrossRef]
40. Collins, L.; Nayiager, T.; Doring, N.; Kennedy, C.; Webber, C.; Halton, J.; Walker, S.; Sala, A.; Barr, R.D. Nutritional Status at Diagnosis in Children with Cancer, I. An Assessment by Dietary Recall—Compared with Body Mass Index and Body Composition Measured by Dual Energy X-ray Absorptiometry. *J. Pediatr. Hematol. Oncol.* **2010**, *32*, e299–e303. [CrossRef]
41. Eys, J.V. Benefits of Nutritional Intervention on Nutritional Status, Quality of Life and Survival. *Int. J. Cancer* **1998**, *78*, 66–68.
42. Gaynor, E.P.T.; Sullivan, P.B. Nutritional Status and Nutritional Management in Children with Cancer. *Arch. Dis. Child.* **2015**, *100*, 1169–1172. [CrossRef] [PubMed]
43. Barr, R.D.; Gomez-Almaguer, D.; Jaime-Perez, J.C.; Ruiz-Argüelles, G.J. Importance of Nutrition in the Treatment of Leukemia in Children and Adolescents. *Arch. Med. Res.* **2016**, *47*, 585–592. [CrossRef] [PubMed]
44. Butturini, A.M.; Dorey, F.J.; Lange, B.J.; Henry, D.W.; Gaynon, P.S.; Fu, C.; Franklin, J.; Siegel, S.E.; Seibel, N.L.; Rogers, P.C.; et al. Obesity and Outcome in Pediatric Acute Lymphoblastic Leukemia. *J. Clin. Oncol..* **2007**, *25*, 2063–2069. [CrossRef]
45. Ethier, M.-C.; Alexander, S.; Abla, O.; Green, G.; Lam, R.; Sung, L. Association between Obesity at Diagnosis and Weight Change during Induction and Survival in Pediatric Acute Lymphoblastic Leukemia. *Leuk. Lymphoma* **2012**, *53*, 1677–1681. [CrossRef] [PubMed]

46. Reilly, J.J.; Odame, I.; McColl, J.H.; McAllister, P.J.; Gibson, B.E.; Wharton, B.A. Does Weight for Height Have Prognostic Significance in Children with Acute Lymphoblastic Leukemia? *Am. J. Pediatr. Hematol. Oncol.* **1994**, *16*, 225–230. [CrossRef]
47. Withycombe, J.S.; Post-White, J.E.; Meza, J.L.; Hawks, R.G.; Smith, L.M.; Sacks, N.; Seibel, N.L. Weight Patterns in Children With Higher Risk ALL: A Report From the Children's Oncology Group (COG) for CCG 1961. *Pediatr. Blood Cancer* **2009**, *53*, 1249–1254. [CrossRef] [PubMed]
48. Paciarotti, I.; McKenzie, J.M.; Davidson, I.; Edgar, A.B.; Brougham, M.; Wilson, D.C. Short Term Effects of Childhood Cancer and Its Treatments on Nutritional Status: A Prospective Cohort Study. *EC Nutr.* **2015**, *3*, 528–540.
49. Brinksma, A.; Roodbol, P.F.; Sulkers, E.; Kamps, W.A.; de Bont, E.S.J.M.; Boot, A.M.; Burgerhof, J.G.M.; Tamminga, R.Y.J.; Tissing, W.J.E. Changes in Nutritional Status in Childhood Cancer Patients: A Prospective Cohort Study. *Clin. Nutr.* **2015**, *34*, 66–73. [CrossRef]
50. Revuelta Iniesta, R.; Paciarotti, I.; Davidson, I.; McKenzie, J.M.; Brougham, M.F.H.; Wilson, D.C. Nutritional Status of Children and Adolescents with Cancer in Scotland: A Prospective Cohort Study. *Clin. Nutr. ESPEN* **2019**, *32*, 96–106. [CrossRef]
51. Schleiermacher, G.; Janoueix-Lerosey, I.; Delattre, O. Recent Insights into the Biology of Neuroblastoma: Biology of Neuroblastoma. *Int. J. Cancer* **2014**, *135*, 2249–2261. [CrossRef]
52. Gómez-Almaguer, D.; Ruiz-Argüelles, G.J.; Ponce-de-León, S. Nutritional Status and Socio-Economic Conditions as Prognostic Factors in the Outcome of Therapy in Childhood Acute Lymphoblastic Leukemia. *Int. J. Cancer* **1998**, *78*, 52–55. [CrossRef]
53. Rogers, P.C. Nutritional Status as a Prognostic Indicator for Pediatric Malignancies. *J. Clin. Oncol.* **2014**, *32*, 1293–1294. [CrossRef]
54. Lange, B.J. Mortality in Overweight and Underweight Children with Acute Myeloid Leukemia. *JAMA* **2005**, *293*, 203. [CrossRef] [PubMed]
55. Aldhafiri, F.K.; McColl, J.H.; Reilly, J.J. Prognostic Significance of Being Overweight and Obese at Diagnosis in Children with Acute Lymphoblastic Leukemia. *J. Pediatr. Hematol. Oncol.* **2014**, *36*, 234–236. [CrossRef]
56. Canner, J.; Alonzo, T.A.; Franklin, J.; Freyer, D.R.; Gamis, A.; Gerbing, R.B.; Lange, B.J.; Meshinchi, S.; Woods, W.G.; Perentesis, J.; et al. Differences in Outcomes of Newly Diagnosed Acute Myeloid Leukemia for Adolescent/Young Adult and Younger Patients: A Report from the Children's Oncology Group. *Cancer* **2013**, *119*, 4162–4169. [CrossRef]
57. Hijiya, N.; Panetta, J.C.; Zhou, Y.; Kyzer, E.P.; Howard, S.C.; Jeha, S.; Razzouk, B.I.; Ribeiro, R.C.; Rubnitz, J.E.; Hudson, M.M.; et al. Body Mass Index Does Not Influence Pharmacokinetics or Outcome of Treatment in Children with Acute Lymphoblastic Leukemia. *Blood* **2006**, *108*, 3997–4002. [CrossRef]
58. Inaba, H.; Surprise, H.C.; Pounds, S.; Cao, X.; Howard, S.C.; Ringwald-Smith, K.; Buaboonnam, J.; Dahl, G.; Bowman, W.P.; Taub, J.W.; et al. Effect of Body Mass Index on the Outcome of Children with Acute Myeloid Leukemia. *Cancer* **2012**, *118*, 5989–5996. [CrossRef] [PubMed]
59. Amankwah, E.K.; Saenz, A.M.; Hale, G.A.; Brown, P.A. Association between Body Mass Index at Diagnosis and Pediatric Leukemia Mortality and Relapse: A Systematic Review and Meta-Analysis. *Leuk. Lymphoma* **2016**, *57*, 1140–1148. [CrossRef]
60. Hunger, S.P.; Sung, L.; Howard, S.C. Treatment Strategies and Regimens of Graduated Intensity for Childhood Acute Lymphoblastic Leukemia in Low-Income Countries: A Proposal. *Pediatr. Blood Cancer* **2009**, *52*, 559–565. [CrossRef]
61. Murphy, A.J.; Mosby, T.T.; Rogers, P.C.; Cohen, J.; Ladas, E.J. An International Survey of Nutritional Practices in Low- and Middle-Income Countries: A Report from the International Society of Pediatric Oncology (SIOP) PODC Nutrition Working Group. *Eur. J. Clin. Nutr.* **2014**, *68*, 1341–1345. [CrossRef]
62. Orgel, E.; Genkinger, J.M.; Aggarwal, D.; Sung, L.; Nieder, M.; Ladas, E.J. Association of Body Mass Index and Survival in Pediatric Leukemia: A Meta-Analysis. *Am. J. Clin. Nutr.* **2016**, *103*, 808–817. [CrossRef]
63. Saenz, A.M.; Stapleton, S.; Hernandez, R.G.; Hale, G.A.; Goldenberg, N.A.; Schwartz, S.; Amankwah, E.K. Body Mass Index at Pediatric Leukemia Diagnosis and the Risks of Relapse and Mortality: Findings from a Single Institution and Meta-Analysis. *J. Obes.* **2018**, *2018*, 1–8. [CrossRef]
64. Weir, J.; Reilly, J.J.; McColl, J.H.; Gibson, B.E.S. No Evidence for an Effect of Nutritional Status at Diagnosis on Prognosis in Children with Acute Lymphoblastic Leukemia. *J. Pediatr. Hematol. Oncol.* **1998**, *20*, 534–538. [CrossRef]

65. Baillargeon, J.; Langevin, A.M.; Lewis, M.; Estrada, J.; Mullins, J.; Pitney, A.; Ma, J.Z.; Chisholm, G.B.; Pollock, B.H. Obesity and Survival in a Cohort of Predominantly Hispanic Children with Acute Lymphoblastic Leukemia. *J. Pediatr. Hematol. Oncol.* **2006**, *28*, 575–578. [CrossRef]
66. Karakurt, H.; Sarper, N.; Kılıç, S.Ç.; Gelen, S.A.; Zengin, E. Screening Survivors of Childhood Acute Lymphoblastic Leukemia for Obesity, Metabolic Syndrome, and Insulin Resistance. *Pediatr. Hematol. Oncol.* **2012**, *29*, 551–561. [CrossRef]
67. Løhmann, D.J.A.; Abrahamsson, J.; Ha, S.-Y.; Jónsson, Ó.G.; Koskenvuo, M.; Lausen, B.; Palle, J.; Zeller, B.; Hasle, H. Effect of Age and Body Weight on Toxicity and Survival in Pediatric Acute Myeloid Leukemia: Results from NOPHO-AML 2004. *Haematologica* **2016**, *101*, 1359–1367. [CrossRef]
68. Joffe, L.; Dwyer, S.; Glade Bender, J.L.; Frazier, A.L.; Ladas, E.J. Nutritional Status and Clinical Outcomes in Pediatric Patients with Solid Tumors: A Systematic Review of the Literature. *Semin. Oncol.* **2019**, *46*, 48–56. [CrossRef]
69. Brown, T.R.; Vijarnsorn, C.; Potts, J.; Milner, R.; Sandor, G.G.S.; Fryer, C. Anthracycline Induced Cardiac Toxicity in Pediatric Ewing Sarcoma: A Longitudinal Study. *Pediatr. Blood Cancer* **2013**, *60*, 842–848. [CrossRef]
70. Altaf, S.; Enders, F.; Jeavons, E.; Krailo, M.; Barkauskas, D.A.; Meyers, P.; Arndt, C. High-BMI at Diagnosis Is Associated with Inferior Survival in Patients with Osteosarcoma: A Report from the Children's Oncology Group. *Pediatr. Blood Cancer* **2013**, *60*, 2042–2046. [CrossRef]
71. Goldstein, G.; Shemesh, E.; Frenkel, T.; Jacobson, J.M.; Toren, A. Abnormal Body Mass Index at Diagnosis in Patients with Ewing Sarcoma Is Associated with Inferior Tumor Necrosis. *Pediatr. Blood Cancer* **2015**, *62*, 1892–1896. [CrossRef] [PubMed]
72. Hingorani, P.; Seidel, K.; Krailo, M.; Mascarenhas, L.; Meyers, P.; Marina, N.; Conrad, E.U.; Hawkins, D.S. Body Mass Index (BMI) at Diagnosis Is Associated with Surgical Wound Complications in Patients with Localized Osteosarcoma: A Report from the Children's Oncology Group. *Pediatr. Blood Cancer* **2011**, *57*, 939–942. [CrossRef] [PubMed]
73. Rodeberg, D.A.; Stoner, J.A.; Garcia-Henriquez, N.; Randall, R.L.; Spunt, S.L.; Arndt, C.A.; Kao, S.; Paidas, C.N.; Million, L.; Hawkins, D.S. Tumor Volume and Patient Weight as Predictors of Outcome in Children with Intermediate Risk Rhabdomyosarcoma: A Report from the Children's Oncology Group. *Cancer* **2011**, *117*, 2541–2550. [CrossRef] [PubMed]
74. Iniesta, R.R.; Paciarotti, I.; Brougham, M.F.H.; McKenzie, J.M.; Wilson, D.C. Effects of Pediatric Cancer and Its Treatment on Nutritional Status: A Systematic Review. *Nutr. Rev.* **2015**, *73*, 276–295. [CrossRef]
75. Donaldson, S.S.; Wesley, M.N.; DeWys, W.D.; Suskind, R.M.; Jaffe, N.; vanEys, J. A Study of the Nutritional Status of Pediatric Cancer Patients. *Am. J. Dis. Child.* **1981**, *135*, 1107–1112. [CrossRef]
76. Lobato-Mendizábal, E.; Ruiz-Argüelles, G.J.; Marín-López, A. Leukaemia and Nutrition I: Malnutrition Is an Adverse Prognostic Factor in the Outcome of Treatment of Patients with Standard-Risk Acute Lymphoblastic Leukaemia. *Leuk. Res.* **1989**, *13*, 899–906. [CrossRef]
77. Mejía-Aranguré, J.M.; Fajardo-Gutiérrez, A.; Reyes-Ruíz, N.I.; Bernáldez-Ríos, R.; Mejía-Domínguez, A.M.; Navarrete-Navarro, S.; Martínez-García, M.C. Malnutrition in Childhood Lymphoblastic Leukemia: A Predictor of Early Mortality during the Induction-to-Remission Phase of the Treatment. *Arch. Med. Res.* **1999**, *30*, 150–153. [CrossRef]
78. Pedrosa, F.; Bonilla, M.; Liu, A.; Smith, K.; Davis, D.; Ribeiro, R.C.; Wilimas, J.A. Effect of Malnutrition at the Time of Diagnosis on the Survival of Children Treated for Cancer in El Salvador and Northern Brazil. *J. Pediatr. Hematol. Oncol.* **2000**, *22*, 502–505. [CrossRef]
79. Brinksma, A.; Sanderman, R.; Roodbol, P.F.; Sulkers, E.; Burgerhof, J.G.M.; de Bont, E.S.J.M.; Tissing, W.J.E. Malnutrition Is Associated with Worse Health-Related Quality of Life in Children with Cancer. *Support. Care Cancer* **2015**, *23*, 3043–3052. [CrossRef]
80. Malihi, Z.; Kandiah, M.; Chan, Y.M.; Hosseinzadeh, M.; Sohanaki Azad, M.; Zarif Yeganeh, M. Nutritional Status and Quality of Life in Patients with Acute Leukaemia Prior to and after Induction Chemotherapy in Three Hospitals in Tehran, Iran: A Prospective Study. *J. Hum. Nutr. Diet.* **2013**, *26* (Suppl. 1), 123–131. [CrossRef]
81. Nathan, P.C.; Furlong, W.; Barr, R.D. Challenges to the Measurement of Health-Related Quality of Life in Children Receiving Cancer Therapy. *Pediatr. Blood Cancer* **2004**, *43*, 215–223. [CrossRef]

82. Tsiros, M.D.; Olds, T.; Buckley, J.D.; Grimshaw, P.; Brennan, L.; Walkley, J.; Hills, A.P.; Howe, P.R.C.; Coates, A.M. Health-Related Quality of Life in Obese Children and Adolescents. *Int. J. Obes.* **2009**, *33*, 387–400. [CrossRef] [PubMed]
83. Varni, J.W.; Limbers, C.; Burwinkle, T.M. Literature Review: Health-Related Quality of Life Measurement in Pediatric Oncology: Hearing the Voices of the Children. *J. Pediatr. Psychol.* **2007**, *32*, 1151–1163. [CrossRef] [PubMed]
84. Varni, J.W.; Burwinkle, T.M.; Jacobs, J.R.; Gottschalk, M.; Kaufman, F.; Jones, K.L. The PedsQL in Type 1 and Type 2 Diabetes: Reliability and Validity of the Pediatric Quality of Life Inventory Generic Core Scales and Type 1 Diabetes Module. *Diabetes Care* **2003**, *26*, 631–637. [CrossRef]
85. Varni, J.W.; Seid, M.; Smith Knight, T.; Burwinkle, T.; Brown, J.; Szer, I.S. The PedsQL in Pediatric Rheumatology: Reliability, Validity, and Responsiveness of the Pediatric Quality of Life Inventory Generic Core Scales and Rheumatology Module. *Arthritis Rheum.* **2002**, *46*, 714–725. [CrossRef]
86. Varni, J.W.; Seid, M.; Kurtin, P.S. PedsQL™ 4.0: Reliability and Validity of the Pediatric Quality of Life Inventory™ Version 4.0 Generic Core Scales in Healthy and Patient Populations. *Med. Care* **2001**, *39*, 800–812. [CrossRef]
87. Ladas, E.J.; Sacks, N.; Meacham, L.; Henry, D.; Enriquez, L.; Lowry, G.; Hawkes, R.; Dadd, G.; Rogers, P. A Multidisciplinary Review of Nutrition Considerations in the Pediatric Oncology Population: A Perspective from Children's Oncology Group. *Nutr. Clin. Pract.* **2005**, *20*, 377–393. [CrossRef]
88. Varni, J.W.; Limbers, C.A.; Burwinkle, T.M. Parent Proxy-Report of Their Children's Health-Related Quality of Life: An Analysis of 13,878 Parents' Reliability and Validity across Age Subgroups Using the PedsQL™ 4.0 Generic Core Scales. *Health Qual. Life Outcomes* **2007**, *5*. [CrossRef]
89. Varni, J.W.; Burwinkle, T.M.; Katz, E.R.; Meeske, K.; Dickinson, P. The PedsQL in Pediatric Cancer: Reliability and Validity of the Pediatric Quality of Life Inventory Generic Core Scales, Multidimensional Fatigue Scale, and Cancer Module. *Cancer* **2002**, *94*, 2090–2106. [CrossRef]
90. Evans, W.J.; Lambert, C.P. Physiological Basis of Fatigue. *Am. J. Phys. Med. Rehabil.* **2007**, *86*, S29–S46. [CrossRef] [PubMed]
91. Mariotto, A.B.; Rowland, J.H.; Yabroff, K.R.; Scoppa, S.; Hachey, M.; Ries, L.; Feuer, E.J. Long-Term Survivors of Childhood Cancers in the United States. *Cancer Epidemiol. Prev. Biomark.* **2009**, *18*, 1033–1040. [CrossRef]
92. Hudson, M.M.; Oeffinger, K.C.; Jones, K.; Brinkman, T.M.; Krull, K.R.; Mulrooney, D.A.; Mertens, A.; Castellino, S.M.; Casillas, J.; Gurney, J.G.; et al. Age-Dependent Changes in Health Status in the Childhood Cancer Survivor Cohort. *J. Clin. Oncol.* **2015**, *33*, 479–491. [CrossRef]
93. Oeffinger, K.C.; Mertens, A.C.; Sklar, C.A.; Kawashima, T.; Hudson, M.M.; Meadows, A.T.; Friedman, D.L.; Marina, N.; Hobbie, W.; Kadan-Lottick, N.S.; et al. Childhood Cancer Survivor Study. Chronic Health Conditions in Adult Survivors of Childhood Cancer. *N. Engl. J. Med.* **2006**, *355*, 1572–1582. [CrossRef] [PubMed]
94. Ladas, E. Nutritional Counseling in Survivors of Childhood Cancer: An Essential Component of Survivorship Care. *Children* **2014**, *1*, 107–118. [CrossRef] [PubMed]
95. Ferlay, J.; Soerjomataram, I.; Dikshit, R.; Eser, S.; Mathers, C.; Rebelo, M.; Parkin, D.M.; Forman, D.; Bray, F. Cancer Incidence and Mortality Worldwide: Sources, Methods and Major Patterns in GLOBOCAN 2012. *Int. J. Cancer* **2015**, *136*, 359–386. [CrossRef]
96. Zhang, F.F.; Kelly, M.J.; Saltzman, E.; Must, A.; Roberts, S.B.; Parsons, S.K. Obesity in Pediatric ALL Survivors: A Meta-Analysis. *Pediatrics* **2014**, *133*, e704–e715. [CrossRef] [PubMed]
97. Zhang, F.F.; Rodday, A.M.; Kelly, M.J.; Must, A.; MacPherson, C.; Roberts, S.B.; Saltzman, E.; Parsons, S.K. Predictors of Being Overweight or Obese in Survivors of Pediatric Acute Lymphoblastic Leukemia (ALL): Predictors of Obesity in ALL Survivors. *Pediatr. Blood Cancer* **2014**, *61*, 1263–1269. [CrossRef]
98. Zhang, F.F.; Liu, S.; Chung, M.; Kelly, M.J. Growth Patterns during and after Treatment in Patients with Pediatric ALL: A Meta-Analysis: Growth Patterns During in Patients with Pediatic All. *Pediatr. Blood Cancer* **2015**, *62*, 1452–1460. [CrossRef]
99. Collins, L.; Beaumont, L.; Cranston, A.; Savoie, S.; Nayiager, T.; Barr, R. Anthropometry in Long-Term Survivors of Acute Lymphoblastic Leukemia in Childhood and Adolescence. *J. Adolesc. Young Adult Oncol.* **2017**, *6*, 294–298. [CrossRef]

100. Karlage, R.E.; Wilson, C.L.; Zhang, N.; Kaste, S.; Green, D.M.; Armstrong, G.T.; Robison, L.L.; Chemaitilly, W.; Srivastava, D.K.; Hudson, M.M.; et al. Validity of Anthropometric Measurements for Characterizing Obesity among Adult Survivors of Childhood Cancer: A Report from the St. Jude Lifetime Cohort Study. *Cancer* **2015**, *121*, 2036–2043. [CrossRef]
101. Marriott, C.J.C.; Beaumont, L.F.; Farncombe, T.H.; Cranston, A.N.; Athale, U.H.; Yakemchuk, V.N.; Webber, C.E.; Barr, R.D. Body Composition in Long-Term Survivors of Acute Lymphoblastic Leukemia Diagnosed in Childhood and Adolescence: A Focus on Sarcopenic Obesity. *Cancer* **2018**, *124*, 1225–1231. [CrossRef]
102. Molinari, P.C.C.; Lederman, H.M.; Lee, M.L.D.M.; Caran, E.M.M. Assessment of The Late Effects on Bones and on Body Composition of Children and Adolescents Treated for Acute Lymphocytic Leukemia According To Brazilian Protocols. *Rev. Paul. Pediatr.* **2017**, *35*, 78–85. [CrossRef]
103. Wang, K.; Fleming, A.; Johnston, D.L.; Zelcer, S.M.; Rassekh, S.R.; Ladhani, S.; Socha, A.; Shinuda, J.; Jaber, S.; Burrow, S.; et al. Overweight, Obesity and Adiposity in Survivors of Childhood Brain Tumours: A Systematic Review and Meta-analysis. *Clin. Obes.* **2018**, *8*, 55–67. [CrossRef] [PubMed]
104. Warner, E.L.; Fluchel, M.; Wright, J.; Sweeney, C.; Boucher, K.M.; Fraser, A.; Smith, K.R.; Stroup, A.M.; Kinney, A.Y.; Kirchhoff, A.C. A Population-Based Study of Childhood Cancer Survivors' Body Mass Index. *J. Cancer Epidemiol.* **2014**, *2014*, 1–10. [CrossRef]
105. Prasad, M.; Arora, B.; Chinnaswamy, G.; Vora, T.; Narula, G.; Banavali, S.; Kurkure, P. Nutritional Status in Survivors of Childhood Cancer: Experience from Tata Memorial Hospital, Mumbai. *Indian J. Cancer* **2015**, *52*, 219.
106. McCarthy, H.D. Body Fat Measurements in Children as Predictors for the Metabolic Syndrome: Focus on Waist Circumference. *Proc. Nutr. Soc.* **2006**, *65*, 385–392.
107. Haddy, T.B.; Mosher, R.B.; Reaman, G.H. Osteoporosis in Survivors of Acute Lymphoblastic Leukemia. *Oncologist* **2001**, *6*, 278–285. [CrossRef]
108. Davies, J.H.; Evans, B.A.J.; Jenney, M.E.; Gregory, J.W. Skeletal Morbidity in Childhood Acute Lymphoblastic Leukaemia. *Clin. Endocrinol. (Oxf.)* **2005**, *63*, 1–9. [CrossRef]
109. Wasilewski-Masker, K.; Kaste, S.C.; Hudson, M.M.; Esiashvili, N.; Mattano, L.A.; Meacham, L.R. Bone Mineral Density Deficits in Survivors of Childhood Cancer: Long-Term Follow-up Guidelines and Review of the Literature. *Pediatrics* **2008**, *121*, 705–713. [CrossRef]
110. Hansen, J.A.; Stancel, H.H.; Klesges, L.M.; Tyc, V.L.; Hinds, P.S.; Wu, S.; Hudson, M.M.; Kahalley, L.S. Eating Behavior and BMI in Adolescent Survivors of Brain Tumor and Acute Lymphoblastic Leukemia. *J. Pediatr. Oncol. Nurs.* **2014**, *31*, 41–50. [CrossRef] [PubMed]
111. Wilson, C.L.; Liu, W.; Yang, J.J.; Kang, G.; Ojha, R.P.; Neale, G.A.; Srivastava, D.K.; Gurney, J.G.; Hudson, M.M.; Robison, L.L.; et al. Genetic and Clinical Factors Associated with Obesity among Adult Survivors of Childhood Cancer: A Report from the St. Jude Lifetime Cohort. *Cancer* **2015**, *121*, 2262–2270. [CrossRef] [PubMed]
112. Brouwer, C.A.J.; Gietema, J.A.; Vonk, J.M.; Tissing, W.J.E.; Boezen, H.M.; Zwart, N.; Postma, A. Body Mass Index and Annual Increase of Body Mass Index in Long-Term Childhood Cancer Survivors; Relationship to Treatment. *Support. Care Cancer* **2012**, *20*, 311–318. [CrossRef]
113. Meacham, L.R.; Gurney, J.G.; Mertens, A.C.; Ness, K.K.; Sklar, C.A.; Robison, L.L.; Oeffinger, K.C. Body Mass Index in Long-Term Adult Survivors of Childhood Cancer: A Report of the Childhood Cancer Survivor Study. *Cancer* **2005**, *103*, 1730–1739. [CrossRef]
114. Lustig, R.H. Hypothalamic Obesity after Craniopharyngioma: Mechanisms, Diagnosis, and Treatment. *Front. Endocrinol.* **2011**, *2*. [CrossRef]
115. Müller, H.L. Craniopharyngioma and Hypothalamic Injury: Latest Insights into Consequent Eating Disorders and Obesity. *Curr. Opin. Endocrinol. Diabetes Obes.* **2016**, *23*, 81–89. [CrossRef]
116. Armstrong, G.T.; Oeffinger, K.C.; Chen, Y.; Kawashima, T.; Yasui, Y.; Leisenring, W.; Stovall, M.; Chow, E.J.; Sklar, C.A.; Mulrooney, D.A.; et al. Modifiable Risk Factors and Major Cardiac Events among Adult Survivors of Childhood Cancer. *J. Clin. Oncol.* **2013**, *31*, 3673–3680. [CrossRef]
117. Elliot, D.L.; Lindemulder, S.J.; Goldberg, L.; Stadler, D.D.; Smith, J. Health Promotion for Adolescent Childhood Leukemia Survivors: Building on Prevention Science and Ehealth. *Pediatr. Blood Cancer* **2013**, *60*, 905–910. [CrossRef] [PubMed]

118. Rock, C.L.; Doyle, C.; Demark-Wahnefried, W.; Meyerhardt, J.; Courneya, K.S.; Schwartz, A.L.; Bandera, E.V.; Hamilton, K.K.; Grant, B.; McCullough, M.; et al. Nutrition and Physical Activity Guidelines for Cancer Survivors. *CA Cancer J. Clin.* **2012**, *62*, 243–274. [CrossRef]
119. Wiseman, M.; Cannon, G. *Food, Nutrition, Physical Activity and the Prevention of Cancer: A Global Perspective: Summary*; World Cancer Research Fund, American Institute for Cancer Research: Washington, DC, USA, 2007.
120. Children's Oncology Group. Long-Term Follow-Up Guidelines for Survivors of Childhood, Adolescent, and Young Adult Cancers. Available online: http://www.survivorshipguidelines.org/pdf/ltfuguidelines_40.pdf (accessed on 13 September 2020).
121. Brinkman, T.M.; Recklitis, C.J.; Michel, G.; Grootenhuis, M.A.; Klosky, J.L. Psychological Symptoms, Social Outcomes, Socioeconomic Attainment, and Health Behaviors Among Survivors of Childhood Cancer: Current State of the Literature. *J. Clin. Oncol.* **2018**, *36*, 2190–2197. [CrossRef]
122. Love, E.; Schneiderman, J.E.; Stephens, D.; Lee, S.; Barron, M.; Tsangaris, E.; Urbach, S.; Staneland, P.; Greenberg, M.; Nathan, P.C. A Cross-Sectional Study of Overweight in Pediatric Survivors of Acute Lymphoblastic Leukemia (ALL). *Pediatr. Blood Cancer* **2011**, *57*, 1204–1209. [CrossRef] [PubMed]
123. Zhang, F.F.; Saltzman, E.; Kelly, M.J.; Liu, S.; Must, A.; Parsons, S.K.; Roberts, S.B. Comparison of Childhood Cancer Survivors' Nutritional Intake with US Dietary Guidelines. *Pediatr. Blood Cancer* **2015**, *62*, 1461–1467. [CrossRef]
124. Landy, D.C.; Lipsitz, S.R.; Kurtz, J.M.; Hinkle, A.S.; Constine, L.S.; Adams, M.J.; Lipshultz, S.E.; Miller, T.L. Dietary Quality, Caloric Intake, and Adiposity of Childhood Cancer Survivors and Their Siblings: An Analysis from the Cardiac Risk Factors in Childhood Cancer Survivors Study. *Nutr. Cancer* **2013**, *65*, 547–555. [CrossRef]
125. Robien, K.; Ness, K.K.; Klesges, L.M.; Baker, K.S.; Gurney, J.G. Poor Adherence to Dietary Guidelines among Adult Survivors of Childhood Acute Lymphoblastic Leukemia. *J. Pediatr. Hematol. Oncol.* **2008**, *30*, 815–822. [CrossRef]
126. Smith, W.A.; Li, C.; Nottage, K.A.; Mulrooney, D.A.; Armstrong, G.T.; Lanctot, J.Q.; Chemaitilly, W.; Laver, J.H.; Srivastava, D.K.; Robison, L.L.; et al. Lifestyle and Metabolic Syndrome in Adult Survivors of Childhood Cancer: A Report from the St. Jude Lifetime Cohort Study. *Cancer* **2014**, *120*, 2742–2750. [CrossRef] [PubMed]
127. Tonorezos, E.S.; Robien, K.; Eshelman-Kent, D.; Moskowitz, C.S.; Church, T.S.; Ross, R.; Oeffinger, K.C. Contribution of Diet and Physical Activity to Metabolic Parameters among Survivors of Childhood Leukemia. *Cancer Causes Control CCC* **2013**, *24*, 313–321. [CrossRef] [PubMed]
128. Zhang, F.F.; Ojha, R.P.; Krull, K.R.; Gibson, T.M.; Lu, L.; Lanctot, J.; Chemaitilly, W.; Robison, L.L.; Hudson, M.M. Adult Survivors of Childhood Cancer Have Poor Adherence to Dietary Guidelines. *J. Nutr.* **2016**, *146*, 2497–2505. [CrossRef]
129. Freycon, F.; Trombert-Paviot, B.; Casagranda, L.; Bertrand, Y.; Plantaz, D.; Marec-Bérard, P. Trends in Treatment-Related Deaths (TRDs) in Childhood Cancer and Leukemia over Time: A Follow-up of Patients Included in the Childhood Cancer Registry of the Rhône-Alpes Region in France (ARCERRA). *Pediatr. Blood Cancer* **2008**, *50*, 1213–1220. [CrossRef]
130. Kaatsch, P. Epidemiology of Childhood Cancer. *Cancer Treat. Rev.* **2010**, *36*, 277–285. [CrossRef]
131. Bauer, J.; Jürgens, H.; Frühwald, M.C. Important Aspects of Nutrition in Children with Cancer1. *Adv. Nutr.* **2011**, *2*, 67–77. [CrossRef]

Publisher's Note: MDPI stays neutral with regard to jurisdictional claims in published maps and institutional affiliations.

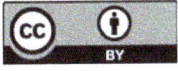

© 2020 by the authors. Licensee MDPI, Basel, Switzerland. This article is an open access article distributed under the terms and conditions of the Creative Commons Attribution (CC BY) license (http://creativecommons.org/licenses/by/4.0/).

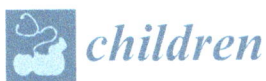

Article

Anthropometric Assessment of Nepali Children Institutionalized in Orphanages

Lucía Fernández [1], Ana Rubini [1], Jose M. Soriano [1,2,*], Joaquín Aldás-Manzano [3] and Jesús Blesa [1,2,4]

1. Food & Health Lab, Institute of Materials Science, University of Valencia, 46980 Paterna, Spain; lucia.fernandez.mol@gmail.com (L.F.); Rubinigimenez@gmail.com (A.R.); jesus.blesa@uv.es (J.B.)
2. Joint Research Unit on Endocrinology, Nutrition and Clinical Dietetics, University of Valencia-Health Research Institute La Fe, 46026 Valencia, Spain
3. Department of Marketing and Market Research, Faculty of Economics, University of Valencia, 46022 Valencia, Spain; joaquin.aldas@uv.es
4. Laboratory of Nutrition, Department of Preventive Medicine and Public Health, Faculty of Pharmacy, University of Valencia, 46100 Burjassot, Spain
* Correspondence: jose.soriano@uv.es; Tel.: +34-963543056

Received: 7 October 2020; Accepted: 5 November 2020; Published: 7 November 2020

Abstract: Nepal is among the world's poorest countries, and it is the third-poorest country in the South Asian region. Asia has the largest number of orphans in the world; in Nepal there are around 13,281 orphan children. The objective of this study is to evaluate the growth status of institutionalized children in Nepal through the analyses of anthropometric measures. The sample was Nepalese children aged 4 to 17, obtained from two different orphanages: in the first one, children with physical and mental disabilities coexist with children without any conditions. In the second one, there were no subjects with disabilities. Significant evidence of an association between mental and physical disability in institutionalized children and undernutrition (wasting and stunting) was found in this study. There is also weak but significant evidence of a relationship between underweight and being male. The study could help reaching a better understanding of growth status of institutionalized children in Nepal.

Keywords: orphanage; Nepal; anthropometry

1. Introduction

In the Asian nation of Nepal, with a population of around 23 million, divided into more than 100 ethnic groups and distributed in 75 different territorial districts, 80% of the population have a sustenance model based on agriculture [1]. In the South Asia region, Nepal is the third-poorest country [2]. Despite being a state where the poverty affects a high percentage of the population, and where some geographic areas could be hostile and even compromise the subsistence of its inhabitants [3], life expectancy is between 67–69 years. It should also be noted that the 35% of the people are under 15 years old and just 7.6% corresponds to people over 60 years of age [4]. On the other hand, Asia has around 60 million children who to have lost one or both parents, being one of the countries in the world with the largest number of orphans [5]. There is no official published government data on the number of children's homes in Nepal since the country currently lacks a complete data-collection system on children in institutional care [6]. However, according to the Central Children Welfare Council, there are around 13,281 abandoned and orphaned children in Nepal, distributed in 610 orphanages [7]. Despite the fact that the majority of orphaned (or abandoned) children in Nepal are cared for in institutions, they would not be excluded from risks generated by poverty, which reflects the need of authorities to be more concerned and proactive to combat this situation. People with disabilities in Nepal face higher incidence of human rights violations, especially discrimination, unequal treatment, disregard for difference, denial of accessibility, and exclusion [8]. Therefore, a child with mental disability living in an institution, would inevitably have greater difficulty attaining an acceptable quality of life. The aim of this study was to evaluate the growth status of children living in Nepali orphanages through the analysis of anthropometric parameters.

2. Materials and Methods

2.1. Participants

Research was conducted in the Nepali town of Hetauda, home of the administrative headquarters of Makwanpur district, placed in the central region of Nepal. This territorial district is mostly rural and is administratively divided in 43 rural and municipal development committees and has a population of around 400,000 [9]. This descriptive study was carried out in collaboration with a Spanish non-governmental organization (NGO) for a one-month period during the summer in 2013 according to the volunteering program of the NGO. The sample was 47 Nepali children (24 girls and 23 boys), who were aged from 4 to 17 years. The sample was taken from two different orphanages: the first one was called Bal Griha 1, where children with physical and mental disabilities coexist with children without any conditions ($n = 24$); the second one, called Bal Griha 2, there were no subjects with disabilities ($n = 23$). In the Bal Griha 1, 12 of the 24 children had no disabilities. The rest of the children of this orphanage had different types of disabilities including burn contractures, posttraumatic amputations, neuromuscular alterations, one cerebral palsy, and different degrees of mental retardation. All subjects gave their informed consent for inclusion before they participated in the study. The study was conducted in accordance with the Declaration of Helsinki, and the protocol was approved by the Ethics Committee of University of Valencia (Spain) (EH-1-2012). The primary caregiver (no aides), who had primary responsibility for children, was informed about the study goals and verbal consent was obtained to take their child's anthropometric measurements.

2.2. Anthropometric Measures

Weight and standing height measurements were performed in triplicate and done according to the Anthropometric Standardization Reference Manual [10]. The subjects wore no shoes and light clothes, and all the measurements were taken by the same trained anthropometrist. A Plenna scale (model MEA 07 400, Plenna®, São Paulo, SP, Brazil; accuracy of 100 g) was used to determine weight and a Seca stadiometer (model 208, Seca, GmbH, Hamburg, Germany; accuracy of 0.5 cm) was used to determine height. Height-for-age Z-scores (HAZ), weight-for-age Z-scores (WAZ) and body mass index (BMI) for age (BAZ) were calculated using the WHO AnthroPlus software developed by the World Health Organization (http://www.who.int/growthref/tools/en), which uses the 2007 WHO reference values [11]. The stunting and underweight are calculated by Z-score: children with a HAZ, WAZ, or BAZ < -2.0 are classified as stunted, underweight, or thin, respectively [11,12]. A low HAZ indicates an incapacity to reach linear growth potential as a result of health and/or nutritional deficient conditions, which is known as stunted growth [13]. Children with a measurement of <-2 standard deviation (SD) from the median of the reference group were classified as short for their age (stunted), while children with measurement of <-3 SD from the median of the reference group were considered to be severely stunted [12]. A low WAZ is considered to indicate whether a subject is underweight (in the absence of wasting). Lastly, BMI is an important index for thinness in children over 10 years of age since weight-for-age can be calculated only for children aged <10 years [13]. To estimate body mass in children with a lack of limbs or other body components (leg, foot, or hand), equations for the assessment of weights status of amputees were used [14–16].

2.3. Statistical Analysis

Values for WAZ, HAZ, and BAZ are presented as means and SD. These means are grouped by sex, orphanage, physical disability, and mental disability. A Kolmogorov–Smirnov test was used to test for normality. To compare the means, the Independent-Samples t-Test was used in case of a normal distribution, otherwise the Mann–Whitney U test was used. All statistical significance was established at a p-value < 0.05. All statistical analyses were performed using the SPSS Statistics 19.0 (SPSS Inc., Chicago, IL, USA).

3. Results

The mean age of all enrolled children into the study was 10.4 ± 3.4 years (range: 4–17 years). The mean of the height was 128.7 ± 18.7 cm and the mean of the weight was 26 ± 10.1 kg. Mean of WAZ, HAZ, and BAZ were all negative (−1.9, −1.9, and−1.4, respectively) (Table 1). This indicates that the average of children was smaller and lighter than the growth standard.

Table 1. Characteristics of the sample. Mean and standard deviation of age, height, weight, and growth-related characteristics.

	Mean	Standard Deviation (SD)
Age (years)	10.4	3.4
Height (cm)	128.7	18.7
Weight (kg)	26.0	10.1
WAZ	−1.9	0.9
HAZ	−1.9	1.2
BAZ	−1.4	1.4

WAZ = Weight-for-age Z-score, HAZ = Height-for-age Z-score, BAZ = Body mass index (BMI) for age.

The prevalence of undernutrition in orphan or abandoned children is the following: 40.4% (total n = 47) were considered stunted, 36% (total n = 25) were underweight and 29.8% (total n = 47) were wasting for children over age 10. The sample used by the underweight indicator is 25 instead of the total (47) because WAZ can be calculated only for children aged < 10 years [16].

Table 2 shows values for WAZ, HAZ, and BAZ presented as means grouped by several parameters as are orphanage, physical disability, mental disability and sex. In the Bal Griha 1, two children had overlapping physical and mental disability.

For orphanage (Table 2), WAZ and BAZ were not significantly different between two groups. HAZ was significantly lower in the Bal Griha 1 (t = −3.47, p < 0.01). The mean of HAZ (−2.03) and WAZ (−2.43), which classifies classify the children of Bal Griha 1 as stunted and underweight, respectively.

For physical disability (Table 2), BAZ and WAZ were not significantly different between the two groups. Despite this, it should be noted that the mean of WAZ (−2.90) classifies the children as underweight. HAZ was significantly lower in the children with a physical disability (t = 3.94, p < 0.01). The mean of HAZ (−3.22) in children with a physical disability is a value below −3.0, which classifies them as severe stunted (moderate and severe based on <−2 Z and <−3 Z score, respectively).

For mental disability (Table 2), HAZ and WAZ were not significantly different between the two groups. Despite this, it should be noted that the mean of HAZ (−2.62) and WAZ (−2.92) classifies the two groups as stunted and underweight, respectively. BAZ was significantly lower in the children with a mental disability (t = 2.53, p < 0.05). The mean of BAZ (−2.70) in children with mental disabilities classifies them as wasted.

For sex (Table 2), HAZ and BAZ were not significantly different between the two groups. WAZ was significantly lower in the boys (t = 2.62, p < 0.05). The mean of WAZ (−2.37) classifies the boys as underweight.

The principal strength of this study is reflected that is the first study carried out in Nepali orphanages. On the other hand, principal limitation is the difficulty in accessing in other orphanages.

Table 2. Mean difference (and standard deviation; SD) for WAZ, HAZ, and BAZ compared with the WHO's standard for age and grouped by orphanage, physical disability, mental disability, and sex.

ORPHANAGE	BAL GRIHA 1 (N = 24)	BAL GRIHA 2 (N = 23)	T	SIG
mean difference (SD) of WAZ	−2.03 (0.84)	−1.87 (0.90)	−0.44	0.663
mean difference (SD) of HAZ	−2.43 (1.20)	−1.33 (0.93)	−3.47 **	0.001
mean difference (SD) of BAZ	−1.26 (1.34)	−1.53 (1.50)	0.65	0.516
PHYSICAL DISABILITY	NO (n = 39)	YES (n = 8)	T	Sig
mean difference (SD) of WAZ	−1.85 (0.72)	−2.90 (2.02)	1.77	0.090
mean difference (SD) of HAZ	−1.62 (1.07)	−3.22 (0.85)	3.94 **	0.000
mean difference (SD) of BAZ	−1.43 (1.44)	−1.18 (1.42)	−0.46	0.650
MENTAL DISABILITY	NO (n = 41)	YES (n = 6)	T	Sig
mean difference (SD) of WAZ	−1.85 (0.96)	−2.92 (1.11)	1.75	0.094
mean difference (SD) of HAZ	−1.78 (1.07)	−2.62 (1.05)	1.62	0.111
mean difference (SD) of BAZ	−1.20 (1.40)	−2.70 (0.91)	2.53 *	0.015
SEX	GIRLS (n = 24)	BOYS (n = 23)	T	Sig
mean difference (SD) of WAZ	−1.54 (0.96)	−2.37 (1.11)	2.62 *	0.020
mean difference (SD) of HAZ	−1.88 (1.07)	−1.90 (1.05)	0.04	0.965
mean difference (SD) of BAZ	−1.12 (0.90)	−1.66 (1.14)	1.30	0.200

* $p < 0.05$; ** $p < 0.01$.

4. Discussion

The analysis of nutritional status of Nepalese children as assessed from WAZ, HAZ, and BAZ showed that undernutrition prevailed in these children compared to the international standard. These institutionalized children had high prevalence of stunting (40.4%), being underweight (36%), and wasting (29.8%). Similar figures were reported in 2011 from the Nepal Demographic Health Survey, where 41% of Nepalese children under five years of age were stunted, 11% were wasted, and 29% were underweight, maintaining that child undernutrition in Nepal is still among the highest in the world [16].

The higher prevalence of wasting found in the present study (29.8%) compared with the data (11%) reported on 2011, could be explained by the fact that our sample includes children with disabilities, who seem to have higher risk of suffering from wasting as supported in our findings; these show that BAZ was significantly lower in the children with a mental disability ($t = 2.53$, $p < 0.05$). This mean of BAZ (−2.70) classifies the children as wasted. Related to this, a study with children with mental disabilities conducted in Turkey showed a decrease in the muscle and fat storages in 38.8% of the sample [17]. Similar results were found in the Egyptian children with mental disabilities [18]. Both research groups ensure to mention that thin musculature indicates low protein and caloric reserve, this could be related with institution living, or could be due to wasting, poor development or both. Even though studies that compare the prevalence of wasting between children with mental and non-mental disabilities were not found, neurologically disabled children are known to be at high risk for developing malnutrition [18]. This could be due to an inadequate nutrient intake produced due to feeding problems or poor feeding knowledge among care providers [19]. In fact, the presence of their poor nutritional status may, in some measure, explain the growth delay commonly manifested in such children [20]. This could also explain that, in the present study, the mean of HAZ of children with mental disabilities (−2.62) classifies them as stunted and the mean of WAZ (2.92) classifies them as underweight, even when HAZ and WAZ were not significantly different between the two groups (mental and non-mental disabilities). In fact, a study conducted in Nepal showed evidence of the increased risk of cognitive delay associated with severe stunting [21], which may negatively affect on the brain development in early life [22].

In any case, even though there have been efforts to cement a causal relationship between stunting and risk of disability, this has proven difficult due to our lack of understanding of the underlying biological mechanisms for childhood mental and physical disability, likely processes controlled by multiple factors [21]. However, it should be also noted that in developing countries, with various degrees and types of malnutrition being common among the entire population [23,24], prevalence of problems on the nutritional status in disabled children could be inevitably higher than the general population [18,25].

Consistent with this, our findings show that HAZ was significantly lower in the children with a physical disability ($t = 3.94$, $p < 0.01$). Further, the mean of WAZ (-2.90) classifies them as underweight, even when WAZ was not significantly different between the two groups (disabled and not disabled). At the same time, the mean of HAZ (-3.22) classifies these children as severely stunted. Similar evidence was found in a study in Iran where the anthropometric assessment showed higher prevalence of malnutrition in disabled children compared to non-disabled children, with the prevalence of stunting being remarkably higher in physically disabled children [25]. These authors ensure that a limited range of motion (a characteristic of physically disabled children) has a much lower lean body mass (LBM). Reduced LBM is also known to be one of the negative functional repercussions of stunting in general [26,27]. As well as the children with mental disabilities, physically disabled children have malnutrition due to feeding problems, but this could also be caused by several other reasons [28]. These unknown reasons would be difficult to determine in our sample given the miscellaneous nature of the physical disabilities of these children. In our study, Bal Griha includes children with disabilities on the sample that could also contribute to increase the prevalence of stunting, given the relationship between poor nutritional status and disability [17,18,21,25,29]. It should also be noted that, in general, children who are not adequately nourished are at risk of failing to reach their developmental potential in cognitive, motor, and socioemotional abilities; two of the key risk factors of this poor development are the severe underweight and stunting [22]. This suggests that underweight or/and stunting could play two different roles in disabilities, they could be a consequence of the disability, but they could also be one of the risk factors of developing a disability.

Regarding the sex, WAZ was significantly lower http://www.unicef.org/publications/files/Africas_Orphaned_and_Vulnerable_Generations_Children_Affected_by_AIDS.pdf among boys ($t = 2.62$, $p < 0.05$). The mean of WAZ (-2.37) classifies boys as underweight. It should also be taken into account that the evaluation of a disabled child's weight may not be accurate seeing as there is no adjusted weight standards available; in fact, studies on disabled children normally use non-disabled healthy children's charts or references [30]. However, a recent study that evaluates the effects of number and sex of siblings on malnutrition of children under 5 years old in Bangladesh, India, and Nepal, reports that a different feeding treatment for girls relative to boys (based on number and sex of siblings) may be occurring in South Asia, advantaging the food access for boys over girls [31]. The same study showed that girls with three or more sisters were at significantly greater risk for severe underweight, where no effect is seen for boys. The differences in the treatment as one of the causes of higher risk malnutrition could not be applicable in this study since differences between sex were not observed in the orphanages. Going back to the Nepal Demographic Health Survey from 2011, we observed that boys under 5 years old are slightly more likely to be underweight (30%) than girls under 5 years old (28%) [16]. Opposite to this, a different study conducted in Nepal with former Kamaya families, who are among the most socioeconomically disadvantaged groups in Nepal [32], showed that girls were more likely to be underweight [33]. This could be due to the sex differences on the treatment mentioned above. However, in a study where the range of age is more like this study (6–10 years old), the prevalence of underweight was slightly higher in boys (52.46%) than in girls (46.09%) [34].

A parallel problem to this study is knowing the prevalence data in Nepal because the current information is very limited. Recently, Bathia et al. [35] proposed a mixed methods study, including large-scale surveys, case data from the police, court system, newspapers, community consultations, and child participation, which can help to know the reality of a situation that affects the child population.

Limitations in our study included the small sample population and the limited reach of the sampling process to the frailest and most vulnerable of children in Nepali orphanages.

5. Conclusions

Evidence of an association between undernutrition and mental and physical disability (wasting and stunting, respectively) was found in this study. There is also weak but significant evidence of a relationship between underweight and being male. Different types and degrees of undernutrition were significantly related with the presence of the disability in institutionalized children. More research about nutritional status of institutionalized disabled children would be necessary to shed more light on their situation, and the fact of being a disabled child living in an institution increasing the vulnerability of poor health conditions. The design and implementation of specific interventions would also contribute to improve their quality of life.

Author Contributions: Conceptualization, methodology, validation and formal analysis, L.F., J.B. and J.M.S.; investigation, L.F., A.R., J.B. and J.M.S.; data curation, L.F., A.R. and J.A.-M.; writing—original draft preparation, L.F., J.A.-M., and J.M.S.; writing—review and editing, J.B.; supervision, J.M.S and J.B. All authors have read and agreed to the published version of the manuscript.

Funding: This research received no external funding.

Conflicts of Interest: The authors declare no conflict of interest.

References

1. Central Bureau of Statics. *Statistical Pocket Book Nepal 2010*; His Majesty's Government: Kathmandu, Nepal, 2010.
2. United Nations Development Programme. Available online: http://www.undp.org/content/undp/en/home/librarypage/hdr/human-development-report-2013/ (accessed on 7 October 2020).
3. Central Bureau of Statics. *Gender Disaggregated Indicators*; Ministry of Women, Children and Social Welfare: Kathmandu, Nepal, 2001.
4. World Health Organization. Available online: http://apps.who.int/gho/data/node.main-searo.WOMENSDG31?lang=en (accessed on 7 October 2020).
5. United Nations Children's Fund (UNICEF). Available online: http://www.unicef.org/publications/files/Africas_Orphaned_and_Vulnerable_Generations_Children_Affected_by_AIDS.pdf (accessed on 7 October 2020).
6. Committee on the Rights of the Child. Available online: http://www.ohchr.org/EN/NewsEvents/Pages/DisplayNews.aspx?NewsID=12218&LangID=E (accessed on 7 October 2020).
7. The Kathmandu Post. Available online: http://www.ekantipur.com/the-kathmandu-post/2012/06/13/metro/inter-country-adoptioncases-fall/235998.html (accessed on 7 October 2020).
8. National Federation of the Disabled. Available online: http://www.nfdn.org.np/news/8/29/Holistic-Report-of-Disability-Rights-Monitoring/d,1.html (accessed on 7 October 2020).
9. Sauvey, S.; Osrin, D.; Manandhar, D.S.; Costello, A.M.; Wirz, S. Prevalence of childhood and adolescent disabilities in rural Nepal. *Indian Pediatr.* **2005**, *42*, 697–702. [PubMed]
10. Lohman, T.G.; Roche, A.F.; Martorell, R. *Anthropometric Standardization Reference Manual*; Human Kinetics Publishers: Champaign, IL, USA, 1988.
11. de Onis, M.; Onyango, A.W.; Borghi, E.; Siyam, A.; Nishida, C.; Siekmann, J. Development of a WHO growth reference for school-aged children and adolescents. *Bull. World Health Organ.* **2007**, *85*, 660–667. [CrossRef] [PubMed]
12. World Health Organization. *WHO Child Growth Standards: Length/Height-For-Age, Weight-For-Age, Weight-For-Length, Weight-For Height and Body Mass Index-For-Age: Methods and Development*; WHO: Geneva, Switzerland, 2006.
13. Ersoy, B.; Günes, H.S.; Gunay, T.; Yilmaz, O.; Kasirga, E.; Egemen, A. Interaction of two public health problems in Turkish schoolchildren: Nutritional deficiencies and goitre. *Public Health Nutr.* **2006**, *9*, 1001–1006. [CrossRef]
14. Lefton, J.; Malone, A. Anthropometric Assessment. In *Pocket Guide to Nutrition Assessment*, 2nd ed.; Charney, P., Malone, A., Eds.; American Dietetic Association: Chicago, IL, USA, 2009; pp. 160–161.
15. Osterkamp, L.K. Current perspective on assessment of human body proportions of relevance to amputees. *J. Am. Diet. Assoc.* **1995**, *95*, 215–218. [CrossRef]
16. Ministry of Health and Population (MOHP); New ERA; ICF International Inc. *Nepal Demographic and Health Survey 2011*; Ministry of Health and Population: Kathmandu, Nepal, 2012.

17. Hakime Nogay, N. Nutritional status in mentally disabled children and adolescents: A study from Western Turkey. *Pak. J. Med. Sci.* **2013**, *29*, 614–618. [PubMed]
18. AbdAllah, A.M.; El-Sherbeny, S.S.A.; Khairy, S. Nutritional status of mentally disabled children in Egypt. *Egypt. J. Hosp. Med.* **2007**, *29*, 604–615.
19. Suzuki, M.; Saitoh, S.; Tasaki, Y.; Shimomura, Y.; Makishima, R.; Hosoya, N. Nutritional status and daily physical activity of handicapped students in Tokyo metropolitan schools for deaf, blind, mentally retarded and physically handicapped individuals. *Am. J. Clin. Nut.* **1991**, *54*, 1101–1111. [CrossRef]
20. Hals, J.; Ek, J.; Svalastog, A.G.; Nilsen, H. Studies on nutrition in severely neurologically disabled children in an institution. *Acta Paediatr.* **1996**, *85*, 1469–1475. [CrossRef]
21. Wu, L.; Katz, J.; Mullany, L.C.; Haytmanek, E.; Khatry, S.K.; Darmstadt, G.L.; West, K.P., Jr.; LeClerq, S.C.; Tielsch, J.M. Association between nutritional status and positive childhood disability screening using the ten questions plus tool in Sarlahi, Nepal. *J. Health Popul. Nutr.* **2010**, *28*, 585–594. [CrossRef]
22. Prado, E.L.; Dewey, K.G. Nutrition and brain development in early life. *Nutr. Rev.* **2014**, *72*, 267–284. [CrossRef]
23. Fernandez, I.D.; Himes, J.H.; de Onis, M. Prevalence of nutritional wasting in populations: Building explanatory models using secondary data. *Bull. World Health Organ.* **2002**, *80*, 282–291.
24. Khuwaja, S.; Selwyn, B.J.; Shah, S.M. Prevalence and correlates of stunting among primary school children in rural areas of southern Pakistan. *J. Trop. Pediatr.* **2005**, *51*, 72–77. [CrossRef]
25. Neyestani, T.R.; Dadkhah-Piraghaj, M.; Haydari, H.; Zowghi, T.; Nikooyeh, B.; Houshyar-Rad, A.; Nematy, M.; Maddah, M. Nutritional status of the Iranian children with physical disability: A cross-sectional study. *Asia Pac. J. Clin. Nutr.* **2010**, *19*, 223–230.
26. Victora, C.G.; Adair, L.; Fall, C.; Hallal, P.C.; Martorell, R.; Richter, L. Maternal and child undernutrition. Consequences for adult health and human capital. *Lancet* **2008**, *371*, 340–357. [CrossRef]
27. Dewey, K.G.; Begum, K. Long-term consequences of stunting in early life. *Matern. Child Nutr.* **2011**, *7*, 5–18. [CrossRef] [PubMed]
28. Kilpinen-Loisa, P.; Pihko, H.; Vesander, U.; Paganus, A.; Ritanen, U.; Makitie, O. Insufficient energy and nutrient intake in children with motor disability. *Acta Paediatr.* **2009**, *98*, 1329–1333. [CrossRef]
29. United Nations Children's Fund. *Monitoring Child Disability in Developing Countries: Results from the Multiple Indicator Cluster Surveys*; United Nations Children's Fund: New York, NY, USA, 2008; pp. 84–87.
30. Shabayek, M.M. Assessment of the nutritional status of children with special needs in Alexandria. Part II: Anthropometric measures. *J. Egypt. Public Health Assoc.* **2004**, *79*, 363–382.
31. Raj, A.; McDougal, L.P.; Silverman, J.G. Gendered effects of siblings on child malnutrition in South Asia: Cross-sectional analysis of demographic and health surveys from Bangladesh, India, and Nepal. *Matern. Child Health J.* **2015**, *19*, 217–226. [CrossRef] [PubMed]
32. Chhetri, R.B. The plight of the Tharu Kamaiyas in Nepal: Are view of the social, economic and political facets. *Occas. Pap. Sociol. Anthropol.* **2005**, *9*, 22–46. [CrossRef]
33. Khatri, R.B.; Mishra, S.R.; Khanal, V.; Choulagai, B. Factors associated with underweight among children of former-Kamaiyas in Nepal. *Front. Public Health* **2015**, *3*, 11. [CrossRef]
34. Ghosh, A.; Adhikari, P.; Chowdhury, S.D.; Ghosh, T. Prevalence of undernutrition in Nepalese children. *Ann. Hum. Biol.* **2009**, *36*, 38–45. [CrossRef]
35. Bhatia, A.; Krieger, N.; Victora, C.; Tuladhar, S.; Bhabha, J.; Beckfield, J. Analyzing and improving national and local child protection data in Nepal: A mixed methods study using 2014 Multiple Indicator Cluster Survey (MICS) data and interviews with 18 organizations. *Child Abuse Negl.* **2020**, *101*, 104292. [CrossRef] [PubMed]

Publisher's Note: MDPI stays neutral with regard to jurisdictional claims in published maps and institutional affiliations.

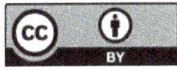

© 2020 by the authors. Licensee MDPI, Basel, Switzerland. This article is an open access article distributed under the terms and conditions of the Creative Commons Attribution (CC BY) license (http://creativecommons.org/licenses/by/4.0/).

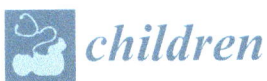

Article

Assessment of the Nutritional Status, Diet and Intestinal Parasites in Hosted Saharawi Children

Mónica Gozalbo [1,*], Marisa Guillen [2], Silvia Taroncher-Ferrer [3], Susana Cifre [4], David Carmena [5], José M Soriano [6,7] and María Trelis [4,7]

[1] Area of Nutrition and Bromatology, Department of Preventive Medicine and Public Health, Food Sciences, Toxicology and Forensic Medicine, University of Valencia, 46100 Burjassot, Spain
[2] Area of Preventive Medicine and Public Health, Department of Preventive Medicine and Public Health, Food Sciences, Toxicology and Forensic Medicine, University of Valencia, 46010 Valencia, Spain; marisa.guillen@uv.es
[3] Clínica Universitària de Nutrició, Activitat física i Fisoteràpia (CUNAFF) , Lluís Alcanyís Foundation-University of Valencia, 46010 Valencia, Spain; silvia.taroncher@fundacions.uv.es
[4] Parasites and Health Research Group, Department of Pharmacy and Pharmaceutical Technology and Parasitology, University of Valencia, 46100 Burjassot, Spain; sucimar@alumni.uv.es (S.C.); maria.trelis@uv.es (M.T.)
[5] Parasitology Reference and Research Laboratory, National Centre for Microbiology, Carlos III Health Institute, 28222 Majadahonda, Madrid, Spain; dacarmena@isciii.es
[6] Observatory of Nutrition and Food Safety for Developing Countries, Food & Health Lab, Institute of Materials Science, University of Valencia, 46980 Paterna, Spain; jose.soriano@uv.es
[7] Joint Research Unit on Endocrinology, Nutrition and Clinical Dietetics, University of Valencia-Health Research Institute La Fe, 46026 Valencia, Spain
* Correspondence: monica.gozalbo@uv.es

Received: 15 October 2020; Accepted: 27 November 2020; Published: 29 November 2020

Abstract: Since the early 1990s, Spanish humanitarian associations have welcomed Saharawi children from the refugee camps in Tindouf (Argelia). These children are the most affected by the lack of food, water, hygienic measures and health care. The main objective of this study was to analyze the anthropometric, nutritional and parasitological data of 38 Saharawi boys and girls (from 10 to 13 years old) under a holiday host program in the city of Valencia. Our results confirm that malnutrition and multiparasitism are highly frequent, so it is understood that living conditions in refugee camps continue to be precarious with a lack of proper hygiene and nutrition. Furthermore, biochemical alterations, lactose malabsorption and the risk of celiac disease, also detected in our study as a secondary objective, will complicate nutritional management and restoration of health. For this reason, sustainable feeding alternatives and interventions from a hygienic and nutritional point of view are proposed, emphasizing in an improvement in the education of parents and children.

Keywords: Sahara; malnutrition; lactose malabsorption; celiac disease; intestinal parasites; hygiene; diet; health

1. Introduction

Western Sahara, located in the African continent, is bordered in the north by Morocco, in the south by Mauritania, in the east by Algeria, and in the west by the Atlantic Ocean. Its population has suffered several episodes of military and political conflicts, which has led to refugee status. Refugee Saharawi families have been staying in the Tindouf (Algeria) camps for 43 years (since 1976), waiting for a political agreement allowing them to return to the Sahara. It was estimated that more than 40,000 Saharawis fled after conflict to Algerian camps (Laayoune, Auserd, Smara, Dajla, Rabunni and Bojador), and today around 180,000 Saharawis live there, according to the census of the United Nations High

Commissioner for Refugees (UNHCR) and the government of the Saharawi Democratic Arab Republic (RASD). It should be noted that these camps distributed in the Algerian desert are located in one of the most inhospitable and arid areas of the world, with very harsh living conditions with a situation of total dependence on humanitarian aid. They lack vegetation and animals for their sustainability, as well as electrical installation and running water. Sirocco, violent and dry sandstorms, are characteristic of the place. The population lives in *jaimas* (canvas shops), in adobe houses and, in recent years, in cement constructions that have been built that include a latrine located outside the central unit. In the educational field, unprecedented success has been achieved moving from an illiteracy rate of 85% of the population to the total schooling of the children between 3 and 12 years with mandatory and free character [1]. With regard to health conditions in the camps, there are numerous factors with a direct negative impact on the health of the population: overcrowding, food and nutritional deficiencies, lack of water and in-unit medical care, and limited access to medicines. Food depends almost entirely on the help of international organizations that provide long-lasting staple foods, such as starch-rich foods and legumes, but few fresh vegetables and fruits, which is causing the double burden of malnutrition: overweight households versus those with malnutrition [2].

Regarding the general economic situation, it should be noted that it does not go beyond the stage of mere subsistence. As a people in exile, the population does not have the financial assistance of non-governmental institutions and humanitarian organizations, and its economic and productive activities focus on planting small orchards, raising some animals such as goats and workshops of textiles and traditional crafts. In the summer of 1979, thanks to the collaboration between the Front Polisario and the PCE (Communist Party of Spain), the first 100 Saharawi children arrived in Spain for a welcoming experience for Spanish families during the summer holidays. This program emerged so that Saharawi children could temporarily distance the very reality of refugee camps, the main objective being to provide good health care and treat diseases (both infectious and nutritional) during the months of stay. The experience was so beneficial that in the mid-1980s the "Holidays in Peace" program was launched, which consists of hosting a Saharawi child (7–13 years old) from the Saharawi Refugee Camp of Tindouf, during the months of July and August [3].

Several international projects have been carried out to collect anthropometric, nutritional and parasitological data of the Saharawi population, especially at-risk groups such as children and pregnant women. Most studies agree on the high prevalence of growth retardation and low weight [2,4–7]. Bilbao et al. [8] wrote a food guide called *"Food Jaima"* for host families in Spain about foods and the recommended daily amount, in order to improve their nutritional status. Other field implementation projects aimed to educate Saharawi mothers about dietary habits to make them protagonists of the improvements in the diet and nutrition of their sons and daughters [9].

On the other hand, data collection on intestinal parasitism in the Saharawi population, within the same host program, was carried out by Paricio-Talayero et al. [4], who observed that enteroparasites were present in 75% of the samples examined. Further studies were conducted over the years and confirmed that hygienic, personal and community measures remained insufficient for the control of parasitic infections and to prevent their long-term effects [4–6,10–13]. Medical examinations and antiparasitic campaigns were carried out in each of these studies through the administration of antiprotozoal and anthelmintic drugs during their stay in Spain. Most children had multiple infections, suggesting a general situation of lack of hygiene, food security and access to safe drinking water, in conjunction with children neglecting hygienic habits and the inability to generate an adequate immune response [12].

The aim of the present study is to verify if there have been changes with respect to previous studies on the parasitological, nutritional and health status of the hosted children in staying into the "Holidays in Peace" program, to design interventions that may improve their living conditions in the short and long term.

2. Materials and Methods

2.1. Design and Subjects of Study

This cross-sectional study was conducted with 38 Saharawi children: 16 boys and 22 girls (42.1% and 57.9%, respectively) with a mean age of 11.1 years (10–13 years), who were hosted in Valencia (Spain) during the summers of 2016 and 2017. The participants in this study were from the following Saharawi refugee camps: Smara (60.5%), Auserd (21.1%) and Laayoune (18.4%). For 60.5% of the participants, it was their first visit to Spain while the rest had already been to the country before. A percentage of 73.7% of the Saharawis interviewed had between 3 and 5 siblings and the place they occupied in their family was, in 55.3% of the cases, the first or the second, and in 31.6%, the third or the fourth. These were boys and girls who lived in generally large families, which, including parents, 58.4% of them had between 5 and 7 members. In 79.0% of the participants, they believed that their parents worked but did not know exactly what work they did.

The criteria for inclusion in the study were: to be a member of the host program and to obtain informed consent from Spanish families (as legal representatives) after being informed of the study and the data protection procedure. The intervention consisted of: (a) a physical and anthropometric examination; (b) a collection of personal data, sociodemographic variables (age, sex, camp of origin, number of siblings, professional occupation of parents), clinical and medical family history, frequency of consumption of food and hygienic habit as a risk factors for parasitic infection (hand washing, contact with animals, source of consumption water, etc.), all in the presence of a healthcare professional and with the help of a translator; (c) a coproparasitological analysis; (d) an analysis of lactose malabsorption using the breathed air test; € a determination of biochemical analytical variables related to nutritional status; and (f) a study of genetic markers associated with risk of celiac disease and primary lactose intolerance.

This study was approved by the Ethics Committee for Human Research of the University of Valencia (procedure number: HI48709978679, 2 March 2017) as part of the project "Promotion of hygienic-health habits for the prevention of intestinal parasites in the Saharawi population" ensuring that the fundamental principles established by the Helsinki Declaration and Spanish legislation in the field of biomedical research, data protection and bioethics are respected.

2.2. Anthropometric Assessment

The physical examination was performed by doctors from the Paediatrics Service of the University Hospital Clinic of Valencia (Spain) and was evaluated for the presence of lax skin, loss of muscle mass in limbs and buttocks, bloating and pubertal development. An Omrom® electronic scale (accuracy, 100 g) and a Cescorf® narrow and inextensible metal tape (accuracy, 1 mm) were used to obtain the weight and height. The height was determined, without shoes or socks, with a non-extensible tape measure, a blank sheet fixed on the wall and a carton; and body weight with participants dressed only in underwear. Height-for-Age and Body Mass Index-for-Age Z-scores (HAZ and BMIZ) were calculated using with WHO Anthro and AnthroPlus software (World Health Organization, 2009, Anthro for Personal Computers, Version 3.01: Software for Assessing Growth and Development of the World's Children), using the WHO child growth standard 2005 version for children aged 0–5 years and the 2007 version for children and adolescents aged 5–19 years. These indicators classified children to varying degrees and types of malnutrition based on WHO reference data [14], which enable the analysis and interpretation of growth patterns of children of any population in the world.

2.3. Dietary Assessment

Data were collected on participants' eating habits, such as the number of meals per day, schedules, food consumed and weekly frequency of consumption. For the assessment of the Saharawi child diet, the foods consumed were grouped together and the frequency of daily consumption of each was calculated. Dietary Diversity Score was determined using a modification of the food groups defined in FAO's Minimum-Women's Food Diversity (MDD-W) and the Food and Nutrition Technical

Assistance Project [15]. The following food groups were considered: (1) Farinaceous ("All starchy foods"); (2) Legumes ("Beans and Peans"); (3) Dairy; (4) Protein foods ("Flesh foods"); (5) Vegetables and (6) Fruits (groups 5 and 6 corresponding to "Vitamin A-rich dark Green leafy vegetables," "Other vitamin A-rich vegetables and fruits," "Other vegetables" and "Other fruits"). It should be noted that this study did not take into account the consumption of vitamin A-rich vegetables, so this detail was obviated and only two groups were determined to collect the information these four points determined in FANTA [15]. With regard to the groups "Nuts and Seeds" and "Eggs," they were not included because they were not consumed by the participating population. According to this indicator, consumption of at least 5 of the 10 established food groups indicates a higher likelihood of reaching micronutrient needs. In addition, the consumption frequencies obtained were compared to those recommended by Bilbao et al. [8] and Estruch et al. [16,17] and are able to assess their suitability.

2.4. Coproparasitological Assessment

For parasitological analysis, one sample of fresh stool per participant was taken. After the filtration and concentration of the samples, they were observed by optical microscopy for the identification of forms of resistance of intestinal parasites in general (cysts or eggs); molecular diagnostic techniques (conventional and real-time polymerase chain reaction or qPCR) were also applied to some specific parasites (*Giardia intestinalis* and *Blastocystis* sp.).

Starting from 3 g of fecal sample, they were filtered and concentrated by centrifugation (2500 rpm, 5 min) in Midi Parasep tubes® (Apacor Ltd., Wokingham, UK). The sediment obtained was divided into two microtubes, one for extraction of total stool DNA for qPCR, and the other with 10% formalin for microscopic observation. The QIAmp DNA Stool Mini Kit (QIAGEN®, Hilden, Germany) was used for DNA extraction according to the manufacturer's instructions.

For the diagnosis of *G. intestinalis* DNA, a qPCR was performed. This protocol specifically amplifies a fragment of the gene that encodes the parasite's small ribosomal subunit RNA (*SSU* rRNA) showing high sensitivity [18]. A commercial assay with the specific primers and probe (LightMix Modular Assays Giardia, Roche®, Basel, Switzerland) was used, together with the mastermix (dNTPS, thermostable Taq polymerase and buffer) (PerfeCTa qPCR ToughMix, Quanta Biosciences, Gaithersburg, MD, USA) for a mix reaction final volume of 15 µL. To each well, 5 µL of sample and positive control DNA was added, and instead water for negative control. The analysis was performed with the StepOne Plus real-time PCR thermocycler® (Applied Biosystems®, Foster City, CA, USA). Any sample that manages to amplify before 43 cycles was considered positive.

Positive samples for *G. intestinalis* by qPCR were subsequently analyzed by multilocus genotyping based on the sequences of genes encoding the parasite's glutamate dehydrogenase (*gdh*) and β-giardine (*bg*) proteins [19]. A semi-nested PCR protocol proposed by Read et al. [20] with minor modifications was used to amplify a fragment of 432 bp of the *gdh* gene with the GDHeF/GDHiR primer pair in the primary reaction and GDHiF/GDHiR in secondary. In parallel, a fragment of 511 bp of the *bg* gene of *G. intestinalis* was amplified using the nested PCR protocol described by Lalle et al. [21] with G7F/G759R primers in the primary reaction and G99F/G609R in secondary [21]. In the case of *Blastocystis* sp., a direct PCR assay was used, targeting the *SSU* rRNA gene using the *Blastocystis* barcode primer pair RD5/BhRDr to amplify a product of 600 bp as previously described [19,22].

All the direct, semi-nested and nested PCR protocols described above were conducted on a 2720 thermal cycler (Applied Biosystems®). Reaction mixes always included 2.5 units of MyTAQ—DNA polymerase (Bioline®, London, UK), and 5 MyTAQ-Reaction Buffer containing 5 mM dNTPs and 15 mM MgCl$_2$. Laboratory-confirmed positive and negative DNA isolates for each parasitic species investigated were routinely used as controls and included in each round of PCR. PCR amplicons were visualized on 2% agarose gels stained with SafeView Nucleic Acid Stain (NBS Biologicals®, Huntingdon, UK).

Positive-PCR products were directly sequenced in both directions using the internal primer set described above. DNA sequencing was conducted by capillary electrophoresis using the BigDye®

Terminator chemistry (Applied Biosystems®, USA) on an ABI PRISM 3130 automated DNA sequencer. Raw sequencing data in both directions, back and forth, was determined using the Chromas Lite version 2.1 sequence analysis program (https://technelysium.com.au/wp/chromas/). The BLAST tool (http://blast.ncbi.nlm.nih.Gov/Blast.cgi) was used to compare nucleotide sequences with sequences retrieved from the NCBI GenBank database. Finally, generated sequences samples were aligned with appropriate reference sequences using MEGA6: Molecular Evolutionary Genetics Analysis Version 6.0 [23] software to identify *G. intestinalis* assemblages and sub-assemblages. Generated *Blastocystis* sp. sequences were submitted to the publicly available database *Blastocystis* 18S (http://pubmlst.org/blastocystis/) for subtype confirmation and allele calling [23]. The sequences generated in this study have been deposited in GenBank under accession numbers MW265975-MW265987 (*G. intestinalis*) and MW265003-MW265005 (*Blastocystis* sp.).

2.5. Laboratory Evaluations

Fasting venous blood samples were obtained from each of the participants for the determination of blood cells, leukocytes, leukocyte formula and platelets. Glucose, creatinine, urea, transaminase (GOT and GPT), alkaline phosphatase, LDH, Immunoglobulins (A, G and E), anti-transglutaminase and anti-endomysium antibodies were also analyzed [24].

The method used for the diagnosis of lactose malabsorption is called "Expired air test" or "Breathtracker gas chromatograph" (QuinTron Instrument Company Inc., Milwaukee, WI, USA), which allows the measurement of hydrogen (H_2) and methane (CH_4) levels contained in the exhaled air after the intake of a sugary substrate. These gases are volatile compounds formed from the bacterial colonic fermentation of sugars that remain in the gut due to their incomplete digestion. To prepare the test, food should be taken in normal quantity the day before, but by restricting the intake of carbohydrates and sugars, the patient should also be fasting for at least the previous 8 h (ideally 12 h) and can only drink water until 4 h before performing it. At the beginning of the test, the patient must breathe into the apparatus to obtain the "basal" gases (ppm) data. The patient then takes an aqueous solution of lactose (25 g of lactose dissolved in 250 mL of water). After that, samples of breathed air are taken every half hour (30, 60, 90, 120, 150, 180, 210 and 240 min) to measure the evolution of the gas content. The "basal" level of H_2 must be less than 10 ppm, and less than 6–8 ppm for CH_4, for the test to be valid and consider its production to be related to the administered substrate. The test is positive when, in any of the measurement points before minute 90, the 20 ppm in hydrogen is exceeded with respect to the "basal" value or the lower of the previous ones, and between 10–15 ppm in the case of methane [25,26].

For the genetic analysis of risk of celiac disease and primary lactose intolerance, were carried out in a small representation of the studied population, oral mucosa samples were obtained using a sterile swab and analyzed in Overgenes S.L. laboratory (Valencia, Spain) for analysis. The presence of celiac disease risk markers (HLA-DQA1 and HLA-DQB1 alleles) were determined. Regarding primary lactose intolerance, five genetic single nucleotide polymorphisms (SNPs) associated with the persistent lactase phenotype were analyzed, two of them more frequent in Caucasian populations and the other three in populations of African origin, all of them present in the sequence of the MCM6 gene, known to regulate lactase expression. The risk genotypes for the 5 SNPs of the MCM6 gene associated with primary lactose intolerance analyzed were: C/T_13910, G/A_22018, G/C_14010, T/G_13915 o G/C_13915 and C/G_13907, which determine the persistent lactose status [7,24,27,28].

2.6. Statistical Analysis

Descriptive statistics were calculated including measures of central tendency (mean and median), measures of dispersion (standard deviation, range and coefficient of variation) and measures of shape (asymmetry and pointing) for quantitative variables, as well as the absolute and relative frequencies for the qualitative variables. Association analyses were performed stratifying by sex and age to observe possible heterogeneity in the results according to these factors. Due to the sample size, non-parametric tests were used (Fisher's exact test and Mann-Whitney U test). Any p value less than 0.05 was considered as statistically significant. All the variables were analyzed using SPSS software (Statistical Package for Social Sciences for Windows, version 26.0, SPSS Inc., Chicago, IL, USA).

3. Results

3.1. Anthropometric Assessment

Table 1 shows HAZ and BMIZ values from Saharawi children. In comparison with WHO standards [14,29–31], HAZ data reflected moderate and severe chronic malnutrition (or stunting) in 10.5% and 5.3%, respectively, of the studied children, and 28.9% of them had increased risk of child stunting. In fact, high presence of chronic malnutrition (with impaired height and even lower cognitive development) could be explained by the lack of an adequate, balanced and sufficient diet for prolonged periods, as well as recurrent infections that hinder progression towards normal growth values. The data were analyzed stratifying by sex, but no statistically significant differences ($p > 0.05$) were found for any of the variables.

Table 1. Percentages for the different types of affectation according to the values of weight, height and BMIZ in the Saharawi children studied.

Z-Score	Height-for-Age Z-Score (HAZ)			Body Mass Index-for-Age Z-Score (BMIZ)		
	Total $n = 38$ (%)	Female $n = 22$ (%)	Male $n = 16$ (%)	Total $n = 38$ (%)	Female $n = 22$ (%)	Male $n = 16$ (%)
<−3	2 (5.3%)	1 (4.5%)	1 (6.3%)	0	0	0
From <−2 to ≥−3	4 (10.5%)	3 (13.6%)	1 (6.3%)	2 (5.3%)	1 (4.5%)	1 (6.3%)
From <−1 to ≥−2	11 (28.9%)	6 (27.3%)	5 (31.3%)	12 (31.6%)	8 (36.4%)	4 (25.0%)
From ≥−1 to ≤+1				24 (63.2)	13 (59.1%)	11 (68.8%)
From ≥+1 to ≤+2	21 (55.3%)	12 (54.5%)	9 (56.3%)	0	0	0
From ≥+2 to ≤+3				0	0	0
>+3	0	0	0	0	0	0

n = number of individuals in each group; % = percentage of individuals in each group.

For BMIZ, the characteristics of malnutrition are characterized by insufficient intake combined with nutrient malabsorption by infectious factors or recurrent diseases. The prevalence of mild and moderate malnutrition as defined was observed in 31.6% and 5.3%, respectively. No statistically significant differences were found when the distribution of the BMIZ by sex was analyzed. However, if obtained results were stratified by age, it was observed that the group with the highest risk of mild malnutrition was that of 10 years of age (4 girls and 3 boys) (70% vs. 6.7% in 11 years, 27.3% in 12 years and 50% in 13 years; $chi^2 = 22.296$; $p = 0.001$). The joint assessment of the BMIZ of all Saharawi boys and girls is represented in Figure 1 as a Gaussian curve with a standard deviation of 0.75 and with an average of −0.6. This curve is displaced to the left (noir-colored line) compared to what would be a normal distribution (gray-colored line). The conclusion that is drawn is that a significant percentage of children are in negative values, with a risk of emaciation, presenting an impairment of growth in both weight and height with respect to the reference values. Therefore, actions should be aimed at reducing the average as close to zero as possible.

3.2. Dietary Assessment

The analysis of the information collected in the surveys showed that all the participants ate between 3 and 4 meals per day. Regarding the times of these meals, 84.6% had breakfast between 7:00 and 8:00 a.m., 76.9% claimed to eat between 1:00 p.m. and 1:30 p.m. For snacks, 75.1% had it between 5:00 p.m. and 6:00 p.m.; 46.2% of the participants commented on having dinner between 9:30 p.m. and 10 p.m.; and 38.5% declared to carry out late night snack. The main foods consumed by the Saharawi child population were those known as basic foods, such as rice (97.4%), couscous (86.8%), milk (81.6%)

or lentils (86.8%), but other foods, with low nutritional value, were occasionally consumed including biscuits, chocolate, Coke beverage and candy (Table 2).

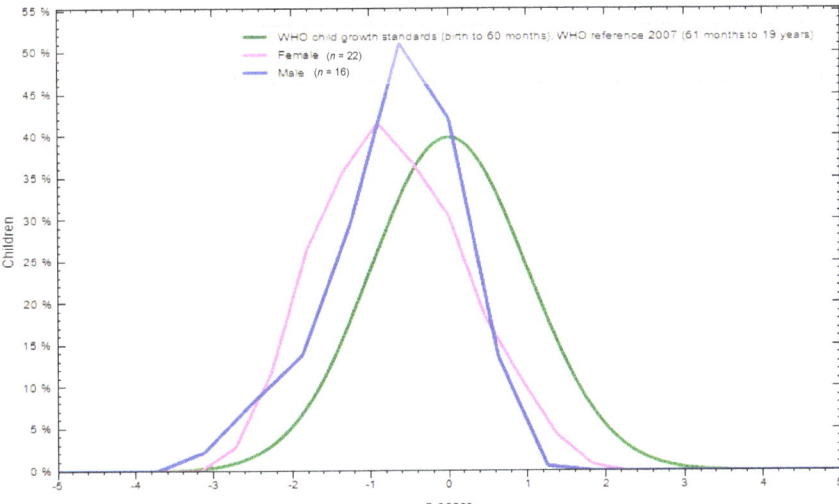

Figure 1. Body Mass Index-for-Age Z-scores (BMIZ) distribution of the Saharawi population (blue: male children; purple: female children; green: World Health Organization (WHO) reference standard).

Table 2. Foods and food groups according to the FANTA classification [14] consumed by the studied Saharawi child population.

	Total n = 38 (%)	Male n = 22 (%)	Female n = 16 (%)
FARINACEOUS	37 (97.4%)	22 (100%)	15 (93.8%)
Couscous	33 (86.8%)	19 (86.3%)	14 (87.5%)
Rice	37 (97.4%)	22 (100%)	15 (93.8%)
Pasta	8 (21.1%)	5 (19.1%)	3 (18.8%)
Bread	7 (18.4%)	5 (19.1%)	2 (12.5%)
DAIRY PRODUCTS	37 (97.4%)	22 (100%)	15 (93.8%)
Milk	31 (81.6%)	21 (95.5%)	10 (62.5%)
Yogurt	33 (86.8%)	20 (90.9%)	13 (81.3%)
Cheese	6 (15.8%)	5 (19.9%)	1 (6.3%)
LEGUMES	34 (89.5%)	20 (90.9%)	14 (87.5%)
Lentils	33 (86.8%)	20 (90.9%)	13 (81.3%)
Chickpeas	20 (52.6%)	12 (54.5%)	8 (50.0%)
VEGETABLES	0 (0%)	0 (0%)	0 (0%)
FRUITS	31 (81.6%)	19 (86.3%)	12 (75.0%)
PROTEIN FOODS (Meat)	38 (100%)	22 (90.9%)	16 (100%)
OCCASIONAL FOODS	38 (100%)	22 (90.9%)	16 (100%)
Biscuits	37 (97.4%)	22 (90.9%)	5 (31.3%)
Chocolate	33 (86.4%)	18 (81.8%)	15 (93.8%)
Coke beverage	33 (86.4%)	19 (86.3%)	14 (87.5%)
Tea	13 (34.2%)	6 (27.3%)	7 (43.8%)
Candy	38 (100%)	22 (100%)	16 (100%)

n = number of individuals in each group; % = percentage of individuals in each group.

According to the classification of food group from FAO FANTA project [14], an average daily consumption frequency of 2.78 ± 1.82, 0.96 ± 0.87, 2.38 ± 1.96, 0.80 ± 0.70 and 1.02 ± 0.67 servings of farinaceous, legumes, dairy products, fruits and protein per day, respectively, were observed in our study. Surprisingly, vegetables were not eaten by any children. Number of consumed food groups is shown in Table 3.

A percentage of 7.9% consumed foods from a single food group, 13.2% consumed from 3 and 5 food groups, 18.4% from 2 food groups, and practically half of the children (47.4%) consumed foods from 4 food groups. No participant consumed at least 5 food groups to ensure correct micronutrient needs. No significant differences were obtained in the consumption of the different food groups between sexes. Furthermore, our group asked about the possibility that some foods caused them gastrointestinal problems (vomiting and/or diarrhea) and found that 47.1% experienced such, with milk (37.5%) and fruit (12.5%) as the causative food.

Table 3. Dietary diversity of the Saharawi child population.

Number of Consumed Food Groups	Total $n = 38$ (%)	Male $n = 22$ (%)	Female $n = 16$ (%)
1	3 (7.9%)	2 (9.1%)	1 (6.3%)
2	7 (18.4%)	4 (18.2%)	3 (18.8%)
3	15 (13.2%)	3 (13.6%)	2 (13.2%)
4	18 (47.2%)	11 (50.0%)	7 (47.4%)
5	5 (13.2%)	2 (9.1%)	3 (13.2%)

n = number of individuals in each group; % = percentage of individuals in each group.

On the other hand, all the children participating in the study declared to always wash their hands before going to eat and after going to the bathroom. Furthermore, 87.5% of the children declare that they brush their teeth and, when asked about the frequency of brushing, 37.5% do it once a day, 12.5% twice a day and 37.5% three times a day or more. When the frequency of toothbrushing stratified by sex was analyzed, no statistically significant differences were observed between boys and girls in tooth brushing. A percentage of 56.3% of the children declared that they had animals at home, of which 55.5% are cats, 33.3% are goats and 11.1% claimed to have contact with dogs.

3.3. Coproparasitological Evaluation

Results of the parasitological analysis are shown in Table 4. Overall, 97.4% of the participants presented intestinal parasites. Of them, 97.4% of parasitization was by protists and 26.3% by helminths (the prevalence of combined protist-helminth infection was also 26.3%). Multiparasitism was the most frequent, highlighting 5.3% of cases harboring seven enteroparasitic species. The most prevalent intestinal protist parasites were, from highest to lowest: *G. intestinalis* (92.1%), *Blastocystis* sp. (86.8%), *Endolimax nana* (52.6%), *Entamoeba coli* (47.4%), *Entamoeba hartmanni* (36.8%), *E. histolytica/E. dispar/E. moshkovskii/E. bangladeshi* (13.2%), *Iodamoeba butschlii* (13.2%) and *Dientamoeba fragilis* (5.3%). Regarding helminths, only two species were detected, *Hymenolepis nana* (18.4%) and *Enterobius vermicularis* (10.5%). Most of these parasitic species are ingested as cysts or eggs (infectious forms) present in food or water by fecal contamination. No statistically significant differences were obtained when stratifying by sex.

The overall prevalence of *G. intestinalis* and *Blastocystis* sp. varied according to the method employed. By direct diagnosis (light microscopy), the occurrence of both species was estimated at 52.6% and 71.1%, respectively. In addition, a prevalence of 60.5% for *G. intestinalis* was obtained by indirect ELISA using anti-*Giardia* (IgA) antibodies, and 81.6% by qPCR. The latter prevalence was also obtained for *Blastocystis* sp. by conventional PCR. Mixed infections involving these two parasitic species were common (81.6%) in the studied Saharawi population. No association analysis could be performed between nutritional status and the presence of intestinal parasites since the entire sample was infected by one or more parasite species.

Furthermore, a total of 31 DNA isolates were positive for *G. intestinalis* by qPCR, providing Ct values ranging from 19.0 to 37.0 (median: 26.3). Of them, 25.8% (8/31) and 16.1% (5/31) were successfully amplified at the *gdh* and *bg* loci, respectively. A total of eight isolates were genotyped and/or sub-genotyped for either of the two markers. Multilocus genotyping data were available for 25.8% (8/31) of the characterized isolates. Only seven *gdh* and six *bg* PCR amplicons were obtained from *G. intestinalis* isolates, highlighting that the low amplification rates obtained for both markers were highly dependent on the Ct qPCR values. Table 5 shows the diversity, frequency and main characteristics of the *G. intestinalis* sequences generated at the *gdh* and *bg* loci.

Sequence analysis revealed the presence of assemblages A (25.0%; 2/8) and B (75.0%; 6/8). Canine (C, D), feline (F) or ruminant (E) assemblages were not detected. Of the two assemblage A sequences, one was assigned to the sub-assemblage AII at the gdh locus and the remaining showed an ambiguous AI/AII result when the two *gdh* and *bg* loci were considered. Similarly, the sequence analysis of the six isolates assigned to assemblage B allowed the identification of sub-assemblages BIII (37.5%; 3/8) and BIV (12.8%; 1/8). Ambiguous BIII/BIV results were determined in 25.0% (2/8) of the isolates at the *gdh* locus. The sequences of the genotyped parasites have been also deposited in GenBank for subsequent molecular epidemiological studies in the future (Table 5).

Table 4. Frequency of infection/carriage by detected species (protists and helminths) analyzed in the total sample and by sex.

Detected Species	Total $n = 38$ (%)	Male $n = 2$ (%)	Female $n = 16$ (%)
Giardia intestinalis	35 (92.1%)	20 (90.9%)	15 (95.8%)
Blastocystis sp.	33 (86.8%)	19 (86.4%)	14 (87.5%)
Endolimax nana	20 (52.6%)	11 (59.0%)	9 (56.3%)
Entamoeba coli	18 (47.4%)	9 (40.9%)	9 (56.3%)
Entamoeba hartmanni	14 (36.8%)	6 (27.3%)	8 (50.0%)
Entamoeba histolytica/E. dispar/E. moshkovskii/E. bangladeshi	5 (13.2%)	2 (9.1%)	3 (18.8%)
Iodamoeba butschlii	5 (13.2%)	3 (13.6%)	2 (12.5%)
Dientamoeba fragilis	2 (5.3%)	1 (4.5%)	0 (0)
Total Parasitization by Protists	37 (97.4%)	21 (95.5%)	16 (100%)
Hymenolepis nana	7 (18.4%)	1 (4.5%)	6 (37.5%)
Enterobius vermicularis	4 (10.5%)	2 (9.1%)	2 (12.5%)
Total Parasitization by Helminths	10 (26.3%)	3 (13.6%)	7 (43.8%)
Total Parasitization	37 (97.4%)	21 (95.5%)	16 (100%)

n = number of individuals in each group; % = percentage of individuals in each group.

Table 5. Diversity, frequency and molecular features of *Giardia intestinalis* sequences at the *gdh* and *bg* loci obtained in the Saharawi children population under study. GenBank accession numbers are provided.

Gene	Assemblage	Sub-Assemblage	Isolates (n)	Reference Sequence	Stretch	Single Nucleotide Polymorphisms	GenBank ID
gdh	A	AI	1	L40509	78–484	None	S16
		AII	1	L40510	64–491	None	S6
	B	BIII	1	AF069059	102–394	T147C	S3
			1	AF069059	41–447	C309T	S12
			1	AF069059	40–454	C87Y, G93R, C99T, T147C, G150A, T276Y, C309T, C336Y, G402R	S10
		BIV	1	L40508	74–496	T183C, T387C, C396T, C423T	S15
		BIII/BIV	1	L40508	76–491	C123Y, T135Y, T183C, G186R, C345Y, T366Y, T387C, C396Y, G408R, C423Y, A438R	S2
		BIII/BIV	1	L40508	76–496	T183Y, C255Y, C273Y, C345Y, T366Y, T387C, C396Y, C423Y, A438R	S9
bg	A	AII	1	AY072723	141–594	T561C	S16
		B	–	AY072727	97–590	C165T, G180A, C309T, C366T, C450T, C567T	S10
			–	AY072727	102–591	C165T, C309T	S2
			–	AY072727	93–590	C309T	S3
			–	AY072727	102–590	C309Y, G320R, C321Y, C543Y, G552R	S9

R = A/G; Y = C/T.

Regarding the molecular characterization of *Blastocystis* sp., from the 31 positive isolates by PCR, 41.9% were successfully subtyped by sequence analysis in the *SSU* rDNA gene. BLAST searches allowed the identification of three subtypes, including ST1 (46.2%; 6/13), ST2 (7.7%; 1/13), and ST3 (42.6%; 6/13). Neither mixed infections involving different STs of the parasite nor infections caused by animal-specific ST10-ST17, ST21 or ST23-26 were recorded.

3.4. Analytical Test Results

The most frequent analytical alterations occurred at the enzymological level in transaminases (ALAT and ASAT), alkaline phosphatase (ALP) and lactate dehydrogenase (LDH). All those that showed high values of any of them (5.3%, 10.5% and 2.6%, respectively) were parasitized by *G. intestinalis*. Although no association of any of them with parasitosis has been reported, there is an association of increased transaminases with cases of untreated celiac disease.

For determinations of total antibodies, immunoglobulins IgG and IgE were elevated in 5.3% and 2.6% of the studied population, respectively. High values of IgG could be a consequence of natural immunization state or vaccination, while elevated IgE is used to be related to infections with intestinal parasites and allergic reactions.

Regarding hematic alterations, for mononuclear leukocytes, it showed high values in terms of monocytosis (7.9% of cases) and lymphocytosis (15.8%). As for polynuclear leukocytes, eosinophilia was detected in 15.8% and neutropenia in 13%. In relation to the red series, an erythrocytic count decreased by 21.1%, with low plasma concentrations of ferritin in 5.3%, of haemoglobin in 21.1% and serum iron in 5.3% of the participants, and, finally, highlighted an increased platelet count in 10.5% of the cases. When the analysis of the association between haematological alterations and nutritional status (HAZ and BMIZ) was carried out, no statistically significant results were obtained for any of the variables.

Lactose malabsorption test was positive in 26.3% of the studied children, 12.5% and 36.4% for male and female, respectively, but without significant differences between sexes. The association between lactose malabsorption and nutritional status assessed by the BMIZ was analyzed, and no statistically significant result was found. However, it was observed in malabsorbers a BMIZ (15.9 ± 1.5 kg/m^2) lower than in absorbers (16.1 ± 1.5 kg/m^2) without significant differences. On the other hand, there was no association between lactose malabsorption state and eating habits, especially with the group of dairy products and derivatives, and no reduction in intake was observed in malabsorbers. Of the participants, 97.4% regularly ingested dairy products and derivatives, although 18.4% reported digestive discomfort after consuming them. Malabsorption could be a cause of intolerance and rejection of these foods. Furthermore, two of them (5.2%), coinciding with the ones with digestive disorders, shared lactose malabsorption and genetic risk of celiac disease.

According to the results obtained about lactase activity in the Saharawi population, by the expired air test measuring the intestinal capacity of absorption of the sugar, the prevalence of children with malabsorption was 26.3%. Meanwhile, by determination of genetic predisposition to develop a deficiency of the enzyme, 50% of the group of children analyzed showed an absence of the protective five polymorphisms of the lactase gene (MCM6).

For determination of the genetic risk of celiac disease, genes HLA-DQ8B1 and HLA-DQA1 were analyzed. A percentage of 62.5% of the genetically studied Saharawi population presented genetic (haplotype) combinations associated with the risk of developing celiac disease, with no significant differences between sexes. The predominant phenotypes detected were: DQ2.2/DQ8 (high risk) (25%), DQ2.2/DQ-(moderate high risk) (12.5%) and DQ8/DQ-(moderate risk) (25%). The association between the risk of developing celiac disease and the nutritional status assessed through the BMIZ was analyzed and no statistically significant results were found. However, it was observed that those at risk had a BMIZ of 15.5 ± 0.7 kg/m^2, lower than that of children who were not at risk, whose BMIZ was 16.1 ± 1.6 kg/m^2 ($p > 0.05$). According to eating habits, those with a predisposition to celiac disease reported consuming less than 1 time/day of food from the farinaceous group, specifically bread or pasta, although without statistical significance.

4. Discussion

Saharawi children are a population that, due to a series of cultural, social and political characteristics, have a high probability of suffering parasitic diseases. These parasites are a problem in developing countries, since they are generally underestimated for being asymptomatic, but they represent an important morbidity factor when associated with malnutrition [32]. Furthermore, it is interesting to reflect that our study has a series of limitations that occurred during data collection from the participating children. The collection of the anamnesis was very difficult not only because of the ignorance of their previous pathologies, but also because of the difference in language and the young age of the girls and boys, and even the difference in customs made during data collection, but the use of interpreter was very helpful. For the physical examination, the children were extremely modest since the factor of age is added to the mistrust generated by another cultural environment, making it convenient that they be assessed by a pediatrician of the same sex. The collection of feces for parasite testing was particularly problematic for host families due to the frequent refusal of children.

For the physical examination and the collected anthropometric data, our study demonstrated that the children, being in the growth and development stage, were, in general, included in Z-scores ≥ -2 SD and $< +1$ SD (between normal weight and risk of chronic malnutrition) according to the growth indicators of BMIZ. The WHO Growth Pattern confirmed that all children born anywhere in the world who receive optimal care from the beginning of their lives have the potential to develop in the same range of height and weights. Of course, there are individual differences between boys and girls, but regionally and globally, the average population growth is remarkably similar. The pattern shows that differences in child growth depend more on nutrition, feeding practices, environment and health care than on generic or ethnic factors. The WHO Child Growth Standards have worldwide validity. Its purpose is to monitor the growth of all children throughout the world regardless of their ethnicity, socioeconomic status and type of diet [14]. Thus, of the study participants, only two children (a boy and a girl) exceeded this limit due to a weight deficit. According to the HAZ, a high presence of low stature was determined (six children in total), a fact that could be explained considering that the sample studied, whose mean age was 11.1 years, had been lacking adequate nutrition for many years, thus presenting a chronic malnutrition that at the same time increases the probabilities of infections by parasites, in particular, which hinders the progression towards normal growth values. It should be noted that the results of this study are similar to those observed in previous studies of this population that showed that chronic malnutrition is frequent (percentages between 20% and 33%) [2,4–6].

According to eating habits, it is worth highlighting the data obtained in the study on the diet of Saharawi boys and girls with respect to the high consumption of sugary drinks, specifically Coke beverage, which 44.7% claim to consume daily, and of candy, which in this case, the percentage rises to 55.2%. This is in contrast with the Aladino study where 12.1% of Spanish children indicate consuming them between 1 and 3 days/week [33]. Leone et al. [34] observed in a Saharawi adult female population that the consumption of sugary beverages was by 62.5% of those surveyed, so the adult population is not a good reference of children towards this beverage consumption. On the other hand, observing the low contribution of fruits, it is common to think about possible deficiencies of vitamins and micronutrients, so increasing the consumption of these foods is important to reverse the high rates of anemia observed in this population [4–6,12,35]. Surprisingly, the consumption of vegetables is null, suggesting that they may not have any type of crop due to the aridity of the land or even a limited supply. It can also be observed that the consumption of oil (olive, sunflower, etc.) and nuts is infrequent, which can be considered as a deficiency of monounsaturated and polyunsaturated fatty acids. Furthermore, if energy inputs and fiber are reduced, it is reflected in the anthropometric assessment. Leone et al. [34] determined that the consumption of vegetables is frequent, although the variety of vegetables consumed is low (tomatoes, onions and carrots represent 90%). Further, sunflower oil is the most consumed, but it is noteworthy that only peanuts, from the nut groups, are part of their diet, and cereals and derivatives are consumed by 50% of those surveyed. If our data are compared with the food Jaima [8], it can be seen that it is an inverted style. Foods that should be at the base of the Jaima are at the peak, with very low or almost zero consumption, as is the case of fruits and vegetables, while sugary foods or drinks, which should be consumed occasionally, occupy the base of the pyramid with a very high consumption. It is highlighted that the number of food groups consumed by the participating children, according to the FANTA [15] distribution, is similar to the study carried out by Morseth et al. [36], in which aspects related to the dietary diversity of Saharawi refugees were evaluated, although the study comprised adults aged between 18 and 82 years. Therefore, it is necessary to provide tools that allow the development of a population (both children and adults), promote personal and work growth, facilitate access to education and better living conditions, as well as increase the availability and variety of food, facilitate food education and minimize nutritional deficiencies.

For hygienic-sanitary habits, it should be mentioned that children know very well what the appropriate response is, although the reality is different, so it can be observed that 100% of children say they wash their hands before eating and after going to the bathroom, when they do not even have enough running water to carry out these tasks on a regular basis. Hygienic measures are considered a key preventive measure against oral-fecal infectious diseases. Washing your hands after using the bathroom and before eating or preparing a meal can reduce childhood diarrhea. A report published by UNICEF [37] revealed that global rates of hand washing with soap and water before and after using the bathroom or handling food vary between 0% and 24%, which concluded that a significant part of the world's population does not comply with basic hygiene measures, with children being the most vulnerable group.

Parasitic intestinal infections mainly affect the child population, which is the most susceptible to the development of acute symptoms, especially when the infectious form penetrates orally. Even at these ages, reinfections are usually more frequent than in adulthood, where parasitic infections are usually chronic [32,38]. The results of the coproparasitological analysis stand out from those obtained in other studies carried out in the same area or with children sheltered in different places in Spain [4–7,10–13]. In this study, higher prevalence of parasites is observed in general, although it should be noted that the most prevalent parasitic species are the same in practically all studies. According to Paricio-Talayero et al. [4] and Martínez and Pérez [11], *G. intestinalis* in 17.6% and 13.5%, *Blastocystis* sp. in 21.8% and 24%, and *E. nana* in 17.1% and 2.7%, respectively, were determined in host children in Spain, while among helminths: *H. nana* in 10.6% and 24%, and *E. vermicularis* in 4.7% and 35%, respectively, were determined in the same mentioned studies. In the two studies carried out in the field (Tindouf) [5,6], prevalence of parasites by protists of 60% and 45% were obtained, respectively, while that in the studies of Sarquella et al. [10] and Seseña del Olmo et al. [13] were determined as a total 19.6% and 37.3% parasitization, respectively. It is worth mentioning the fact that there is a high degree of intestinal parasitization by *G. intestinalis* and *Blastocystis* sp., maybe due to the use of different coprodiagnosis techniques in this study that had complemented the information. Since the emission of cysts along with the feces seems to be intermittent, microscopic diagnosis as a gold standard technique is not effective; therefore, the combination with molecular methods (such as PCR) that evaluate the intestinal presence of a certain parasite improve the diagnostic sensitivity [38]. Furthermore, the origin of the high prevalence of both protists can be due to poor health of drinking water [39] and the hygienic-sanitary habits (it is usually eaten from the same container with the hands), which facilitates oral-fecal transmission [40]. In addition, these parasitic infections, which are often asymptomatic [32], may be a trigger for secondary food malabsorption/intolerance (in particular, to carbohydrates), dyspepsia or irritable bowel syndrome [38,41–44]. Moreover, the alterations that they cause are related to cases of anemia, acute and chronic diarrhea and malabsorption syndrome can be explained by the presence of *G. intestinalis*. This parasitic protozoan is known to cause the activation of CD8 lymphocytes in the intestinal villi in the absorbent mucosa, which affects the growth and cognitive development of the child affected population [43,45]. Recent studies have associated this protozoan with alterations in iron absorption, decreased serum iron, low levels of Hb in the blood and, in general, with iron deficiency anemia [33,45–49]. Iron is absorbed in the duodenum, specifically in the enterocytes, and the mechanism of action of G. *intestinalis* is to line the intestinal mucosa and prevent the absorption of this mineral. Malnutrition, due to a diet that is not balanced or varied, is the result of the living conditions to which they are subjected. Therefore, this is the cause that affects the Saharawi, iron deficiency due to a diet deficient in this micronutrient. Host parents are advised to intensify their intake of iron-rich foods as well as oral iron supplementation if necessary. Serum iron, transferrin saturation index (TSI) and decreased ferritin appear in these children.

Human giardiasis is considered a zoonotic infection. The molecular characterization of *G. intestinalis* in the recent years has revealed significant genetic diversity. Assemblages from A to H have been identified, with assemblages A and B being the most diverse with at least four types of sub-assemblages (AI-AIII and BIII-BIV). Assemblages A and B are the most common in humans and have also been documented in wildlife and domestic animals. Assemblages C and D are found in dogs, and assemblages E, F and G in domestic ruminants, cats and rodents respectively, while assembly H has been described in marine pinnipeds [50]. *Blastocystis* sp. can remain in the body without causing symptoms but secretes proteases that are the cause of abdominal spasms, vomiting and diarrhea, with the consequent malabsorption of nutrients and the rejection of certain types of food [42]. There are hypotheses that support that this variation in host symptoms is related to the *Blastocystis* subtype [44,51,52]. Presently, 10 subtypes (ST1-ST9 and ST12) have been found in humans, 4 of which are the most frequently found: ST1, ST2, ST3 and ST4, coinciding with those determined in the participating Saharawi population. In addition, various studies attribute *Blastocystis* sp. controversial pathogenicity, even suggesting that the native microbiota or the immune status of the host may determine the pathogenicity and virulence of the protist [44,50,51].

On the other hand, *E. histolytica* destroys tissues through adherence to cells, leading to amoebic colitis and acute diarrhea, anorexia and low weight. *Entamoeba hartmanni, E. nana* or *E. coli*, although they have less relevance from the clinical point of view, may be useful indicators of poor personal and community hygienic-sanitary conditions in the population studied (especially in children) and its environment, as they are also transmitted through the fecal-oral route [53]. For helminth infections, they also produce nutrient malabsorption, and the relationship between anemia and the presence of helminths is frequently observed. Therefore, it is associated with an altered nutritional and cognitive status [54,55]. Finally, multiple infections or multiparasitism may be due to previous malnutrition, differences in children's hygienic-sanitary behavior, the irregular distribution of infective stages in the environment, differences in the ability to generate an adequate immune response to basic differences between parasites and, also, genetic differences between hosts [12].

The participants underwent a blood test that estimated low levels of some indicators of anemia such as haemoglobin, haematocrit and red blood cell count, and also highlighted the presence of other values such as high levels of eosinophils and monocytes, indicators of parasitic infections and low levels of IgA, which favors intestinal colonization. These indicators were altered in previous studies in the refugee population and are related to signs of malnutrition in those parasitized, in particular, with *G. intestinalis* [5,35,47,56].

The breath test, despite being a non-invasive test and considered the reference method for the diagnosis of carbohydrate malabsorption, has its limitations [25,57]. In our study, more than a quarter of the host children were positive to the secondary lactose malabsorption/intolerance, and half of the children analyzed had primary lactose intolerance. Naturally after weaning, and depending on race, ethnicity and genetics, lactase activity persists or does not for a longer or shorter period of time, also depending on the lactose that is ingested. In cases of absent or reduced synthesis of lactase, this substrate reaches the colon where the bacteria metabolize it, generating abdominal pain or diarrhea. The relationship between symptoms and diet in patients with functional digestive disorders may lead to a suppression of dairy consumption, with the risk of a calcium and vitamin D deficiency in children [28]. Some of the Saharawi children studied reported abdominal pain after ingestion of milk. However, a history of post-ingestion symptoms is of little use in determining that a patient has lactase deficiency or lactase malabsorption [58]. Chaud et al. [59] obtained 90.8% of lactose malabsorption of the parasitized by *G. intestinalis*, compared to 7.5% in the control group. More studies are needed to link carbohydrate malabsorption in the general population, and in childhood and adolescence, in particular, with intestinal parasitization, which is not well documented. Another study in African and Finnish children suggested that decreased enzyme activity may be earlier in African children [60]. The study carried out by Rollán et al. [28] determined a high frequency of lactase deficiency associated with the C/T_13910 polymorphism of the MCM6 gene, as well as a high diagnostic yield of the genetic test, comparable or superior to the expiratory test, as observed in the data obtained in the Saharawi child population.

To detect celiac disease, two types of tests are performed to diagnose it: serological tests and genetic tests. Serological samples are focused for high levels of certain antibodies in the blood that reveal an immune reaction triggered after the consumption of foods containing gluten, although it should be noted that a negative result does not totally rule out the existence of celiac disease. On exposure to gluten, plasma cells produce IgA class anti-human tissue transglutaminase antibodies (IgA-TG2) and deaminated peptides (IgA-DGP70 and IgA-DGP71) [24,61]. In our analyzed blood samples, some of the participants had IgA-TG2, although the interpretation of the results of the genetic predictive test for celiac disease did not reveal the probability of suffering from the disease, nor were they statistically significant to establish any relationship. Regarding genetic tests, the presence of certain HLA-DQ heterodimers and their association were detected, which indicated a risk of suffering from the disease in 62.5% of the analyzed participants, and that they can make them more susceptible to intestinal parasites due to the damage caused to the intestinal mucosa. Previous studies suggest that gluten sensitivity is one of the common disorders in North Africa and the Eastern Mediterranean, determining a high frequency of celiac disease in the Saharawi population, and its consequent delay in physical and mental growth [10,62–66].

5. Conclusions

Low height was in approximately one-fifth of the children in foster care, and the prevalence of parasites was almost 100%, with multiparasitic infections being the most frequent. It should be noted that intestinal parasitosis is a contributing factor to malnutrition and iron deficiency; therefore, it is common to find problems such as anemia, celiac disease and growth retardation among the child population. The diet of the Saharawi children in the camp is deficient in terms of quantity and quality, highlighting the scarce contribution of fruits, vegetables and protein foods, while sugary foods are excessively high. It should be noted that it is a culture where eating with your hands and from the same container is part of their way of life. This complicates the quantification of consumption rations for each stage of life, as, for the children who are going to enter adolescence and are in full growth, their nutritional needs are not met. In addition, malnutrition affecting height, nutritional deficiencies and multiple infections with frequent intestinal parasites are related to insufficient hygienic measures, water shortages and the difficulty of access to basic food, especially fresh. Thus, since the main problems derive from a lack of adequate hygiene and incorrect nutrition, it is proposed for future editions of the "Holidays in Peace" program, and for field interventions, that sustainable food alternatives and health education programs and nutrition be made available to parents and children. It should even be noted that since the population selected for the program is exposed to very harsh lifestyles, among which is the scarcity of water that is responsible for poor personal and community hygiene, the probability of presenting intestinal parasites is very high, since the route of transmission is oral-fecal. The greater the shortage of hygienic measures, the greater the number of parasitic infections, which aggravates the low caloric intake, thus ending in malnutrition. Increasing programs on hygiene and food education for parents and children in less fortunate regions reduces the risk of infections and health problems. The prevalence of intestinal parasites in Saharawi host children is very high, especially in the case of the protist *G. intestinalis* and *Blastocystis* sp. In most cases, it is multiparasitism combining pathogenic protists with other commensal amoeba or helminths. The combination of direct and indirect diagnostic techniques has allowed the diagnosis of a greater number of cases. Real-time PCR for *G. intestinalis* and conventional PCR for *Blastocystis* sp. have been more sensitive in diagnosis than light microscopy, but microscopy has given us broader species identification. It is convenient to establish a protocol for the diagnosis and treatment of parasites as far as possible because, when they return to their country, reinfections take place; therefore, the objective is to reduce the parasite load and improve the quality of life. With the high prevalence of parasites in children in foster care, empirical treatment of children in foster care is considered appropriate, always under the supervision of visiting pediatricians. All the boys and girls participating in the study present some type of intestinal parasitosis that can be caused by the deficient hygienic sanitary measures of the place. For this reason, hygiene-sanitary education must continue annually to try to change habits that, upon return to their country, can be useful to prevent fecal-oral transmission diseases. A high prevalence of lactose malabsorbers or intolerant participants was found, and those conditions could be a cause of or lead to the aggravation of intestinal parasites, as well as celiac disease. The coexistence of trionomial, malnutrition, intestinal parasites and food intolerances has to be considered for proper nutritional and parasitological management to try to restore children's health status. All the information of this study will provide us a better point of view of the health status of these children and help to create health education policies for the Saharawi population.

Author Contributions: Conceptualization, M.T.; data curation, M.G. (Mónica Gozalbo) and M.G. (Marisa Guillen); formal analysis, M.G. (Mónica Gozalbo), M.G. (Marisa Guillen), S.T.-F., S.C., D.C., J.M.S. and M.T.; funding acquisition, M.G. (Marisa Guillen) and M.T.; investigation, M.G. (Mónica Gozalbo), M.G. (Marisa Guillen), S.T.-F., S.C., D.C., J.M.S. and M.T.; methodology, M.G. (Mónica Gozalbo), M.G. (Marisa Guillen), S.T.-F., S.C., D.C., J.M.S. and M.T.; project administration, M.G. (Marisa Guillen) and M.T.; Supervision, M.T.; writing—original draft, M.G. (Mónica Gozalbo), S.T.-F., D.C., J.M.S. and M.T.; writing—review & editing, M.G. (Marisa Guillen) and S.C. All authors have read and agreed to the published version of the manuscript.

Funding: This study was part of the project "Promotion of hygienic-health habits for the prevention of intestinal parasites in the Saharawi population" promoted by the University of Valencia in collaboration with the Nutrition Clinic of the University of Valencia (CUNAFF), the Federation of Solidarity Associations with the Saharawi People of the Valencian Country (FASPS-PV) and the Ministry of Sanitat de la Comunitat Valenciana, in addition to being funded by the UNESCO Chair.

Acknowledgments: We thank the Paediatrics Service of the University Hospital Clinic of Valencia (Spain) for conducting physical examinations.

Conflicts of Interest: The authors declare no conflict of interest.

References

1. Besenyö, J. Saharawi refugees in Algeria. *AARMS* **2010**, *6*, 67–78.
2. Grijalva-Eternod, C.S.; Wells, J.C.K.; Cortina-Borja, M.; Salse-Ubach, N.; Tondeur, M.C.; Dolan, C.; Meziani, C.; Wilkinson, C.; Spiegel, P.; Seal, A.J. The double burden of obesity and malnutrition in a protracted emergency setting: A cross-sectional study of Western Sahara refugees. *PLoS Med.* **2012**, *9*, e1001320. [CrossRef] [PubMed]
3. Obokata, R.; Veronis, L.; McLeman, R. Empirical research on international environmental migration: A systematic review. *Popul. Environ.* **2014**, *36*, 111–135. [CrossRef] [PubMed]
4. Paricio-Talayero, J.M.; Santos, L.; Fernández, A.; Ferriol, M.; Rodríguez, F.; Brañas, P. Health examination of children from the Democratic Sahara Republic (Northwest Africa) on vacation in Spain. *An. Pediatr.* **1998**, *49*, 33–38.
5. Lopriore, C.; Guidoum, Y.; Briend, A.; Branca, F. Spread fortified with vitamins and minerals induces catch-up growth and errdicates severe anemia in stunted refugee children aged 3–6 years. *Am. J. Clin. Nutr.* **2004**, *80*, 973–980. [CrossRef]
6. Doménech, G.; Escortell, S.; Gilabert, R.; González-Osnaya, L.; Lucena, M.; Martínez, M.C.; Soriano, J.M. Dietary intake and food pattern of Saharawi children refugee in Tindouf (Algeria). *Proc. Nutr. Soc.* **2008**, *67*, E174. [CrossRef]
7. Soriano, J.M.; Domènech, G.; Mañes, J.; Catalá-Gregori, A.I.; Barikmo, I.E. Disorders of malnutrition among the Saharawi children. *Rev. Esp. Nutr. Hum. Diet.* **2011**, *15*, 10–19. [CrossRef]

8. Bilbao, L.; Soriano, J.M.; Doménech, G.; Martínez, C. La Jaima Alimentaria, guía alimentaria para las familias de acogida de los niños/niñas saharauis. *Nutr. Hosp.* **2014**, *30*, 1384–1390.
9. Arroyo-Izaga, M.; Andia, V.; Demon, G. Diseño de un programa de educación nutricional destinado a mujeres saharauis residentes en los campamentos de Tindouf (Argelia). *Nutr. Hosp.* **2016**, *33*, 91–97. [CrossRef]
10. Sarquella, G.; Asso, L.; García, A.M.; Álvarez, A. Use the brief visit for hosted Saharawi children to detect nutritional disorders. *An. Pediatr.* **2004**, *60*, 134.
11. Martínez, M.; Pérez, E. Health test for children from Saharawi refugee camps hosted during the summer. In *Annual Meeting European Society for Social Paediatric*; Annual Meeting European Society for Social Pediatric: Oxford, UK. Available online: http://www.pediatriasocial.com/Documentos/LIBRO%20ESSOP.pdf (accessed on 10 October 2020).
12. Soriano, J.M.; Doménech, G.; Martínez, M.C.; Mañes, J.; Soriano, F. Intestinal parasitic infections in hosted Saharawi children. *Trop. Biomed.* **2011**, *28*, 557–562. [PubMed]
13. Seseña del Olmo, G.; Rodríguez, M.J.; Martínez, M.C.; Pérez, J.A. Prevalencia de parasitosis intestinales en niños de acogida saharauis. *Rev. Del Lab. Clin.* **2011**, *4*, 42–44. [CrossRef]
14. WHO. *Training Course on Child Growth Assessment*; WHO: Geneva, Switzerland. Available online: http://www.who.int/childgrowth/training/en/ (accessed on 10 October 2020).
15. FANTA. Introducing the Minimum Dietary Diversity-Women (MDD-W) Global Dietary Diversity Indicator for Women 2014. Available online: http://www.fsnnetwork.org/sites/default/files/minimum_dietary_diversity_-_women_mdd-w_sept_2014.pdf (accessed on 10 October 2020).
16. Estruch, R.; Ros, E.; Salas-Salvadó, J.; Covas, M.I.; Corella, D.; Arós, F.; Gómez-Gracia, E.; Ruiz-Gutiérrez, V.; Fiol, M.; Lapetra, J.; et al. Primary prevention of cardiovascular disease with a Mediterranean Diet. *N. Engl. J. Med.* **2013**, *368*, 1279–1290. [CrossRef] [PubMed]
17. Estruch, R.; Ros, E.; Salas-Salvadó, J.; Covas, M.I.; Corella, D.; Arós, F.; Gómez-Gracia, E.; Ruiz-Gutiérrez, V.; Fiol, M.; Lapetra, J.; et al. Primari prevention of cadiovascular disease with a Mediterranean Diet supplemented with extra-virgin olive oil or nuts. *N. Engl. J. Med.* **2018**, *378*, e34. [CrossRef]
18. Verweij, J.J.; Schinkel, J.; Laeijendecker, D.; van Rooyen, M.A.A.; van Lieshout, L.; Polderman, A.M. Real-time PCR for detection of Giardia lamblia. *Mol. Cell. Probes* **2003**, *17*, 223–225. [CrossRef]
19. Dacal, E.; Saugar, J.M.; de Lucio, A.; Hernández-de-Mingo, M.; Robinson, E.; Köster, P.C.; Aznar-Ruiz-de-Alegría, M.L.; Espasa, M.; Ninda, A.; Gandasegui, J.; et al. Prevalencia and molecular characterization of *Strongyloides stercoralis, Giardia duodenalis, Cryptosporidium* spp., and *Blastocystis* spp. Isolates in school children in Cubal, Western Angola. *Parasites Vectors* **2018**, *11*, 67. [CrossRef]
20. Read, C.M.; Monis, P.T.; Thompson, R.C. Discrimination of all genotypes of *Giardia duodenalis* at the glutamate dehydrogenase locus using PCR-RFLP. *Infect. Genet. Evol.* **2004**, *4*, 125–130. [CrossRef]
21. Lalle, M.; Pozio, E.; Capelli, G.; Bruschi, F.; Crotti, D.; Cacciò, S.M. Genetic heterogeneity at the beta-giardin locus among human and animal isolates of *Giardia duodenalis* and identification of potentially zoonotic subgenotypes. *Int. J. Parasitol.* **2005**, *35*, 207–213. [CrossRef]
22. Scicluna, S.M.; Tawari, B.; Clark, C.G. DNA barcoding of *Blastocystis. Protist* **2006**, *157*, 77–85. [CrossRef]
23. Tamura, K.; Stecher, G.; Peterson, D.; Filipski, A.; Kumar, S. MEGA6: Molecular Evolutionary Genetics Analysis version 6.0. *Mol. Biol. Evol.* **2013**, *30*, 2725–2729. [CrossRef]
24. Ludvigsson, J.F.; Bai, J.C.; Biaqi, F.; Card, T.R.; Ciacci, C.; Ciclitira, P.J.; Green, P.H.R.; Hadjisvassiliou, M.; Holdoway, A.; van Heel, D.A.; et al. Diagnosis and management of adult coeliac disease: Guidelines from the Bristish Society of Gastroenterology. *Gut* **2014**, *63*, 1210–1228. [CrossRef] [PubMed]
25. Ghosal, U. How to interpret Hydrogen Breath Test. *J. Neurogastroenterol. Motil.* **2011**, *17*, 312–317. [CrossRef] [PubMed]
26. Hinojosa-Guadix, J.H.; Gamarro, M.P.; Sánchez, I.M. Malabsortion and fructose: Fructose-sorbitol intolerance in functional pathology. *Rev. Andal. Patol. Dig.* **2017**, *40*, 119–124.
27. Sollid, L.M.; Markussen, G.; Ek, J.; Gjerde, H.; Vartdal, F.F.; Thorsby, E. Evidence for a primary association of celiac disease to a particular HLA-DQ alpha/beta heterodimer. *J. Exp. Med.* **1989**, *169*, 345–350. [CrossRef] [PubMed]
28. Rollan, A.; Vial, C.; Quesada, S.; Espinoza, K.; Hatton, M.; Puga, A.; Repetto, G. Comparative performance of symptoms questionnaire, hydrogen test and genetic test for lactose intolerance. *Rev. Med. Chile* **2012**, *140*, 1101–1108.

29. De Onis, M. The use of anthropometry in the prevention of childhood overweight and obesity. *Int. J. Obes.* **2004**, *28*, S81–S85. [CrossRef]
30. De Onis, M.; Onyango, A.W.; Borghi, E.; Garza, E.; Yang, H. Comparison of the World Heallth Organitzation (WHO) Child Growth Standerds and the National Center for Health Statistics/WHO international growth reference: Implications for child health programmes. *Public Health Nutr.* **2006**, *9*, 942–947. [CrossRef]
31. De Onis, M.; Onyango, A.W.; Borghi, E.; Siyam, A.; Nishida, C.; Siekman, J. Development of a WHO growth reference for school-children and adolescents. *Bull. World Heath Organ.* **2007**, *85*, 660–667. [CrossRef]
32. Solano, L.; Acuña, I.; Barón, M.; Morón de Salim, A.; Sánchez, A. Influencia de las parasitosis intestinales y otros antecedentes infecciosos sobre el estado nutricional y antropométrico en niños en situación de pobreza. *Parasitol. Latinoam.* **2008**, *63*, 12–19. [CrossRef]
33. Agencia Española de Seguridad Alimentaria y Nutrición. Estudio ALADINO. Estudio de vigilancia del crecimiento, alimentación, actividad física, desarrollo infantil y obesidad en España. 2015. Available online: http://www.aecosan.msssi.gob.es/AECOSAN/docs/documentos/nutricion/observatorio/Estudio_ALADINO_2015.pdf (accessed on 10 October 2020).
34. Leone, A.; Battezzati, A.; Sara Di Lello, S.; Ravasenghi, S.; Mohamed-Iahdih, B.; Saleh, S.M.L.; Bertoli, S. Dietary habits of Saharawi type ii diabetic women living in Algerian refugee camps: Relationship with nutritional status and glycemic profile. *Nutrients* **2020**, *12*, 568. [CrossRef]
35. Seal, A.J.; Creeke, P.I.; Mirghani, Z.; Abdalla, F.; McBurney, R.P.; Pratt, L.S.; Brookes, D.; Ruth, L.J.; Marchand, E. Iron and vitamin A deficiency in long-term African refugee. *J. Nutr.* **2005**, *135*, 808–813. [CrossRef] [PubMed]
36. Morseth, M.; Grewal, N.; Kaasa, I.; Harloy, A.; Barikmo, I.; Henjum, S. Dietary diversity is related to socioeconomic status among adult Saharawi refugees living in Algeria. *BMC Public Health* **2017**, *17*, 621. [CrossRef] [PubMed]
37. UNICEF (United Nations Children's Foundation). *The Child Care Transition: Innocenti Report Card 8*; UNICEF Innocenti Research Centre: Florence, Italy, 2008.
38. Trelis, M.; Taroncher-Ferrer, S.; Gozalbo, M.; Ortiz, V.; Soriano, J.M.; Osuna, A.; Merino-Torres, J.F. *Giardia intestinalis* and fructose malabsorption: A frequent association. *Nutrients* **2019**, *11*, 2973. [CrossRef] [PubMed]
39. Aakre, I.; Henjum, S.; Gjengedal, E.L.F.; Haugstad, C.R.; Vollset, M.; Moubarak, K.; Ahmed, T.S.; Alexander, J.; Kjellevold, M.; Molin, M. Trace element concentrations in drinking water and urine among saharawi women and young children. *Toxics* **2018**, *6*, 40. [CrossRef]
40. Torgerson, P.R.; de Silva, N.R.; Fevre, E.M.; Kasuga, F.; Rokni, M.B.; Zhou, X.N.; Sripa, B.; Gargouri, N.; Willingham, A.L.; Stein, C. The global burden of foodborne parasitic diseases: An update. *Trends Parasitol.* **2014**, *30*, 20–26. [CrossRef]
41. Moya-Camarena, S.Y.; Sotelo, N.; Valencia, M.E. Effects of asymptomatic *Giardia intestinalis* infection on carbohydrate absorption in well-nourished Mexican children. *Am. J. Trop. Med. Hyg.* **2002**, *66*, 255–259. [CrossRef]
42. Grazioli, B.; Matera, G.; Laratta, C.; Schipani, G.; Guarnieri, G.; Spiniello, E.; Imeneo, M.; Amorosi, A.; Focà, A.; Luzza, F. *Giardia lamblia* infection in patients with irritable bowel syndrome and dispepsia: A prospective study. *World J. Gastroenterol.* **2006**, *12*, 1941–1944. [CrossRef]
43. Halliez, M.C.M.; Buret, A.G. Extraintestinal and long-term consequences of *Giardia duodenalis* infections. *World J. Gastroenterol.* **2013**, *19*, 8974–8985. [CrossRef]
44. Cifre, S.; Gozalbo, M.; Ortiz, V.; Soriano, J.M.; Merino, J.F.; Trelis, M. *Blastocystis* subtypes and their association with Irritable Bowel Syndrome. *Med. Hypotheses* **2018**, *116*, 4–9. [CrossRef]
45. Cotton, J.A.; Beatty, J.K.; Buret, A.G. Host parasite interactions and phatophysiology in *Giardia* infections. *Internat. J. Parasitol.* **2011**, *4*, 925–933. [CrossRef]
46. Sackey, M.E.; Weigel, M.M.; Armijos, R.X. Predictors and nutritional consequences of intestinal parasitic infections in rural ecuadorian children. *J. Trop. Pediatr.* **2003**, *49*, 17–23. [CrossRef] [PubMed]
47. Ponce-Macotela, M.; González-Maciel, A.; Reynoso-Robles, R.; Martínez-Gordillo, M. Goblets cells: Are they an unspecific barrier against *Giardia intestinalis* or a gate. *Parasitol. Res.* **2008**, *102*, 509–513. [CrossRef] [PubMed]
48. Mihai, C.M.; Balasa, A.; Mihai, L.; Stroia, V.; Stoicescu, M.R. Parasitic infection in children under 2 years old from rural áreas and their relationship with micronutrients deficiencies. *Pediatr. Res.* **2010**, *68*, 509. [CrossRef]

49. Motta de Oliveira, C.L.; Ferreira, W.A.; Da Mata, A.; Vale-Barbosa, M.G. Anemia of iron deficiency and your correlation with intestinal parasites in a population of the area near urban of Manaus. *Rev. Ibero Latinoam. Parasitol.* **2011**, *70*, 93–100.
50. Feng, Y.; Xiao, L. Zoonotic potential and molecular epidemiology of *Giardia* species and giardiasis. *Clin. Microbiol. Rev.* **2011**, *24*, 110–140. [CrossRef] [PubMed]
51. Skotarczak, B. Genetic diversity and pathogenicity of *Blastocystis*. *Ann. Agric. Environ. Med.* **2018**, *25*, 411–416. [CrossRef] [PubMed]
52. Kök, M.; Çekin, Y.; Çekin, A.H.; Uyar, S.; Harmandar, F.; Şahintürk, Y. The role of *Blastocystis hominis* in the activation of ulcerative colitis. *Turk. J. Gastroenterol.* **2019**, *30*, 40–46.
53. Gozalbo, M. Estudio Epidemiológico de las Parasitosis Intestinales en Población Infantil del Departamento de Managua (Nicaragua). Ph.D. Thesis, Universitat de València, Valencia, Spain, 2012.
54. Crompton, D.W.T.; Nesheim, M.C. Nutritional impact of intestinal helmintiasis during the human life cycle. *Annu. Rev. Nutr.* **2002**, *22*, 35–59. [CrossRef]
55. Sayasone, S.; Utzinger, J.; Akkhavong, K.; Odermatt, P. Multiparasitism and intensity of helmints infections in relation to simptoms and nutritional status among children: A cross-sectional study in southern Lao People's Democratic Republic. *Acta Trop.* **2015**, *141*, 322–331. [CrossRef]
56. Alparo, I. Giardiasis and malnutrition. *Rev. Soc. Bol. Ped.* **2005**, *44*, 166–173.
57. Gasbarrini, A.; Corazza, G.R.; Gasbarrini, G.; Montalto, M.; Di Stefano, M.; Basilisco, G. Methodology and indications of H2-breath testing in gastorintestinal diseases: The Rome Consensus Conference. *Aliment. Pharmacol. Ther.* **2009**, *9*, 82.
58. Casellas, F.; Aparici, A.; Casaus, M.; Rodríguez, P.; Malagelada, J.R. subjective perception of lactose intolerance does not always indicate lactose malabsorption. *Clin. Gastroenterol. Hepatol.* **2010**, *8*, 581–586. [CrossRef] [PubMed]
59. Chahud, A.; Zegarre, C.; Díaz, A.; Pichilingue, O. Lactose intolerance and giardiasis. *Rev. Gastroenterol. Perú.* **1982**, *2*, 39–43.
60. Rasinperä, H.; Savilahti, E.; Enattah, N.S.; Koukkanen, M.; Tötterman, N.; Lindahl, H.; Järvela, i.; Kolho, K.L. A genetic test which can be used to diagnose adult-type hypolactasia in children. *Gut* **2004**, *53*, 1571–1576. [CrossRef] [PubMed]
61. Fasano, A.; Catassi, C. Current approaches to diagnosis and treatment of celiac disease: An evolving spectrum. *Gastroenterology* **2001**, *120*, 636–651. [CrossRef] [PubMed]
62. Khuffash, F.A.; Barakat, M.H.; Shaltout, A.A.; Farwana, S.S. Coeliac disease among children in Kuwait: Difficulties in diagnosis and management. *Gut* **1987**, *28*, 1595–1599. [CrossRef]
63. Rawashdah, M.O.; Khalil, B.; Raweily, E. Celiac disease in Arabs. *J. Pediatr. Gastroenterol. Nutr.* **1996**, *23*, 415–418. [CrossRef]
64. Catassi, C.; Rätsch, I.M.; Gandol, L.; Pratesi, R.; Fabiani, E.; Al Asmar, R.; Frijia, M.; Bearzi, I.; Vizzoni, L. Why is celiac disease endemic in the people of the Sahara? *Lancet* **1999**, *354*, 647–648. [CrossRef]
65. López-Vázquez, A. MHC class I region plays a role in the development of diverse clinical forms of celiac disease in a Saharawi population. *Am. J. Gastroenterol.* **2004**, *99*, 662–667. [CrossRef]
66. Rästch, I.M.; Catassi, C. Coeliac disease: A potentially treatable health problem of Saharawi refugee children. *Bull. World Heath Organ.* **2007**, *79*, 541–545.

Publisher's Note: MDPI stays neutral with regard to jurisdictional claims in published maps and institutional affiliations.

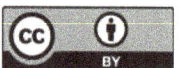

© 2020 by the authors. Licensee MDPI, Basel, Switzerland. This article is an open access article distributed under the terms and conditions of the Creative Commons Attribution (CC BY) license (http://creativecommons.org/licenses/by/4.0/).

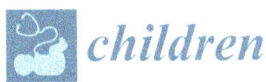

Article

Triage for Malnutrition Risk among Pediatric and Adolescent Outpatients with Cystic Fibrosis, Using a Disease-Specific Tool

Dimitrios Poulimeneas [1,2], Maria G. Grammatikopoulou [3], Argyri Petrocheilou [4], Athanasios G. Kaditis [4,5] and Tonia Vassilakou [1,*]

1. Department of Public Health Policy, School of Public Health, University of West Attica, 196, Alexandras Avenue, GR-11521 Athens, Greece; dpoul@hua.gr
2. Department of Nutrition and Dietetics, Harokopio University, E. Venizelou 70, GR-17671 Athens, Greece
3. Department of Nutritional Sciences & Dietetics, Alexander Campus, International Hellenic University, GR-57001 Thessaloniki, Greece; maria@ihu.gr
4. Cystic Fibrosis Department, Agia Sophia Children's Hospital, Thivon 1, GR-11527 Athens, Greece; apetroch@gmail.com (A.P.); kaditia@hotmail.com (A.G.K.)
5. Division of Pediatric Pulmonology and Sleep Disorders Laboratory, First Department of Pediatrics, National and Kapodistrian University of Athens School of Medicine and Aghia Sophia Children's Hospital, Thivon 1, GR-11527 Athens, Greece
* Correspondence: tvasilakou@uniwa.gr

Received: 4 November 2020; Accepted: 1 December 2020; Published: 4 December 2020

Abstract: Malnutrition prevails in considerable proportions of children with Cystic Fibrosis (CF), and is often associated with adverse outcomes. For this, routine screening for malnutrition is pivotal. In the present cross-sectional study, we aimed to assess the risk for malnutrition in pediatric outpatients with CF. A total of 76 outpatients (44 girls, 11.9 ± 3.9 years old, 39.5% adolescents) were recruited and anthropometric, clinical, dietary and respiratory measures were collected. All outpatients were screened for malnutrition risk with a validated disease-specific instrument. Most children exhibited a low risk for malnutrition (78.9%), whereas none of the participants were characterized as having a high malnutrition risk. In the total sample, malnutrition risk was positively associated with age ($r = 0.369$, $p = 0.001$), and inversely related to the body mass index ($r = -0.684$, $p < 0.001$), height z-score ($r = -0.264$, $p = 0.021$), and forced expiratory volume (FEV$_1$%, $r = -0.616$, $p < 0.001$). Those classified as having a low malnutrition risk were younger ($p = 0.004$), heavier ($p < 0.001$) and taller ($p = 0.009$) than their counterparts with a moderate risk. On the other hand, patients in the moderate risk group were more likely pubertal ($p = 0.034$), with a reduced mid-upper arm fat area ($p = 0.011$), and worse pulmonary function ($p < 0.001$). Interestingly, none of the children attaining ideal body weight were classified as having a moderate malnutrition. risk, whereas 37.5% of the patients allocated at the moderate risk group exhibited physiological lung function. In this cohort of outpatients with CF that were predominantly well-nourished and attained physiological lung function, malnutrition risk was identified only in small proportions of the sample. Our data support that patients that are older, pubertal, or have diminished fat mass are at greater risk for malnutrition.

Keywords: children; pulmonary disease; forced expiratory volume; pulmonary infection; nutritional assessment; screening; underweight; pulmonary function; pancreatic insufficiency; PERT

---

1. Introduction

Cystic fibrosis (CF) is a chronic condition characterized by an increased risk of malnutrition. Poor nutritional intake due to increased energy loss and demands, inadequate caloric intake, malabsorption and maldigestion, exacerbations of the disease, genetic susceptibility and the often underlying infections, increase the risk of malnutrition among patients with CF [1–6]. Between adults and children, the latter appear to be more vulnerable to the development of malnutrition, due to their yet underdeveloped system, further increasing their nutrient demands and susceptibility to infection [5]. Nevertheless, malnutrition during childhood has also been associated with an increased malnutrition risk during adult years and a greater probability of requiring lung transplantation [7].

Although several research projects have revealed a high degree of malnourishment among children with CF [8–10], early identification of such cases, through screening, is pivotal for early intervention and improved outcomes. In parallel, today, malnutrition identification practice is mainly reliant on anthropometric data, the subjective assessment and clinical judgement of each pediatrician, with the mainstay of this approach being biased by the often-inadequate nutritional expertise of pediatricians [11]. Severe cases of malnutrition might be more evident to the untrained eye, however, children at risk, or milder forms of malnutrition, often remain undiagnosed [12]. With this in mind, a variety of screening tools have been developed for pediatric patients, most of which can be used among hospitalized children, with the majority exhibiting good sensitivity and specificity [13].

With regards to CF however, disease-specific screening tools for malnutrition are limited, especially for pediatric patients, with only two existing in the literature to date, the first being published during 2008 [14] and the more recent one presented in the year 2016 [15]. The use of malnutrition screening tools specifically for each underlying disease, in this case CF, is important, as the pathophysiology of the disease contributing to the development of malnutrition is considered, all factors contributing to the development of malnutrition in the condition are accounted for and a more accurate triage of patients is enabled.

With this in mind, the aim of the present study was to assess the risk for malnutrition among pediatric patients with CF, using a disease-specific tool.

2. Materials and Methods

2.1. Sample Recruitment

The GreeCF study is an observational study, aiming to assess the relationship between growth indices, clinical and dietary parameters among school-aged children with CF. The study was conducted during the last quarter of 2015, in the outpatient Clinic for CF, situated in Aghia Sophia Children's Hospital, in metropolitan Athens, Greece. Details concerning the recruitment have been previously reported [10,16]. All children were screened for eligibility, during their routine appointment at the clinic. Inclusion criteria involved (1) having an age between 6–18 years, (2) having a confirmed CF diagnosis and (3) willingness to participate. Exclusion criteria included (1) being < 6 years old, or being an adult, (2) having a concurrent disease affecting growth, and (3) refusal of the parents/guardians to provide informed consent for participation. A total of 114 children/adolescents with CF met the inclusion criteria. For the purposes of the present paper, we analyzed the data of 76 patients (response rate 66.7%, mean age 11.9 ± 3.9 years old, 44 girls, 39.5% adolescents) with complete answers on all measures required for the analyses.

The parents/guardians of all patients provided informed written consent prior to participation. The study was conducted in accordance with the Declaration of Helsinki, and the protocol was approved by the Ethics Committees of both Aghia Sophia Children's Hospital, and University of West Attica (reference number 16084/14-07-15).

2.2. Anthropometric Measures

Anthropometry was conducted during morning hours, with patients wearing light clothing and having bare feet, by the same experienced dietician (DP). Body weight was measured at the nearest 0.1 kg (SECA 874 portable digital scale, Hamburg, Germany) and height to the nearest 0.5 cm (SECA 214 portable stadiometer, Hamburg, Germany), and then body mass index (BMI) was computed. Height-for-age (HAZ) and BMI-for age (BAZ) z-scores were calculated for each patient, based on the

Centers for Disease Control (CDC) growth charts [17]. According to the BAZ, patients were classified as underweight (BAZ < −2.0), or normal body weight (−2.0 ≤ BAZ < 1.0), overweight or obese (BAZ ≥ 1.0, and BAZ ≥ 2.0, respectively). CF-specific classification was used to assess ideal body weight (IBW) (BAZ ≥ 0.0) and possible nutritional failure (BAZ < −1.04). Children with an HAZ < −2.0 were considered chronically malnourished (stunting).

On the left side of the body, mid-upper arm circumference (MUAC) was measured at the mid-point between the olecranon process and the acromium, while triceps' skinfold thickness (TSF) values were taken three times (Harpenden Skinfold Calipers, Batty International, Burgess Hill, England) in order to attain a median value. MUAC, TSF, mid upper arm muscle (MUAMA) and fat area (MUAFA) z-scores were calculated according to the NHANES III survey [18].

Dietary intake was assessed at the day of the visit, through a multiple-pass, 24-h dietary recall, by the same experienced dietician (D.P.). For children aged below 9 years old, parental consensus during the interview was sought. Recall data were then analyzed for total energy intake (TEI) using the Food Processor software (ESHA, Portland, Oregon). TEI was then converted in % of the recommended daily intake.

2.3. Patients' Medical History, Physical and Clinical Parameters and CF-Related Comorbidities

Individual medical records were searched for age at diagnosis and diagnostic criteria, presence of pancreatic insufficiency (PI), CF-related diabetes (CFRD), intermittent and/or chronic infection by pathogens (*Pseudomonas Aeruginosa*, methicillin resistant *Staphylococcus Aureus*, *Burkholderia cepacia*), enteral feeding, and serum albumin levels. Pulmonary function was assessed during the day of each patient's visit to the clinic, through the Forced Expiratory Volume at 1 s (FEV_1). Pulmonary function was compared against predicted values ($FEV_1\%$) using the equations suggested by Wang et al. [19] (for boys aged 6–17 years old and girls 6–15 years old) and Hankinson et al. (for boys aged 18 years old and girls exceeding the 16 years of age) [20].

Measurements of weight and height collected during previous visits were also recorded to evaluate impaired weight gain and/or weight loss, and failure to thrive. Puberty was defined after physical examination (and/or menarche in girls) by the team of medical doctors; no specific data regarding the pubertal stages of the patients were recorded.

2.4. Malnutrition Risk

Malnutrition Risk was assessed by the validated CF-specific tool, developed by dos Santos Simon and associates [15]. In more detail, this tool assigns ratings based on 10 risk factors including: (i) BMI status, (ii) presence of PI and (iii) CFRD, (iv) colonization by specific pathogens, (v) reduced dietary intake, (vi) impaired weight gain or involuntary weight loss, (vii) impaired height gain, (viii) enteral feeding, (ix) impaired lung function as evidenced by $FEV_1\%$, and (x) low serum albumin levels. A composite score is then computed by summing up the ratings of each risk factor. The score ranges from 0 to 14, with higher values indicative of higher nutritional risk. Furthermore, ratings between 0–3 indicate low malnutrition risk, ratings of 4–7 suggest medium risk, whereas a score ≥ 8 is indicative of increased risk for malnutrition [15].

2.5. Statistical Analyses

Data distribution was visually explored with Q-Q plots; all continuous variables but age at diagnosis (months) were normally distributed. Therefore, continuous variables are presented as means ± standard deviation, whereas age at diagnosis is presented as a median with its respective interquartile ranges (1st and 3rd IQR). Categorical variables are presented as relative frequencies and percentages. Differences between continuous variables were assessed with independent *t*-test (or Mann–Whitney test for age at diagnosis). Chi-square or the Fisher's exact test was employed to explore differences between categorical variables. Association between continuous variables was examined through

Spearman's r correlation co-efficient. The level of significance was set at $\alpha = 0.05$. All analyses were performed with SPSS version 25.0 (IBM, SPSS Inc., Chicago, IL, USA).

3. Results

3.1. Assessment of Malnutrition Risk

A total of 32 boys and 44 girls were recruited for the purposes of this study (aged 11.9 ± 3.9 years old, 39.5% adolescents). Their mean BAZ was 0.05 ± 1.13, whereas their mean HAZ was -0.28 ± 1.09. Referring to their pulmonary function, patients exhibited a mean FEV1% of 98.0 ± 19.8%.

Risk factors for malnutrition, and malnutrition risk are presented in Table 1. None of the patients exhibited suboptimal albumin levels, or received enteral feedings. Only a small minority of the examined children failed to reach linear growth, or had impaired lung function. On the contrary, most children (59.2%) attained IBW for CF, and reached the recommended targets for energy intake (71.1%). A great proportion of participants had pancreatic insufficiency (86.8%), whereas none of the children were on enteral nutrition or exhibited low serum albumin levels. Most patients exhibited a low risk for malnutrition (78.9%), whereas none of the participants were characterized as having high malnutrition risk. No significant differences between the examined risk factors, or total malnutrition risk and malnutrition risk categories was observed according to the sex of the participants ($p > 0.05$ for all comparisons, data not shown).

Table 1. Prevalence of malnutrition risk factors, and total malnutrition risk score among participating children, according to the Nutrition Screening Tool for Pediatric Patients with Cystic Fibrosis [15] (N = 76).

Risk Factor		n (%) *
1	BMI < 50th percentile	31 (40.8)
	BMI < 10th percentile	10 (13.2)
2	Pancreatic Insufficiency	66 (86.8)
3	*Pseudomonas, Burkholderia cepacia* or MRSA colonization	29 (38.2)
4	Dietary Intake < 100% RDA	22 (28.9)
5	Weight gain less than minimum, zero weight gain or weight loss	6 (7.9)
6	Height gain less than minimum, or zero height gain	4 (5.3)
7	Enteral feeding	0 (0.0)
8	CFRD	4 (5.3)
9	FEV_1% (<80% predicted)	13 (17.1)
10	Serum albumin < 3.5 mg/dL	0 (0.0)
Mean total Malnutrition Score		2.43 ± 1.52
	Patients at low risk for malnutrition (n, %)	60 (78.9)
	Patients at average risk for malnutrition (n, %)	16 (21.1)
	Patients at high risk for malnutrition (n, %)	0 (0.0)

BMI, body mass index; CFRD, Cystic-fibrosis-related diabetes; FEV_1, forced expiratory volume at 1 s; MRSA, methicillin-resistant *Staphylococcus aureus*; PI, pancreatic insufficiency; RDA, recommended dietary allowance; * Values presented as n (%), or mean ± standard deviation.

3.2. Factors Associated with Malnutrition Risk

In the total sample, a moderate positive association was noted between malnutrition risk and age ($r = 0.369$, $p = 0.001$). Malnutrition risk was inversely associated with BAZ ($r = -0.684$, $p < 0.001$), HAZ ($r = -0.264$, $p = 0.021$), and FEV1% ($r = -0.616$, $p < 0.001$). Referring to arm anthropometrics, malnutrition risk was not associated with TSF, MUAC, MUAMA or MUAFA z-scores ($p > 0.05$ for all comparisons). When the aforementioned indices were examined according to sex, similar results were revealed, with the exception of age. In further detail, malnutrition risk did not significantly associate with the age of boys (data not shown).

When patients were stratified according to malnutrition risk, several differences between the groups were identified (Table 2). Patients classified as having a low malnutrition risk were younger ($p = 0.004$), heavier ($p < 0.001$) and taller ($p = 0.009$) than their moderate-risk counterparts. Significantly more patients in the medium-risk group were in puberty ($p = 0.034$), whereas patients in the moderate-risk group exhibited smaller mean mid upper arm fat area ($p = 0.011$), and overall worse pulmonary function ($p < 0.001$).

Table 2. Associations between anthropometry and clinical parameters, by malnutrition risk strata ($N = 76$).

Variable	Malnutrition Risk		p-Value
	Low ($n = 60$)	Medium ($n = 16$)	
Sex (% girls)	58.3	56.3	0.881
Age (years)	11.2 ± 3.8	14.4 ± 3.4	0.004
Adolescence (%)	33.3	62.5	0.034
BAZ	0.41 ± 0.92	−1.28 ± 0.78	<0.001
Underweight (%)	3.3	18.8	0.027
Nutritional Failure (%)	8.3	56.3	<0.001
Ideal Body Weight (%)	75.0	0.0	<0.001
HAZ	−0.10 ± 1.04	−0.93 ± 1.03	0.009
Stunting (%)	3.3	12.5	0.145
MUACz	−0.41 ± 0.96	−0.46 ± 1.05	0.885
TSFz	1.56 ± 0.80	1.82 ± 1.07	0.371
MUAMAz	0.16 ± 2.77	−0.29 ± 2.54	0.562
MUAFAz	1.24 ± 1.45	0.23 ± 0.90	0.011
FEV_1%	103.4 ± 15.4	77.7 ± 21.8	<0.001
Dietary Intake (% RDA)	137 ± 49	125 ± 42	0.384
$FEV_1 > 90$% (%)	80.4	37.5	0.001
Homozygote F508del (%)	43.3	31.3	0.382
Age at diagnosis (months)	3.5 (1.0, 8.8)	5.0 (1.0, 9.5)	0.627
Meconium Ileus (%)	16.7	25.0	0.445
Diagnosis by NBS (%)	13.3	6.3	0.436

BAZ, body mass index for age; FEV_1, forced expiratory volume at 1 s; HAZ, height-for age; MUAC, mid upper arm circumference; MUAFA, mid upper arm fat area; MUAMA, mid upper arm muscle area; NBS, new-born screening; RDA, recommended dietary allowance; TSF, triceps skinfold.

None of the other clinical parameters were associated with any of the nutritional risk strata. Interestingly, among the children attaining ideal body weight, none were categorized as being of moderate risk for malnutrition. On the other hand, 37.5% of the participants stratified as being at moderate risk for malnutrition exhibited physiological lung function.

4. Discussion

In the present study, participants with CF were predominantly well-nourished and exhibited adequate physiological lung function, with a moderate risk for malnutrition prevailing only in small proportions (1/5) of the sample, and none of the patients were classified as being of high malnutrition risk. Malnutrition risk was inversely associated with patients' anthropometry and lung function. Although none of the patients attaining ideal body weight for CF were at nutritional risk, this was not the case for physiological lung function, with 38% of the children with $FEV_1 > 90$% being allocated in the moderate risk for malnutrition group.

Throughout the literature, BMI z-scores have been extensively employed to identify malnutrition in pediatric CF patients, using a variety of cut-offs (Table 3). Most of the studies suggest that attaining a BMI below the 10th percentile (roughly corresponding to a z-score $< −1.0$) is indicative of malnutrition. With this in mind, published data suggest that malnutrition prevails in 12–74% of pediatric patients with CF [21–26]. Some earlier studies using the stricter cut-off of the 15th BMI percentile to identify malnutrition support similar findings, with malnutrition being diagnosed in 20–30% of pediatric patients [27–30]. Nevertheless, very few studies have examined the risk for malnutrition among pediatric patients with CF. In the validation study of the screening tool employed in the present study, dos Santos Simon and colleagues [15] reported a moderate malnutrition risk in 36.6% of their sample and a high malnutrition risk at 7.3% of their pediatric patients.

Table 3. The existing literature on the prevalence of malnutrition among children and adolescents with CF.

First Author	Country	Population		Cut-off Used for Malnutrition Diagnosis	Prevalence of Malnutrition (%)
		N (% Girls)	Age (Years)		
Barni [24]	Brasil	73 (55%)	25.6 ± 7.3	BMI < 10th percentile	24.7
Chaves [26]	Brasil	48 (NR)	10.8 ± 3.3	BMI < 10th percentile	29
Isa [23]	Bahrain	47 (43%)	<18	BMI < 10th percentile	22.1
Kilinc [22]	Turkey	143 (47%)	0–18	BMI < 10th percentile	74
Lucidi [28]	Italy	82 (49%)	13 (5–30)	BMI < 15th percentile	20.9
Panagopoulou [25]	Greece	68 (49%)	19.81 ± 8.98	BMI < 10th percentile	45.5
Phong [21]	USA	49 (27%)	9.4 ± 5.2	BMI < 10th percentile	12
				MUACz < −1.0	49
Poulimeneas [16]	Greece	84 (58%)	11.8 ± 3.9	BMI < 15th percentile	17.9
Wiedemann [27]	Germany	4557 (NR)	0–18	BMI < 15th percentile	30.4
Wiedemann [30]	Germany	2688 (NR)	0–18	BMI < 15th percentile	28.6
Zhang [29]	USA	13,021 (NR)	2–18	BMI < 15th percentile	10–30

BMI, body mass index; CF, cystic Fibrosis; MUAC, mid upper arm circumference; NR, not reported.

In the present analysis, patients at risk for malnutrition were shorter and exhibited a lower BMI than their counterparts with low-malnutrition risk. While malnutrition is a known effector impeding linear growth, weight and height measures have also been critiqued for not providing early signs of malnutrition in children with CF [31].

A similar case might also apply for FEV_1. Consistent with the existing literature [32], patients at malnutrition risk exhibited worse pulmonary function. Notably, even though the moderate malnutrition risk group demonstrated an impaired mean pulmonary function than the low-risk group, 38% of the patients with moderate malnutrition risk exhibited an adequate lung function (predicted $FEV_1 \geq 90\%$). At the same time, 1/5 of the children with low malnutrition risk demonstrated impaired lung function (predicted $FEV_1 < 90\%$). These observations may indicate that in response to malnutrition, lung function is delayed, or that FEV_1 measures may not be sensitive enough during the early phase and signs of malnutrition (given that in a large proportion of the patients, malnutrition risk was "masked" under adequate lung function). For this reason, triage for malnutrition using CF-specific tools is required in all cases and one should not rely on anthropometric indices or pulmonary function alone. It may also be that these measures are more sensitive in identifying malnutrition risk when their secular trends are taken into account, such as when using CF-specific screening tools for malnutrition, like in the present study.

Other risk factors for malnutrition identified in the present study include ascending age, puberty, and diminished fat mass. In our sample, age was positively correlated with malnutrition risk, a finding more profound among girl participants. Regardless of sex, BMI has been previously shown to decline with age [27], while, on the other hand, age has been associated with malnutrition [24]. The fact that this association was more apparent among girls may be attributed to the worse influence of the disease in the girls as compared to the boys, as previously documented in the literature [33,34].

With regards to puberty, it remains a grey area in CF-research. Girls with CF have been reported to enter puberty with a two year delay as compared to their healthy counterparts [35,36]. In parallel, a delay in reaching peak height velocity in adolescence has been reported to take place [36], and for this, a greater proportion of adolescents with CF are underweight as compared to the children [16]. This delay in puberty has also been reported to influence bone health and mineralization [37], making patients with CF more vulnerable to fractures and osteoporosis [38].

With regards to the relationship between low fat mass and malnutrition risk, very few studies have assessed body composition among children with CF. Although a variety of tools have been proposed for the assessment of body composition in CF [39], the majority of studies have used adult samples. In parallel, a consensus on body composition measurements, diagnoses and thresholds is required to attain a uniform core set of outcomes [40]. Case-control studies have revealed a greater visceral adipose tissue mass among patients with CF as compared to healthy controls, and this was associated with poorer diet quality [41]. In parallel, according to many cross-sectional studies, reduced fat-free mass has been associated with reduced pulmonary function assessed by FEV_1 and frequency of exacerbations in both children and adults with CF [42–44]. All studies agree that fat-free mass is more sensitive than BMI for assessing malnutrition and compromised pulmonary function. Overall, our findings, combined with the current literature, call for the need for routine measurements of multiple auxological indices (body height and weight, along with body composition measures) in children and adolescents with CF, in order to attain timely assessments of malnutrition risk.

The limitations of the present study include its cross-sectional design, not allowing for the establishment of causality in the observed relationships. The sample might appear as relatively small, however, sampling was performed in the largest CF center in Greece, located in the capital of Greece providing CF-care to a large population with CF. The inclusion of younger children (aged < 6 years old) in our sample may have provided more robust results, given that early-life malnutrition impairs lung function, and this impairment is persistent for over a decade [45]. Although a greater malnutrition risk was identified during adolescence, no data were recorded with regards to the pubertal stage. Stratification by pubertal stage might have provided further insight into the observed relationships, an analysis we were unable to perform and that future studies should elaborate on. Cystic Fibrosis Transmembrane Regulator (CFTR) modulator therapy commenced shortly after the present study was conducted [46], hence no data were reported on the association of malnutrition risk and the specific therapy. This evidence gap should be further examined by future research, given the positive effects of CFTR modulators in anthropometric indices of individuals with CF [47]. Furthermore, no data concerning biochemical parameters and malnutrition risk were recorded. It is highly possible that serum lipid levels or circulating levels of other nutrients might have produced significant associations with malnutrition risk, however, we did not want to cherry-pick associations that were not predefined in advance. On the other hand, the present study is one of the few that have assessed malnutrition risk in the pediatric CF population, further highlighting risk factors for malnutrition that may be masked under optimal clinical outcomes (such as physiological lung function).

5. Conclusions

In this cohort of predominantly well-nourished patients with CF, 1/5 of the patients were at risk for malnutrition, with those that were older, pubertal or with diminished fat-mass being at higher risk. Screening for malnutrition risk in pediatric patients with CF is important, although often neglected. Even in populations with a low prevalence of malnutrition, the risk for malnutrition might be elevated, highlighting the need for more frequent assessments and nutrition interventions.

Author Contributions: Conceptualization, D.P. and T.V.; methodology, D.P., M.G.G. and T.V.; formal analysis, D.P.; investigation, D.P., A.P., and A.G.K.; data curation, D.P.; writing—original draft preparation, D.P. and M.G.G.; writing—review and editing, all authors; supervision and project administration, T.V.; funding acquisition, T.V. All authors have read and agreed to the published version of the manuscript.

Funding: This research did not receive any external funding.

Acknowledgments: The authors wish to express their gratitude to the patients, and their parents/guardians for participating in this study. The authors acknowledge the University of West Attica, Athens, Greece, for funding the present publication.

Conflicts of Interest: The authors declare no conflict of interest.

References

1. Culhane, S.; George, C.; Pearo, B.; Spoede, E. Malnutrition in cystic fibrosis: A review. *Nutr. Clin. Pract.* **2013**, *28*, 676–683. [CrossRef] [PubMed]
2. Pencharz, P.B.; Durie, P.R. Pathogenesis of malnutrition in cystic fibrosis, and its treatment. *Clin. Nutr.* **2000**, *19*, 387–394. [CrossRef] [PubMed]
3. Solomon, M.; Bozic, M.; Mascarenhas, M.R. Nutritional Issues in Cystic Fibrosis. *Clin. Chest Med.* **2016**, *37*, 97–107. [CrossRef] [PubMed]
4. Poulimeneas, D.; Grammatikopoulou, M.G.; Devetzi, P.; Petrocheilou, A.; Kaditis, A.G.; Papamitsou, T.; Doudounakis, S.E.; Vassilakou, T. Adherence to dietary recommendations, nutrient intake adequacy and diet quality among pediatric cystic fibrosis patients: Results from the greecf study. *Nutrients* **2020**, *12*, 3126. [CrossRef]
5. Brownell, J.N.; Bashaw, H.; Stallings, V.A. Growth and Nutrition in Cystic Fibrosis. *Semin. Respir. Crit. Care Med.* **2019**, *40*, 775–791. [CrossRef]
6. Dray, X.; Kanaan, R.; Bienvenu, T.; Desmazes-Dufeu, N.; Dusser, D.; Marteau, P.; Hubert, D. Malnutrition in adults with cystic fibrosis. *Eur. J. Clin. Nutr.* **2005**, *59*, 152–154. [CrossRef]
7. Ashkenazi, M.; Nathan, N.; Sarouk, I.; Aluma, B.E.B.; Dagan, A.; Bezalel, Y.; Keler, S.; Vilozni, D.; Efrati, O. Nutritional Status in Childhood as a Prognostic Factor in Patients with Cystic Fibrosis. *Lung* **2019**, *197*, 371–376. [CrossRef]
8. Kumru, B.; Emiralioğlu, N.; Gökmen Ozel, H. Malnutrition in children with cystic fibrosis. *Clin. Nutr.* **2018**, *37*, S90–S91. [CrossRef]
9. Reilly, J.J.; Edwards, C.A.; Weaver, L.T. Malnutrition in children with cystic fibrosis: The energy-balance equation. *J. Pediatr. Gastroenterol. Nutr.* **1997**, *25*, 127–136. [CrossRef]
10. Poulimeneas, D.; Grammatikopoulou, M.G.; Petrocheilou, A.; Kaditis, A.G.; Troupi, E.; Doudounakis, S.E.; Laggas, D.; Vassilakou, T. Comparison of International Growth Standards for Assessing Nutritional Status in Cystic Fibrosis: The GreeCF Study. *J. Pediatr. Gastroenterol. Nutr.* **2020**, *71*, e35–e39. [CrossRef]
11. Rocha, G.A.; Rocha, E.J.M.; Martins, C.V. The effects of hospitalization on the nutritional status of children. *J. Pediatr. (Rio. J.)* **2006**, *82*, 70–74. [CrossRef] [PubMed]
12. Shaaban, S.; Nassar, M.; El-Gendy, Y.; El-Shaer, B. Nutritional risk screening of hospitalized children aged < 3 years. *EMHJ* **2019**, *25*, 18–23. [PubMed]
13. Klanjsek, P.; Pajnkihar, M.; Marcun Varda, N.; Povalej Brzan, P. Screening and assessment tools for early detection of malnutrition in hospitalised children: A systematic review of validation studies. *BMJ Open* **2019**, *9*, e025444. [CrossRef] [PubMed]
14. McDonald, C.M. Validation of a nutrition risk screening tool for children and adolescents with cystic fibrosis ages 2-20 years. *J. Pediatr. Gastroenterol. Nutr.* **2008**, *46*, 438–446. [CrossRef]
15. Souza Dos Santos Simon, M.I.; Forte, G.C.; da Silva Pereira, J.; da Fonseca Andrade Procianoy, E.; Drehmer, M. Validation of a Nutrition Screening Tool for Pediatric Patients with Cystic Fibrosis. *J. Acad. Nutr. Diet.* **2016**, *116*, 813–818. [CrossRef]
16. Poulimeneas, D.; Petrocheilou, A.; Grammatikopoulou, M.G.; Kaditis, A.G.; Loukou, I.; Doudounakis, S.E.; Laggas, D.; Vassilakou, T. High attainment of optimal nutritional and growth status observed among Greek pediatric cystic fibrosis patients: Results from the GreeCF study. *J. Pediatr. Endocrinol. Metab.* **2017**, *30*, 1169–1176. [CrossRef]
17. Kuczmarski, R.J.; Ogden, C.L.; Guo, S.S.; Grummer-Strawn, L.M.; Flegal, K.M.; Mei, Z.; Wei, R.; Curtin, L.R.; Roche, A.F.; Johnson, C.L. 2000 CDC growth charts for the United States: Methods and development. *Vital Heal. Stat.* **2002**, *11*, 1–190.
18. Frisancho, R.A. *Anthropometric Standards for the Assessment of Growth and Nutritional Status*, 1st ed.; University of Michigan Press: Ann Arbor, MI, USA, 2008.
19. Wang, X.; Dockery, D.W.; Wypij, D.; Fay, M.E.; Ferris, B.G. Pulmonary function between 6 and 18 years of age. *Pediatr. Pulmonol.* **1993**, *15*, 75–88. [CrossRef]
20. Hankinson, J.L.; Odencrantz, J.R.; Fedan, K.B. Spirometric reference values from a sample of the general U.S. population. *Am. J. Respir. Crit. Care Med.* **1999**, *159*, 179–187. [CrossRef]
21. Phong, R.Y.; Taylor, S.L.; Robinson, B.A.; Jhawar, S.; Nandalike, K. Utility of Mid-Upper Arm Circumference in Diagnosing Malnutrition in Children With Cystic Fibrosis. *Nutr. Clin. Pract.* **2020**, *35*, 1094–1100. [CrossRef]

22. Kilinc, A.A.; Beser, O.F.; Ugur, E.P.; Cokugras, F.C.; Cokugras, H. The Effects of Nutritional Status and Intervention on Pulmonary Functions in Pediatric Cystic Fibrosis Patients. *Pediatr. Int.* **2020**. [CrossRef] [PubMed]
23. Isa, H.M.; Al-Ali, L.F.; Mohamed, A.M. Growth assessment and risk factors of malnutrition in children with cystic fibrosis. *Saudi Med. J.* **2016**, *37*, 293–298. [CrossRef] [PubMed]
24. Barni, G.C.; Forte, G.C.; Forgiarini, L.F.; Abrahão, C.L.D.O.; Dalcin, P.D.T.R. Factors associated with malnutrition in adolescent and adult patients with cystic fibrosis. *J. Bras. Pneumol.* **2017**, *43*, 337–343. [CrossRef] [PubMed]
25. Panagopoulou, P.; Fotoulaki, M.; Nikolaou, A.; Nousia-Arvanitakis, S. Prevalence of malnutrition and obesity among cystic fibrosis patients. *Pediatr. Int.* **2014**, *56*, 89–94. [CrossRef] [PubMed]
26. Chaves, C.R.M.D.M.; Britto, J.A.A.D.; Oliveira, C.Q.D.; Gomes, M.M.; Cunha, A.L.P.D. Association between nutritional status measurements and pulmonary function in children and adolescents with cystic fibrosis. *J. Bras. Pneumol.* **2009**, *35*, 409–414. [CrossRef]
27. Wiedemann, B.; Paul, K.D.; Stern, M.; Wagner, T.O.; Hirche, T.O.; German CFQA Group. Evaluation of body mass index percentiles for assessment of malnutrition in children with cystic fibrosis. *Eur. J. Clin. Nutr.* **2007**, *61*, 759–768. [CrossRef]
28. Lucidi, V.; Bizzarri, C.; Alghisi, F.; Bella, S.; Russo, B.; Ubertini, G.; Cappa, M. Bone and body composition analyzed by Dual-energy X-ray Absorptiometry (DXA) in clinical and nutritional evaluation of young patients with Cystic Fibrosis: A cross-sectional study. *BMC Pediatr.* **2009**, *9*, 61. [CrossRef]
29. Zhang, Z.; Lai, H.J. Comparison of the use of body mass index percentiles and percentage of ideal body weight to screen for malnutrition in children with cystic fibrosis. *Am. J. Clin. Nutr.* **2004**, *80*, 982–991. [CrossRef]
30. Wiedemann, B.; Steinkamp, G.; Sens, B.; Stern, M.; German Cystic Fibrosis Quality Assurance Group. The German cystic fibrosis quality assurance project: Clinical features in children and adults. *Eur. Respir. J.* **2001**, *17*, 1187–1194. [CrossRef]
31. Stapleton, D.; Kerr, D.; Gurrin, L.; Sherriff, J.; Sly, P. Height and weight fail to detect early signs of malnutrition in children with cystic fibrosis. *J. Pediatr. Gastroenterol. Nutr.* **2001**, *33*, 319–325. [CrossRef]
32. Mauch, R.M.; Kmit, A.H.P.; de Marson, F.A.L.; Levy, C.E.; de Barros-Filho, A.A.; Ribeiro, J.D. Association of growth and nutritional parameters with pulmonary function in cystic fibrosis: A literature review. *Rev. Paul. Pediatr.* **2016**, *34*, 503–509. [CrossRef] [PubMed]
33. Barr, H.L.; Britton, J.; Smyth, A.R.; Fogarty, A.W. Association between socioeconomic status, sex, and age at death from cystic fibrosis in England and Wales (1959 to 2008): Cross sectional study. *BMJ* **2011**, *343*, d4662. [CrossRef] [PubMed]
34. Jackson, A.D.; Daly, L.; Jackson, A.L.; Kelleher, C.; Marshall, B.C.; Quinton, H.B.; Fletcher, G.; Harrington, M.; Zhou, S.; McKone, E.F.; et al. Validation and use of a parametric model for projecting cystic fibrosis survivorship beyond observed data: A birth cohort analysis. *Thorax* **2011**, *66*, 674–679. [CrossRef] [PubMed]
35. Umławska, W.; Sands, D.; Zielińska, A. Age of menarche in girls with cystic fibrosis. *Folia Histochem. Cytobiol.* **2010**, *48*, 185–190. [CrossRef]
36. Zhang, Z.; Lindstrom, M.J.; Farrell, P.M.; Lai, H.J.; Wisconsin Cystic Fibrosis Neonatal Screening Group. Pubertal Height Growth and Adult Height in Cystic Fibrosis After Newborn Screening. *Pediatrics* **2016**, *137*, e20152907. [CrossRef] [PubMed]
37. Sermet-Gaudelus, I.; Castanet, M.; Retsch-Bogart, G.; Aris, R.M. Update on cystic fibrosis-related bone disease: A special focus on children. *Paediatr. Respir. Rev.* **2009**, *10*, 134–142. [CrossRef] [PubMed]
38. Putman, M.S.; Anabtawi, A.; Le, T.; Tangpricha, V.; Sermet-Gaudelus, I. Cystic fibrosis bone disease treatment: Current knowledge and future directions. *J. Cyst. Fibros.* **2019**, *18* (Suppl. 2), S56–S65. [CrossRef]
39. Calella, P.; Valerio, G.; Brodlie, M.; Taylor, J.; Donini, L.M.; Siervo, M. Tools and Methods Used for the Assessment of Body Composition in Patients With Cystic Fibrosis: A Systematic Review. *Nutr. Clin. Pract.* **2019**, *34*, 701–714. [CrossRef]
40. Declercq, D.; Van Meerhaeghe, S.; Marchand, S.; Van Braeckel, E.; van Daele, S.; De Baets, F.; Van Biervliet, S. The nutritional status in CF: Being certain about the uncertainties. *Clin. Nutr. ESPEN* **2018**, *29*, 15–21. [CrossRef]
41. Bellissimo, M.P.; Zhang, I.; Ivie, E.A.; Tran, P.H.; Tangpricha, V.; Hunt, W.R.; Stecenko, A.A.; Ziegler, T.R.; Alvarez, J.A. Visceral adipose tissue is associated with poor diet quality and higher fasting glucose in adults with cystic fibrosis. *J. Cyst. Fibros.* **2019**, *18*, 430–435. [CrossRef]

42. Gomes, A.; Hutcheon, D.; Ziegler, J. Association Between Fat-Free Mass and Pulmonary Function in Patients With Cystic Fibrosis: A Narrative Review. *Nutr. Clin. Pract.* **2019**, *34*, 715–727. [CrossRef] [PubMed]
43. Calella, P.; Valerio, G.; Thomas, M.; McCabe, H.; Taylor, J.; Brodlie, M.; Siervo, M. Association between body composition and pulmonary function in children and young people with cystic fibrosis. *Nutrition* **2018**, *48*, 73–76. [CrossRef] [PubMed]
44. Alicandro, G.; Bisogno, A.; Battezzati, A.; Bianchi, M.L.; Corti, F.; Colombo, C. Recurrent pulmonary exacerbations are associated with low fat free mass and low bone mineral density in young adults with cystic fibrosis. *J. Cyst. Fibros.* **2014**, *13*, 328–334. [CrossRef] [PubMed]
45. Sanders, D.B.; Zhang, Z.; Farrell, P.M.; Lai, H.J.; Wisconsin CF Neonatal Screening Group. Early life growth patterns persist for 12 years and impact pulmonary outcomes in cystic fibrosis. *J. Cyst. Fibros.* **2018**, *17*, 528–535. [CrossRef] [PubMed]
46. Loukou, I.; Moustaki, M.; Plyta, M.; Douros, K. Longitudinal changes in lung function following initiation of lumacaftor/ivacaftor combination. *J. Cyst. Fibros.* **2020**, *19*, 534–539. [CrossRef]
47. Bailey, J.; Rozga, M.; McDonald, C.M.; Bowser, E.K.; Farnham, K.; Mangus, M.; Padula, L.; Porco, K.; Alvarez, J.A. Effect of CFTR Modulators on Anthropometric Parameters in Individuals with Cystic Fibrosis: An Evidence Analysis Center Systematic Review. *J. Acad. Nutr. Diet.* **2020**. online ahead of print. [CrossRef]

Publisher's Note: MDPI stays neutral with regard to jurisdictional claims in published maps and institutional affiliations.

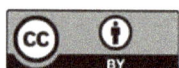

© 2020 by the authors. Licensee MDPI, Basel, Switzerland. This article is an open access article distributed under the terms and conditions of the Creative Commons Attribution (CC BY) license (http://creativecommons.org/licenses/by/4.0/).

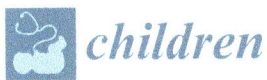

Article

Sociodemographic Correlates of Obesity among Spanish Schoolchildren: A Cross-Sectional Study

José Francisco López-Gil [1,*], Alba López-Benavente [2], Pedro Juan Tárraga López [3] and Juan Luis Yuste Lucas [2]

1. Departamento de Actividad Física y Deporte, Facultad de Ciencias del Deporte, Universidad de Murcia (UM), San Javier, 30720 Murcia, Spain
2. Departamento de Expresión Plástica, Musical y Dinámica, Facultad de Educación, Universidad de Murcia (UM), Espinardo, 30100 Murcia, Spain; alba.lopez3@um.es (A.L.-B.); jlyuste@um.es (J.L.Y.L.)
3. Departamento de Ciencias Médicas, Facultad de Medicina, Universidad Castilla-La Mancha (UCLM), 02008 Albacete, Spain; pjtarraga@sescam.jccm.es
* Correspondence: josefranciscolopezgil@gmail.com

Received: 4 September 2020; Accepted: 22 October 2020; Published: 28 October 2020

Abstract: Some studies have been conducted in order to assess the association between weight status (assessed by body mass index) and socio-demographic factors. Nevertheless, only a few of them have indicated these associations by other anthropometric parameters (e.g., skinfolds). The aim of this study was to determine, compare, and examine the influence of age, sex, type of the schooling, per capita income, area of residence, and immigrant status on obesity parameters in schoolchildren aged 6–13 from the Region of Murcia. A cross-sectional study was carried out in six different Primary schools of the Region of Murcia (Spain). A total sample of 370 children (166 girls) aged 6–13 (8.7 ± 1.8) were selected. In order to determine participants' body composition, body mass index, waist circumference, waist-to-height ratio, and skinfold measurements were calculated. Higher associations of excess of weight (OR = 1.96; 95%CI = 1.19–3.20) and abdominal obesity (OR = 3.12; 95CI% = 1.49–6.94) were shown in the case of children from public schools. A greater association of high trunk fat mass was found in children from municipalities with high per capita income (OR = 3.20; 95%CI = 1.05–9.77). Therefore, lower association of having an inadequate %BF was found in the participants aged 6–9 (OR = 0.38; 95%CI = 0.24–0.54), and immigrant students (OR = 2.63; 95%CI = 1.69–4.10). Our study suggested that overweight/obesity among schoolchildren in the Region of Murcia is higher than the overall prevalence of Spain. The results of the adjusted analyses showed that age, type of schooling, per capita income, and immigrant status were associated with obesity parameters.

Keywords: adiposity; waist circumference; anthropometry; children; socioeconomic factors; health inequality indicators

1. Introduction

Globally, overweight and obesity have reached worryingly high levels [1], especially in Europe, where this situation represents a major public health threat [2]. Thus, the last World Health Organization (WHO) European Childhood Obesity Surveillance (COSI) study has ranked Spain with the highest obesity prevalence rate in Europe (17.7%) [2]. The risk of morbidity and mortality in adult life increases in those who are overweight or obese (understood as excess weight) in their childhood or adolescence [3], which also increases the likelihood of having worse risk parameters for cardiovascular disease [4]. This is why the WHO Member States have committed to ensuring that childhood obesity figures do not increase by 2025 [5].

Regarding obesity identification, body mass index (BMI) is the most applied anthropometric parameter in children; existing several reference cut-off points, both internationally [6–8] and nationally [9]. However, even though BMI can be an assessment tool to help detect overweight or obese children, it has been advised that it does not identify the majority of children who will develop morbidities related to obesity in adult life [10]. Also, there is a great variability in the association of BMI and fat mass, which could be due to physiological changes, the level of pubertal maturation, and the sex of the children [11]. In the same way, during the process of growth and development, several changes occur in body composition, mainly in the storage and distribution of fat, muscle, and bone mass according to age and sex [12]. Thus, a recent systematic review performed by Orsso et al. [13] has suggested that skinfold measurements are one of the possible reliable methodologies for determining body composition in paediatric obesity. At the same time, Schröder et al. [14] found a large proportion of normal-weight Spanish children who present abdominal obesity. For these reasons, evaluation accompanied by other body composition variables is highly recommended, such as waist-to-height ratio (WHtR), waist circumference (WC), or skinfolds in order to effectively determine the risk in participants [15].

Following this line, some studies have been conducted in order to assess the association between weight status (assessed by BMI) and socio-demographic factors, such as sex [16], type of schooling [17], area of residence [18], immigrant status [19], or per capita income [20]. For example, children from public schools have been associated with a higher prevalence of overweight or obesity [17], as well as children belonging to an immigrant family [21]. Equally, the prevalence of obesity is significantly higher in school children from families with lower incomes compared to those with higher ones in Spain [22], being so in the case of children from rural areas [23]. Hence, some of these studies have shown certain degree of association between these variables. Notwithstanding, only a few of them have indicated these associations by other anthropometric parameters (e.g., skinfolds) [24], and there is a gap of knowledge in this sense.

In addition to this, children and adolescents who have obesity are about five times as likely to be obese in adulthood than their counterparts who do not present obesity [25]. Thus, because of the long-term implications of childhood obesity and the influence on their health in adulthood, studies to clarify the relationship between sociodemographic characteristics and the risk of overweight and obesity merits further consideration [26]. As a result, identifying those children at high risk of being obese in adulthood and its related factors could be a useful matter; particularly in the Region of Murcia, where the greatest figures of excess weight children has been pointed out [27].

According to the worrying situation of childhood obesity in Spain, particularly in the Region of Murcia, as well as the lack of information about those sociodemographic factors that could be related to childhood obesity, the aim of this research was to determine, compare and examine the influence of age, sex, type of the schooling, area of residence, immigrant status, and per capita income on obesity parameters in schoolchildren aged 6–13 from the Region of Murcia.

2. Materials and Methods

2.1. Sample

This study had a cross-sectional design. All nine primary schools from the Valley of Ricote (Region of Murcia, Spain) were invited to take part, with six schools agreeing to participate. Out of 972 possible participants, a total of 370 schoolchildren (166 girls and 204 boys) with ages between 6–13 years old (8.7 ± 1.8) participated, representing a response rate of 38.1%. For this study we used the non-probability sampling technique. In spite of this, all schoolchildren were likewise offered to join.

All the children involved in the study had to provide a signed consent form by their parents/legal guardians. Before the performance of the study, both parents and children were informed about the purpose of the research and the type of tests that would be carried out. Data was obtained in the 2017/2018 academic year. All the measurements were performed during Physical Education classes. As an inclusion criterion, only schoolchildren aged 6–13 who had obtained positive informed consent from their parents or legal guardians were included.

Regarding the origin of the immigrant students ($n = 71$), 61.1% are of South American origin, 29.1% of Arab origin, 5.6% from other European countries, 2.8% born in Asia, and 1.4% of African origin.

The Bioethics Committee of the University of Murcia (ID 2218/2018) approved the present study. It has been executed respecting the human rights of the participants and following the Helsinki Declaration.

2.2. Data Collection

Sex and age were self-reported. The type of schooling was dichotomised into two categories: (1) public and (2) private with public funds. Area of residence was divided into (1) urban (>5000 inhabitants) and (2) rural (≤5000 inhabitants) [28]. Students who met at least one of the following conditions were considered to be immigrant: (a) born outside Spain, (b) immigrant parents, or (c) at least one of their parents comes from another country. The socio-economic characteristics were determined by the per capita income of the different municipalities. Thus, this variable was dichotomised into two groups: (1) high per capita income (€20,000 or more) and (2) low per capita income (under €20,000). A portable height rod with an accuracy of 0.1 cm (Leicester Tanita HR 001, Tokyo, Japan) was used so as to determine participants' height. Their bodyweight was measured with an electronic scale with an accuracy of 0.1 kg (Tanita BC-545, Tokyo, Japan). BMI was calculated from the ratio between body weight (kg) and the height squared of the participants (m^2). Besides, weight status was determined using the age-specific and sex-specific thresholds provided by the WHO [6]. WC was measured with a precision of 0.1 cm at the level of the intersection between the last rib and the border of the iliac crest, using a constant tension tape. Children were split by "no high trunk fat mass" and "high trunk fat mass" according to sex- and age-specific cut-off values [29]. Moreover, the WHtR was calculated in order to determine the prevalence of abdominal obesity and children were classified as "no abdominal obesity" and "abdominal obesity" [30]. Skinfold measurements (subscapular, iliac crest, biceps and triceps) were taken using pre-calibrated steel callipers with a precision of 0.2 mm (Holtain, Crosswell, Crymych, United Kingdom) and following the guidelines of the International Society for the Advancement of Kinanthropometry (ISAK) [31]. To calculate the body density, the log of the sum of skinfolds measurements was considered [32]. Siri formula was used in order to compute body fat from body density [33], and fat-free mass was then determined minus total body mass and body fat (BF) mass. Likewise, participants were divided into "adequate adiposity" and "high adiposity" [34].

All the measurements were performed by the same trained researcher. Two measurements were taken and, if existed discrepancies exceeding 0.1 centimetres (cm) between measurements the procedure, was performed again. The relative technical error of measurement (TEM) was obtained by performing a number of repeated measurements on the same participant, taking the differences and inserting them into a correct equation. For intra-observer TEM of the two measurements taken the following equation was applied: $\sqrt{\Sigma D/2N}$, where "D" is the difference between measurements and "N" is the number of participants measures. Also, the absolute TEM was multiplied by 100 and divided by the variable average value in order to provide the relative TEM (%TEM). The %TEM were 0.3%, 0.2%, 0.5%, and 2.3%, for weight, height, WC, and skinfolds, respectively.

2.3. Data Management and Statistical Analysis

For all continuous variables, data was shown as mean (M) and standard deviation (SD). Conversely, all categorical variables were expressed as number (n) and percentage (%). Likewise, the confidence intervals (95%) were calculated. To assess the differences between groups of age, sex, type of schooling (public/private), per capita income (high/low), area of residence (urban/rural), and immigrant status (native/immigrant), the Chi-squared test was used or, if expected values were lower than 5, Fisher's Exact test was applied. Furthermore, binary logistic regression analyses were performed to determine the association between sociodemographic characteristics and the different obesity parameters. Finally, data analysis was performed using the software SPSS (IBM Corp, Armonk, NY, USA) for Windows (v.24.0). Statistical significance was maintained at p-value ≤ 0.050.

3. Results

Data of age and continuous variables of anthropometric characteristics are shown in Table 1, as well as, the prevalence according to different obesity parameters are presented in Table 2. According to BMI, the prevalence of excess weight was 52.4% (WHO criteria). Moreover, when WC was considered, the values ranged from 14.6% to 20.3%, for abdominal obesity and high trunk mass fat, respectively. Conversely, a 45.4% presented high adiposity based on %BF.

Table 1. Characteristics of age and anthropometric parameters of the analysed sample ($n = 370$).

Variables	Mean	SD	CI$_{95\%}$
Age (years)	8.7	1.8	(8.5–8.9)
Weight (kg)	35.7	10.9	(34.6–36.8)
Height (cm)	1.36	0.12	(1.35–1.37)
BMI (kg/m^2)	19.05	3.71	(18.67–19.43)
WC (cm)	62.1	8.2	(61.3–62.9)
WHtR (WC/Height (cm))	0.46	0.05	(0.45–0.47)
BF (%)	29.63	7.13	(28.90–30.36)
BF (kg)	11.17	5.93	(10.56–11.78)
FFM (%)	70.37	7.13	(69.64–71.10)
FFM (kg)	24.54	5.58	(23.97–25.11)

Data expressed as mean, standard deviation and confident intervals (95%). BMI: body mass index; BF (%): Body fat percentage; BF (kg) = Body fat in kilograms; FFM: free-fat mass; WC: waist circumference; WHtR: waist-to-height ratio.

Table 2. Prevalence of different obesity parameters in the analysed simple.

Variables	n	%	CI$_{95\%}$
BMI (WHO)			
Overweight	104	28.1	(23.8–32.9)
Obesity	90	24.3	(20.2–29.0)
Excess weight	194	52.4	(47.3–57.5)
WHtR			
Abdominal obesity	54	14.6	(11.4–18.6)
WC			
High trunk fat mass	75	20.3	(16.5–24.7)
%BF			
High adiposity	168	45.4	(40.4–50.5)

Data expressed as frequencies, percentages and confident intervals (95%). BMI: body mass index; BF: body fat; WHO: World Health Organization; WC: waist circumference; WHtR: waist-to-height ratio.

Figure 1 shows the differences between the prevalence of obesity parameters according to the sociodemographic factors analysed. In relation to sex, boys had higher excess weight (43.6%) than girls (42.2%), with no statistically significant differences found. This absence of statistically significant differences was also shown in the case of WC, WHtR and %BF. On the other hand, no statistically significant differences were obtained for BMI, WC, and WHtR with regard to age group; not being so in the case of %BF ($p < 0.001$). So, a greater number of children aged 10–13 with great levels of %BF (22.3% higher) was identified. Regarding the type of schooling, children from public school showed greater values in all variables of obesity. Likewise, statistically significant differences were shown in most of obesity parameters that were examined (except for %BF). Also, higher prevalence of excess weight, abdominal obesity, high trunk fat mass, and high adiposity was found in the case of high per capita income group (only statistically significant for BMI). Finally, according to the area of residence, children from urban areas showed greater association with having higher obesity parameter (except for

WC) without showing statistically significant differences for any obesity parameter. Data on absolute and relative frequencies is available in Table S1.

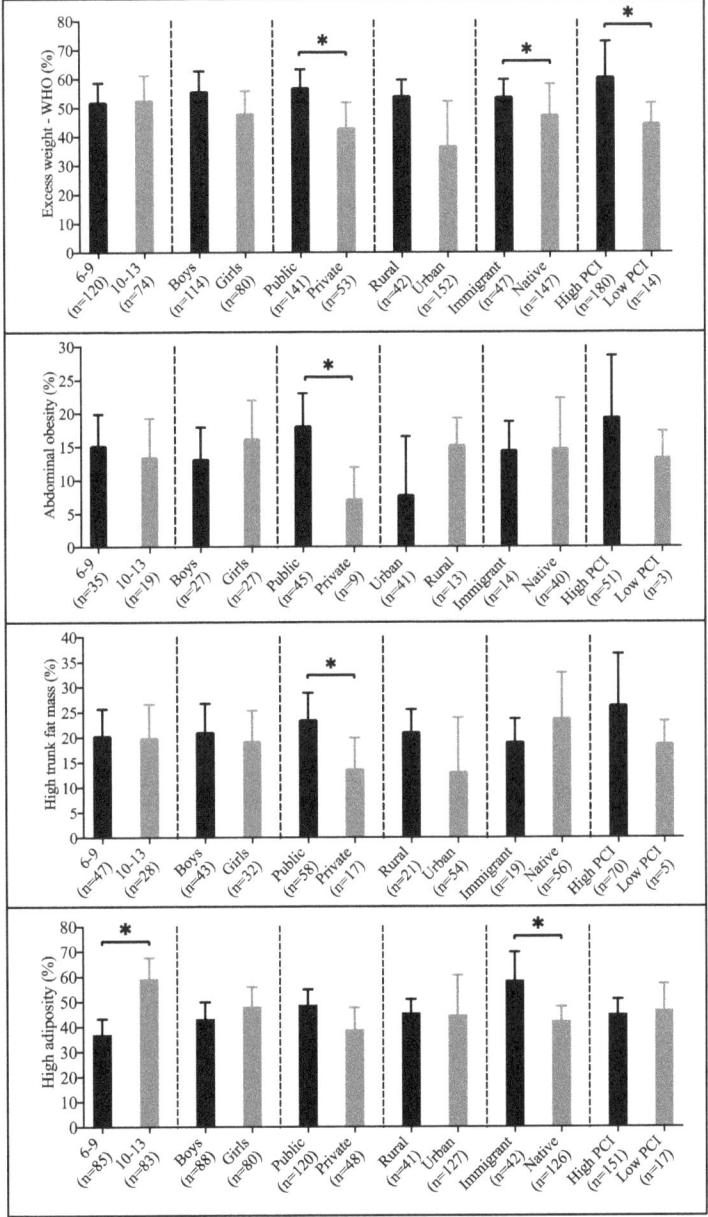

Figure 1. Prevalence of having excess weight, abdominal obesity, high trunk fat mass, and high adiposity according to the different sociodemographic factors. Data presented as number (*n*) and percentage (%). PCI: per capita income. * $p < 0.050$.

Figure 2 indicates the association between different status in the anthropometric categorical variables of the study and the age group, sex, type of schooling, per capita income, area of residence and immigrant status. Therefore, no statistically significant association was shown in the case of BMI, WC, and WHtR according to age group and sex. Conversely, a higher association of excess weight was found in children from public schools, as well as of having abdominal obesity. Lower association of having an inadequate %BF were found in the participants aged 6–9 and in boys, in those from private schools, in the low per capita income group, in children from rural areas, and in native students (only statistical significance in the case of age group and immigration). Information on odds ratio and 95% confident intervals is presented in Table S2.

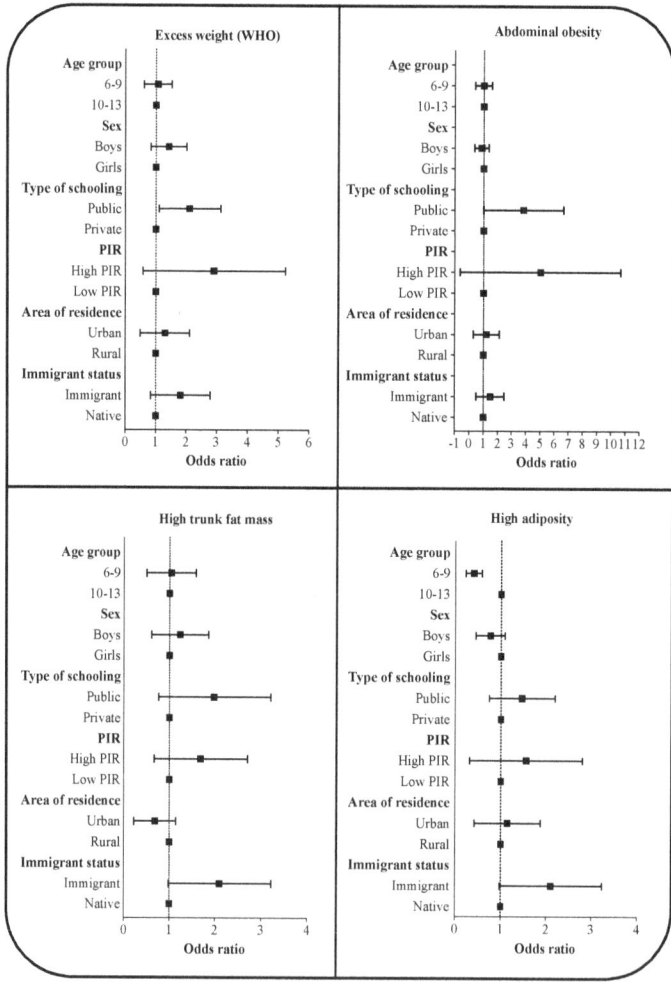

Figure 2. Association of having excess weight, abdominal obesity, high trunk fat mass, and high adiposity according to the different sociodemographic factors. Data expressed as odds ratio (confident intervals 95%). BMI: body mass index; BF: body fat; PIR: per capita income; WHO: World Health Organization; WC: waist circumference; WHtR: waist-to-height ratio. Adjusted by age group, sex, type of schooling, PIR, area of residence, and immigrant status.

4. Discussion

The aim of the present study was to determine, compare, and examine the influence of age, sex, type of the schooling, per capita income, area of residence, and immigrant status on obesity parameters in schoolchildren aged 6–13 from the Region of Murcia. In this line, this study revealed that a great number of schoolchildren are overweight/obese in the analysed sample. Our results are higher than those reported by the last Estudio ALADINO [22], which reported a prevalence of excess weight of 41.3% for boys and 39.7% for girls, and by the Estudio PASOS [35], which reported an 34.9% of excess weight. According to the Estudio ALADINO (2019), the obesity trends seem to be stabilising in Spain. However, despite this apparent stabilisation, Spain has been pointed out as the European country with the highest prevalence rate of obesity in children (17.7%) in the latest data (2015–2017) from the Childhood Obesity Surveillance Initiative (COSI) led by the WHO [2]. One possible reason for this higher prevalence could be the fact that the municipality with greater per capita income of this study was slightly over 20,000€ and it has been recently shown that the prevalence of obesity is significantly greater in schoolchildren with family incomes below €18,000 per year [22]. Also, a further explanation could be that one out of three children is at risk of child poverty and social exclusion in the Region of Murcia [27], which could at least partially explain these superior figures. However, we must consider that, as reported in the scientific literature, the etiology of obesity is multifactorial [3], so other factors could influence this greater prevalence.

In addition, in relation to age, our adjusted model did not show statistical significance in order to have excess weight. Obesity prevalence rises as children grow older [36], and age is the single major predictor of obesity in children [37]. However, it was remarkable that we did not observe any association between obesity (assessed by BMI) and age in contrast to the findings of other authors who reported that obesity significantly increased with age [38,39]. This fact was not verified in the case of %BF, which indicated higher prevalence of older children (aged 10–13) with high adiposity. These differences among methods could be explained by the different procedures that they use to examine the obesity levels. For example, BMI is not able to differentiate the amount of fat mass and free-fat mass to body weight and could cause the wrong identification of obesity status when used in children [40]. At the same time, the so-called "adiposity rebound" phenomenon in the scientific literature, characterised by an increase in body fat at around the age of 8, continues until the end of the growth process [41].

Concerning sex, the categorisation of BMI reported very close prevalence of excess weight between boys and girls. Thus, we observed that being a girl or boy did not predict the likelihood of having excess weight/obesity, a finding that is consistent with some previous studies conducted [42,43]. However, contrary to our results, some other studies either reported differences in obesity prevalence between the sexes [17,21,44] or found girls to be at increased risk for childhood obesity [39]. In the case of %BF, we found a greater number of girls with higher adiposity than boys. Our results agree with other previous studies [45,46] and was able to verify the long differences well-known for %BF [47]. Nevertheless, we must consider that we used the Siri's equation [33] that measures four skinfolds of upper body (biceps, triceps, subscapular, and suprailiac) without considering the lower body, which could modify this results. At the same time, another aspect that could have influenced this is the fact that the Siri's equation [33] seems to overestimate the %BF between boys and girls, according to some studies [46,48].

Regarding the type of schooling, children from public school were more likely to have excess weight when compared to children of private schools. This fact matches with the findings of other studies which evaluated children and adolescent's excess weight in different countries [49,50] and in Spain [17]. Therefore, it must be remarkable that public school children were more than three times likely to have abdominal obesity. These results seem to point out to the remarkable difference between public and private schools. This might be due to the fact that, in Spain, public schools are funded by the government, while private schools can charge considerably higher fees (tuition, uniform, or school materials). For this reason, only parents who can afford the fees would choose to enrol their children in private schools; the influence of socioeconomic factors in childhood obesity has already been indicated in Spain [22]. At the same time, families with low socioeconomic status may have less access or are not able to afford healthy foods and beverages compared to wealthier homes [51].

Conversely, a higher prevalence of excess weight, abdominal obesity, and especially of high trunk fat mass were shown in children from high per capita income. Our findings match with those reported by Arruda et al. [52], who reported a greater proportion of excess weight among children from families with more favourable living environments (e.g., greater per capita income). Similarly, Beal et al. [20] have recently found that higher per capita income was linked to a greater prevalence of childhood excess weight in Vietnam. Thus, income inequality could affect childhood obesity, through an increase in excessive food intake, as well as in a more sedentary lifestyle which could favour the development of overweight/obesity [1,53,54]. However, caution is needed when interpreting the results because of certain aspects. First, per capita income is referred to the municipality and not to the individual's socioeconomic status. Second, these authors used different criteria to determine per capita income, as well as different cut-off points. Third, the per capita income indicator may vary depending on the analysed country and presents certain limitations to describe wealth inequalities (e.g., gross national income or Gini index) [53].

Concerning the area of residence, the evidence available on this relationship is inconclusive [26]. For example, Bel-Serrat et al. [26] indicated no association with obesity in a large and representative sample of Irish children aged 8–12. In a systematic review of Chinese studies, Guo et al. [18] showed that the prevalence of excess weight was greater in urban areas. Conversely, other studies have indicated that children living in cities with less density of population present higher rates of childhood obesity than children who reside in urban areas, both in North America [39] and Europe [54]. Moreover, one study carried out by Vaquero-Álvarez et al. [23] found a prevalence of 48.5% of excess weight in a sample of Spanish children from rural areas. One explanation could lie in the fact that, although it is thought that a rural life implies physically demanding activities, it is not always the case, and it could have an influence in the greater prevalence of obesity in rural areas [55]. Despite the above, we found higher obesity prevalence in children from urban areas. This fact could be explained (at least in part) because the analysed schools in our study belonged to adjacent cities, so there might not be much differences between the schoolchildren. Furthermore, the total population reached in the city with the largest number of inhabitants was only around 20,000 inhabitants. These aspects, together with the criterion used for the categorisation of the area of residence [28], could have influenced the results obtained. Moreover, obesity rates by area of residence have not yet been well studied in depth [39].

In the case of immigration, we observed that immigrant children had a higher prevalence of excess weight and high adiposity. This fact is consistent with others studies performed both in Europe [56] and Spain [16,57], suggesting that belonging to an immigrant family has a higher prevalence of excess of weight. In this sense, immigrant children are more likely to suffer from social exclusion, which seems to lead to unhealthy behaviour [58] and probably to increased body weight. However, it has been pointed out that the level of adiposity may differ due to the level of integration of the local culture rather than the fact of being an immigrant itself [59]. On the other hand, the recent study by de Bont et al. [19] also found lower figures among children of African and Asian nationalities. Moreover, these same authors showed that the risk of having excess weight increased over time, according to the cumulative ages of residence in Spain. This tendency has been identified in other studies, in which it was considered that exposure and acculturation to the Western lifestyle among the immigrant population led to this increase [60]. Nonetheless, data on childhood obesity in immigrant population in Europe and Spain are limited and may fluctuate considerably in relation to what is described in the United States [19].

In this study, we found some strengths that characterise our study, we assessed several obesity-related parameters such as WC, WHtR, or %BF, apart from the most commonly used BMI. This choice is based on the intention to offer a better understanding of the childhood obesity problem since, according to previously recommendations, BMI should be complemented by other anthropometric parameters (WC, for instance) to establish efficiently the risk in individuals [14,15]. Furthermore, the inclusion of several sociodemographic factors resulted in two essential aspects: on the one hand, a better understanding of the influence of these factors on the differences in childhood obesity in the region of Spain with the highest number of obese children [27]; on the other hand, a call for both regional and national government institutions to assume responsibility, leadership, political commitment, and take action in line with the recommendations of the WHO to address childhood obesity in the long term [5]. Contrariwise, there are certain limitations that must be declared. First, because of the cross-sectional design of this study, we are not able to establish cause-effect associations. Another limitation that we found is related to the lack of information on the individual's developmental stage—for example, Tanner Stage, as an indicator of sexual maturation. In this line, differences in the distribution of BF begin at the age of the puberty, with boys developing a distribution which favours central deposition of fat, irrespective of their total BF [47]. Moreover, although we reported on per capita income of the different cities, information on the individual's socioeconomic status could provide more accurate information about this variable.

Finally, our study suggested that overweight/obesity among schoolchildren in the Region of Murcia is higher than the overall prevalence of Spain. The result of the adjusted analyses showed that age, type of schooling, per capita income, and immigrant status were associated with obesity parameters. The identification of socio-demographic variables related to paediatric obesity can be an appropriate tool for possible early prevention and intervention. Public health policies and interventions aimed at the prevention and treatment of childhood obesity should incorporate a sensitive and clear focus on social and economic inequalities; emphasising on the groups most at risk.

Supplementary Materials: The following are available online at http://www.mdpi.com/2227-9067/7/11/201/s1, Table S1. Prevalence of having excess weight, abdominal obesity, high trunk fat mass, and high adiposity according to the different sociodemographic factors; Table S2. Association of having excess weight, abdominal obesity, high trunk fat mass and high adiposity according to different sociodemographic factors.

Author Contributions: J.F.L.-G. and J.L.Y.L. designed the study; J.F.L.-G. and A.L.-B. contributed to the analysis of the data and writing of the draft; J.F.L.-G. contributed to the analysis and interpretation of the data; A.L.-B., P.J.T.L. and J.L.Y.L. contributed to the revision of the manuscript. All authors have read and agreed to the published version of the manuscript.

Funding: This research received no external funding.

Acknowledgments: We are thankful for the participation of all the students, physical education teachers, parents/legal guardians, schools, and staff members who were involved, as well as the Ayuntamiento de Archena and the Universidad de Murcia for supporting this research.

Conflicts of Interest: The authors declare no conflict of interest.

References

1. Abarca-Gómez, L.; Abdeen, Z.A.; Hamid, Z.A.; Abu-Rmeileh, N.M.; Acosta-Cazares, B.; Acuin, C.; Adams, R.J.; Aekplakorn, W.; Afsana, K.; Aguilar-Salinas, C.A.; et al. Worldwide trends in body-mass index, underweight, overweight, and obesity from 1975 to 2016: A pooled analysis of 2416 population-based measurement studies in 128.9 million children, adolescents, and adults. *Lancet* **2017**, *390*, 2627–2642. [CrossRef]
2. Rito, A.I.; Buoncristiano, M.; Spinelli, A.; Salanave, B.; Kunešová, M.; Hejgaard, T.; García Solano, M.; Fijałkowska, A.; Sturua, L.; Hyska, J.; et al. Association between Characteristics at Birth, Breastfeeding and Obesity in 22 Countries: The WHO European Childhood Obesity Surveillance Initiative—COSI 2015/2017. *Obes. Facts* **2019**, *12*, 226–243. [CrossRef] [PubMed]
3. Kumar, S.; Kelly, A.S. Review of Childhood Obesity. *Mayo Clin. Proc.* **2017**, *92*, 251–265. [CrossRef] [PubMed]
4. Friedemann, C.; Heneghan, C.; Mahtani, K.; Thompson, M.; Perera, R.; Ward, A.M. Cardiovascular disease risk in healthy children and its association with body mass index: Systematic review and meta-analysis. *BMJ* **2012**, *345*, e4759. [CrossRef] [PubMed]
5. World Health Organization; Commission on Ending Childhood Obesity. *Report of the Commission on Ending Childhood Obesity*; World Health Organization: Geneva, Switzerland, 2016; ISBN 978-92-4-151006-6.

6. De Onis, M.; Onyango, A.W.; Borghi, E.; Siyam, A.; Nishida, C.; Siekmann, J. Development of a WHO growth reference for school-aged children and adolescents. *Bull. World Health Organ.* **2007**, *85*, 660–667. [CrossRef] [PubMed]
7. Cole, T.J.; Lobstein, T. Extended international (IOTF) body mass index cut-offs for thinness, overweight and obesity: Extended international BMI cut-offs. *Pediatr. Obes.* **2012**, *7*, 284–294. [CrossRef] [PubMed]
8. Kuczmarski, R.J.; Ogden, C.L.; Guo, S.S. *2000 CDC Growth Charts for the United States: Methods and Development*; Vital and Health Statistics. Series 11, Data from the National Health Survey; National Center for Biotechnology Information: Rockville Pike, MA, USA, 2002.
9. Fernández, C.; Lorenzo, H.; Vrotsou, K.; Aresti, U.; Rica, I.; Sánchez, E. *Estudio de Crecimiento de Bilbao: Curvas y Tablas de Crecimiento (Estudios Longitudinal y Transversal)*; Fundación Faustino Orbegozo: Bilbao, Spain, 2011.
10. Llewellyn, A.; Simmonds, M.; Owen, C.G.; Woolacott, N. Childhood obesity as a predictor of morbidity in adulthood: A systematic review and meta-analysis: Childhood obesity and adult morbidity. *Obes. Rev.* **2016**, *17*, 56–67. [CrossRef]
11. De Arruda, G.A.; Fernandes, R.A.; Christófaro, D.G.D.; de Oliveira, A.R. Relação entre idade cronológica, indicadores de adiposidade corporal e aptidão física relacionada à saúde em meninos e meninas. *Rev. Andal. Med. Deporte* **2013**, *6*, 24–29. [CrossRef]
12. Barnett, T.A.; Maximova, K.; Sabiston, C.M.; Van Hulst, A.; Brunet, J.; Castonguay, A.L.; Bélanger, M.; O'Loughlin, J. Physical activity growth curves relate to adiposity in adolescents. *Ann. Epidemiol.* **2013**, *23*, 529–533. [CrossRef]
13. Orsso, C.E.; Silva, M.I.B.; Gonzalez, M.C.; Rubin, D.A.; Heymsfield, S.B.; Prado, C.M.; Haqq, A.M. Assessment of body composition in pediatric overweight and obesity: A systematic review of the reliability and validity of common techniques. *Obes. Rev.* **2020**, *21*. [CrossRef]
14. Schröder, H.; Ribas, L.; Koebnick, C.; Funtikova, A.; Gomez, S.F.; Fíto, M.; Perez-Rodrigo, C.; Serra-Majem, L. Prevalence of Abdominal Obesity in Spanish Children and Adolescents. Do We Need Waist Circumference Measurements in Pediatric Practice? *PLoS ONE* **2014**, *9*, e87549. [CrossRef] [PubMed]
15. González-Muniesa, P.; Mártinez-González, M.-A.; Hu, F.B.; Després, J.-P.; Matsuzawa, Y.; Loos, R.J.F.; Moreno, L.A.; Bray, G.A.; Martinez, J.A. Obesity. *Nat. Rev. Dis. Primer* **2017**, *3*, 17034. [CrossRef] [PubMed]
16. Serral, G.; Bru, R.; Sánchez-Martínez, F.; Ariza, C. Overweight and childhood obesity according to socioeconomic variables in schoolchildren of third grade in the city of Barcelona. *Nutr. Hosp.* **2019**, *36*, 1043–1048. [CrossRef]
17. Arriscado, D.; Muros, J.J.; Zabala, M.; Dalmau, J.M. Influencia del sexo y el tipo de escuela sobre los índices de sobrepeso y obesidad. *Rev. Pediatría Aten. Primaria* **2014**, *16*, e139–e146. [CrossRef]
18. Guo, Y.; Yin, X.; Wu, H.; Chai, X.; Yang, X. Trends in Overweight and Obesity among Children and Adolescents in China from 1991 to 2015: A Meta-Analysis. *Int. J. Environ. Res. Public Health* **2019**, *16*, 4656. [CrossRef] [PubMed]
19. De Bont, J.; Díaz, Y.; Casas, M.; García-Gil, M.; Vrijheid, M.; Duarte-Salles, T. Time Trends and Sociodemographic Factors Associated with Overweight and Obesity in Children and Adolescents in Spain. *JAMA Netw. Open* **2020**, *3*, e201171. [CrossRef]
20. Beal, T.; Le, T.D.; Trinh, H.T.; Burra, D.D.; Béné, C.; Huynh, T.T.T.; Truong, M.T.; Nguyen, S.D.; Tran, D.T.; Nguyen, K.T.; et al. Child Overweight or Obesity Is Associated with Modifiable and Geographic Factors in Vietnam: Implications for Program Design and Targeting. *Nutrients* **2020**, *12*, 1286. [CrossRef] [PubMed]
21. Hales, C.M.; Fryar, C.D.; Carroll, M.D.; Freedman, D.S.; Ogden, C.L. Trends in Obesity and Severe Obesity Prevalence in US Youth and Adults by Sex and Age, 2007–2008 to 2015–2016. *JAMA* **2018**, *319*, 1723. [CrossRef]
22. *Estudio ALADINO 2019 Estudio de Vigilancia del Crecimiento, Alimentación, Actividad Física, Desarrollo Infantil y Obesidad en España 2019*; Ministerio de Sanidad, Servicios Sociales e Igualdad: Madrid, Spain, 2020.
23. Vaquero-Álvarez, M.; Romero-Saldaña, M.; Valle-Alonso, J.; Llorente Cantarero, F.J.; Blancas-Sánchez, I.M.; Fonseca del Pozo, F.J. Estudio de la obesidad en una población infantil rural y su relación con variables antropométricas. *Aten. Primaria* **2019**, *51*, 341–349. [CrossRef]
24. Vásquez, F.; Diaz, E.; Lera, L.; Vásquez, L.; Anziani, A.; Levton, B.; Burrows, R. Evaluación longitudinal de la composición corporal por diferentes. *Nutr. Hosp.* **2013**, *28*, 148–154. [CrossRef]

25. Simmonds, M.; Llewellyn, A.; Owen, C.G.; Woolacott, N. Predicting adult obesity from childhood obesity: A systematic review and meta-analysis: Adult obesity from childhood obesity. *Obes. Rev.* **2016**, *17*, 95–107. [CrossRef] [PubMed]
26. Bel-Serrat, S.; Heinen, M.M.; Mehegan, J.; O'Brien, S.; Eldin, N.; Murrin, C.M.; Kelleher, C.C. School sociodemographic characteristics and obesity in schoolchildren: Does the obesity definition matter? *BMC Public Health* **2018**, *18*, 337. [CrossRef] [PubMed]
27. Ministerio de Sanidad, Consumo y Bienestar Social. *Encuesta Nacional de Salud de España 2017*; Ministerio de Sanidad, Consumo y Bienestar Social: Madrid, Spain, 2018.
28. Ministerio de Medio Ambiente y Medio Rural y Marino. *Población y Sociedad Rural*; Serie AgrInfo; Unidad de Análisis y Prospectiva; Ministerio de Medio Ambiente y Medio Rural y Marino: Madrid, Spain, 2009.
29. Taylor, R.W.; Jones, I.E.; Williams, S.M.; Goulding, A. Evaluation of waist circumference, waist-to-hip ratio, and the conicity index as screening tools for high trunk fat mass, as measured by dual-energy X-ray absorptiometry, in children aged 3–19 y. *Am. J. Clin. Nutr.* **2000**, *72*, 490–495. [CrossRef] [PubMed]
30. Browning, L.M.; Hsieh, S.D.; Ashwell, M. A systematic review of waist-to-height ratio as a screening tool for the prediction of cardiovascular disease and diabetes: 0.5 could be a suitable global boundary value. *Nutr. Res. Rev.* **2010**, *23*, 247–269. [CrossRef] [PubMed]
31. Stewart, A.; Sutton, L. (Eds.) *Body Composition in Sport, Exercise, and Health*; Routledge: Abingdon, UK; New York, NY, USA, 2012; ISBN 978-0-415-61497-9.
32. Brook, C.G. Determination of body composition of children from skinfold measurements. *Arch. Dis. Child.* **1971**, *46*, 182–184. [CrossRef] [PubMed]
33. Siri, W.E. Body composition from fluid spaces and density: Analysis of methods. In *Techniques for Measuring Body Composition*; National Academy of Sciences: Washington, DC, USA, 1961; pp. 223–244.
34. Weststrate, J.A.; Deurenberg, P. Body composition in children: Proposal for a method for calculating body fat percentage from total body density or skinfold-thickness measurements. *Am. J. Clin. Nutr.* **1989**, *50*, 1104–1115. [CrossRef]
35. *Gasol Foundation Resultados Principales del Estudio PASOS 2019 Sobre la Actividad Física, los Estilos de vida y la Obesidad de la Población Española de 8 a 16 años*; Gasol Foundation: Barcelona, Spain, 2019.
36. Ogden, C.L.; Carroll, M.D.; Curtin, L.R.; McDowell, M.A.; Tabak, C.J.; Flegal, K.M. Prevalence of overweight and obesity in the United States, 1999–2004. *JAMA* **2006**, *295*, 1549–1555. [CrossRef]
37. Long, J.M.; Mareno, N.; Shabo, R.; Wilson, A.H. Overweight and obesity among White, Black, and Mexican American children: Implications for when to intervene. *J. Spec. Pediatr. Nurs. JSPN* **2012**, *17*, 41–50. [CrossRef]
38. Skinner, A.C.; Ravanbakht, S.N.; Skelton, J.A.; Perrin, E.M.; Armstrong, S.C. Prevalence of Obesity and Severe Obesity in US Children, 1999–2016. *Pediatrics* **2018**, *141*, e20173459. [CrossRef]
39. Ogden, C.L.; Fryar, C.D.; Hales, C.M.; Carroll, M.D.; Aoki, Y.; Freedman, D.S. Differences in Obesity Prevalence by Demographics and Urbanization in US Children and Adolescents, 2013–2016. *JAMA* **2018**, *319*, 2410. [CrossRef]
40. Ellis, K.J.; Abrams, S.A.; Wong, W.W. Monitoring Childhood Obesity: Assessment of the Weight/Height2 Index. *Am. J. Epidemiol.* **1999**, *150*, 939–946. [CrossRef] [PubMed]
41. Rolland-Cachera, M.F.; Deheeger, M.; Bellisle, F.; Sempé, M.; Guilloud-Bataille, M.; Patois, E. Adiposity rebound in children: A simple indicator for predicting obesity. *Am. J. Clin. Nutr.* **1984**, *39*, 129–135. [CrossRef] [PubMed]
42. Wang, Y.; Beydoun, M.A. The Obesity Epidemic in the United States Gender, Age, Socioeconomic, Racial/Ethnic, and Geographic Characteristics: A Systematic Review and Meta-Regression Analysis. *Epidemiol. Rev.* **2007**, *29*, 6–28. [CrossRef] [PubMed]
43. Ogden, C.L.; Carroll, M.D.; Kit, B.K.; Flegal, K.M. Prevalence of Obesity and Trends in Body Mass Index among US Children and Adolescents, 1999–2010. *JAMA* **2012**, *307*, 483. [CrossRef]
44. Yusuf, Z.I.; Dongarwar, D.; Yusuf, R.A.; Bell, M.; Harris, T.; Salihu, H.M. Social Determinants of Overweight and Obesity among Children in the United States. *Int. J. MCH AIDS* **2020**, *9*, 22–33. [CrossRef]
45. Arriscado, D.; Muros, J.J.; Zabala, M.; Dalmau, J.M. Relación entre condición física y composición corporal en escolares de primaria del norte de España (Logroño). *Nutr. Hosp.* **2014**, *30*, 385–394. [CrossRef]

46. Tovar-Galvez, M.I.; González-Jiménez, E.; Martí-García, C.; Schmidt-RioValle, J. Composición corporal en escolares: Comparación entre métodos antropométricos simples e impedancia bioeléctrica. *Endocrinol. Diabetes Nutr.* **2017**, *64*, 424–431. [CrossRef]
47. Cowell, C.T.; Briody, J.; Lloyd-Jones, S.; Smith, C.; Moore, B.; Howman-Giles, R. Fat Distribution in Children and Adolescents & ndash; the Influence of Sex and Hormones. *Horm. Res.* **1997**, *48*, 93–100. [CrossRef]
48. Nielsen, D.H.; Cassady, S.L.; Janz, K.F.; Cook, J.S.; Hansen, J.R.; Wu, Y.-T. Criterion methods of body composition analysis for children and adolescents. *Am. J. Hum. Biol.* **1993**, *5*, 211–223. [CrossRef]
49. Mekonnen, T.; Tariku, A.; Abebe, S.M. Overweight/obesity among school aged children in Bahir Dar City: Cross sectional study. *Ital. J. Pediatr.* **2018**, *44*. [CrossRef]
50. Elías-Boneta, A.R.; Toro, M.J.; Garcia, O.; Torres, R.; Palacios, C. High prevalence of overweight and obesity among a representative sample of Puerto Rican children. *BMC Public Health* **2015**, *15*. [CrossRef]
51. Hirvonen, K.; Bai, Y.; Headey, D.; Masters, W.A. Affordability of the EAT–Lancet reference diet: A global analysis. *Lancet Glob. Health* **2020**, *8*, e59–e66. [CrossRef]
52. De Arruda Moreira, M.; Coelho Cabral, P.; da Silva Ferreira, H.; Cabral de Lira, P.I. Prevalence and factors associated with overweight and obesity in children under five in Alagoas, Northeast of Brazil; a population-based study. *Nutr. Hosp.* **2014**, *29*, 1320–1326. [CrossRef]
53. Murphy, R.; Stewart, A.W.; Hancox, R.J.; Wall, C.R.; Braithwaite, I.; Beasley, R.; Mitchell, E.A.; The ISAAC Phase Three Study Group. Obesity underweight and BMI distribution characteristics of children by gross national income and income inequality: Results from an international survey: BMI distribution by GNI and Gini. *Obes. Sci. Pract.* **2018**, *4*, 216–228. [CrossRef]
54. Biehl, A.; Hovengen, R.; Grøholt, E.-K.; Hjelmesæth, J.; Strand, B.H.; Meyer, H.E. Adiposity among children in Norway by urbanity and maternal education: A nationally representative study. *BMC Public Health* **2013**, *13*, 842. [CrossRef]
55. Joens-Matre, R.R.; Welk, G.J.; Calabro, M.A.; Russell, D.W.; Nicklay, E.; Hensley, L.D. Rural–Urban Differences in Physical Activity, Physical Fitness, and Overweight Prevalence of Children. *J. Rural Health* **2008**, *24*, 49–54. [CrossRef]
56. Murer, S.B.; Saarsalu, S.; Zimmermann, J.; Herter-Aeberli, I. Risk factors for overweight and obesity in Swiss primary school children: Results from a representative national survey. *Eur. J. Nutr.* **2016**, *55*, 621–629. [CrossRef]
57. Pardo Arquero, V.P.; Jiménez Pavón, D.; Guillén del Castillo, M.; Benítez Sillero, J.D. Actividad física, condición física y adiposidad: Inmigrantes versus escolares españoles. *Rev. Int. Med. Cienc. Act. Física Deporte* **2014**, *14*, 319–338.
58. On behalf of the IDEFICS Consortium; Iguacel, I.; Fernández-Alvira, J.M.; Bammann, K.; Chadjigeorgiou, C.; De Henauw, S.; Heidinger-Felső, R.; Lissner, L.; Michels, N.; Page, A.; et al. Social vulnerability as a predictor of physical activity and screen time in European children. *Int. J. Public Health* **2018**, *63*, 283–295. [CrossRef]
59. Renzaho, A.M.N.; Swinburn, B.; Burns, C. Maintenance of traditional cultural orientation is associated with lower rates of obesity and sedentary behaviours among African migrant children to Australia. *Int. J. Obes.* **2008**, *32*, 594–600. [CrossRef]
60. Hao, L.; Kim, J.J.H. Immigration and the American Obesity Epidemic. *Int. Migr. Rev.* **2009**, *43*, 237–262. [CrossRef] [PubMed]

Publisher's Note: MDPI stays neutral with regard to jurisdictional claims in published maps and institutional affiliations.

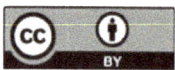

© 2020 by the authors. Licensee MDPI, Basel, Switzerland. This article is an open access article distributed under the terms and conditions of the Creative Commons Attribution (CC BY) license (http://creativecommons.org/licenses/by/4.0/).

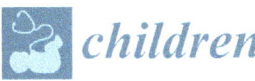

Article

Effects of Nutrition, and Physical Activity Habits and Perceptions on Body Mass Index (BMI) in Children Aged 12–15 Years: A Cross-Sectional Study Comparing Boys and Girls

Vilelmine Carayanni [1,*], Elpis Vlachopapadopoulou [2], Dimitra Koutsouki [3], Gregory C. Bogdanis [3], Theodora Psaltopoulou [4], Yannis Manios [5], Feneli Karachaliou [2], Angelos Hatzakis [4] and Stefanos Michalacos [2]

1. Laboratory of Statistical Modelling and Educational Technology in Public and Environmental Health–sepeh.lab, University of West Attica, 196 Alexandras Avenue, 11521 Athens, Greece
2. Department of Endocrinology, Children's Hospital P. & A. Kyriakou, Thivon & Levadeiasstr, Ampelokipoi T.K., 11527 Athens, Greece; elpis.vl@gmail.com (E.V.); fenkar1@hotmail.com (F.K.); stmichalakos@gmail.com (S.M.)
3. School of Physical Education & Sports Science, National and Kapodistrian University of Athens, 41, EthnikisAntistaseosstr, Daphne, 17237 Athens, Greece; dkoutsou@phed.uoa.gr (D.K.); gbogdanis@phed.uoa.gr (G.C.B.)
4. Department of Hygiene, Epidemiology and Medical Statistics, School of Medicine, National and Kapodistrian University of Athens, 75 MikrasAsias Str., 11527 Goudi, Greece; tpsaltop@med.uoa.gr (T.P.); ahatzak@med.uoa.gr (A.H.)
5. Department of Nutrition & Dietetics, School of Health Science & Education, Harokopio University, 70, El Venizelou Ave Kallithea, 17671 Athens, Greece; manios@hua.gr
* Correspondence: vkaragian@uniwa.gr

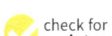

Citation: Carayanni, V.; Vlachopapadopoulou, E.; Koutsouki, D.; Bogdanis, G.C.; Psaltopoulou, T.; Manios, Y.; Karachaliou, F.; Hatzakis, A.; Michalacos, S. Effects of Nutrition, and Physical Activity Habits and Perceptions on Body Mass Index (BMI) in Children Aged 12–15 Years: A Cross-Sectional Study Comparing Boys and Girls. *Children* 2021, *8*, 277. https://doi.org/10.3390/children 8040277

Academic Editor: Carin Andrén Aronsson

Received: 7 February 2021
Accepted: 25 March 2021
Published: 3 April 2021

Publisher's Note: MDPI stays neutral with regard to jurisdictional claims in published maps and institutional affiliations.

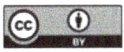

Copyright: © 2021 by the authors. Licensee MDPI, Basel, Switzerland. This article is an open access article distributed under the terms and conditions of the Creative Commons Attribution (CC BY) license (https://creativecommons.org/licenses/by/4.0/).

Abstract: *Background*: The aim of the present study was to examine the effects of socioeconomic status, nutrition and physical activity lifestyle habits and perceptions on Body Mass Index (BMI) in children aged 12–15 years in Greece. Furthermore, to compare the difference between the two sexes. *Methods*: This is a cross-sectional study conducted on a representative secondary school cohort that included 5144 subjects, aged 12 to 15 years. Students and their parents filled in validated questionnaires evaluating socioeconomic status, nutrition and physical activity. International Obesity Task Force cut offs were used to classify the children. Factor analysis of mixed data and partial proportional ordered logistic models were used to analyze BMI distributions. All analyses were stratified by gender. *Results*: Boys were 2.9 (95%CI: 2.592–3.328) times more likely to be overweight/obese than girls. Partial proportional ordinal models indicate significant associations between nutritional and physical habits and perceptions variables but also significant gender differences in socio-demographic, nutritional risk factors as well as physical activity habits and perceptions. *Conclusions*: A clear understanding of the factors that contribute to the sex differences in nutrition and physical activity habits and perceptions may guide intervention efforts.

Keywords: adolescents; nutrition habits; nutrition perceptions; Body Mass Index (BMI) category; overweight; obesity; physical activity habits; physical activity perceptions; Greece

1. Introduction

The prevalence of obesity during childhood and adolescence has risen significantly over the last decades, specifically according to NHANES study the rate of obesity during adolescence has quadrupled [1] The World Health Organization (WHO) has announced that childhood and adolescent obesity is the number one problem of public health and advises on actions needed to halt the progression of obesity epidemic [2].

Greece among other countries of southern Europe has one of the highest prevalence rates of childhood obesity [3]. Obesity is of multifactorial etiology including genetic, environmental such as nutrition and physical activity, and socioeconomic factors [4,5].

Obesity is associated with short-and long-term complications and comorbidities including metabolic syndrome, diabetes mellitus type 2 and premature cardiovascular disease [6,7].

In order to implement prevention strategies, it is very important to define the modifiable factors that contribute to the increase of body mass index (BMI). These factors can be recognized at an individual, family, community or national level [1,4,5]. In regards to sex there are several biological (sex specific) factors that have to do with the timing of puberty, body composition and growth patterns and social and cultural factors (gender specific) that reflect the ways in which boys and girls react to their physical and social environment [5]. Previous observational studies have examined associations of gender with behaviors linked to obesity and have observed gender related differences, namely that participation in vigorous exercise and in school sports had a protective effect for boys while drinking milk had a protective effect for girls [8]. It has also been reported that there are certain behaviors, especially eating disordered behaviors, as well as perceptions, such as fear of negative evaluation and weight shape concerns, that are gender dimorphic [9,10]. Furthermore, prevalence of components of metabolic syndrome and lifestyle behaviors may vary among the two sexes [11].

To our knowledge, there is limited information concerning the differences among boys and girls in adolescence, in regard to nutrition and physical habits and perceptions and their influence on BMI. The sex differences in acquired behaviors and perceptions vary across cultures and their impact on childhood obesity remains unclear. Previous research indicates that girls naturally require less energy intake than boys and that girls may be more attentive to food as well as to its effects on health and weight control [12].

The aim of the present study was to examine the effects of nutrition and physical activity lifestyle habits and perceptions on BMI in a large representative sample of children aged 12–15 years in Greece and to examine possible differences between the two sexes.

2. Materials and Methods

The "Hellenic Action Plan for the Assessment, Prevention and Treatment for Childhood Obesity" was a school-based survey, financed by the National Strategic Reference Framework, conducted at a national level in Greece and provided the data that were used in the present analysis. The study was conducted according to the guidelines of the Declaration of Helsinki, and approved by the Greek Ministry of National Education and the Greek Ministry of Health and the Hellenic Data Protection Authority (ethical code MIS 301205). Data were collected between January2015 and June 2015. The study population comprised schoolchildren attending secondary schools located in several municipalities in Greece (urban, semi-urban and rural areas, including islands). Semi-urban population includes the population of municipalities and communities, whose most populous settlement has 2000–9999 inhabitants, except those belonging to urban planning. Details for all regions and prefectures selected into the sample and their participation rate were given in Appendix A (Table A1).

Probability proportional to size (PPS) sampling was applied. The sampling of schools was stratified by region, proportionally to the total number of pupils attending these schools. Following this procedure, an appropriate number of schools were randomly selected from each one of these regions. Specifically, 73 secondary schools were included. Prior to signing an informed consent, an extended letter explaining the objectives of the study was provided to all parents or guardians whose children were attending these schools. Parents who approved participation of their children to the study proceeded to sign the informed consent form. Pupils with severe chronic illnesses i.e., malignancies, diabetes mellitus, rheumatoid arthritis or systemic lupus erythematosusor receiving chronic therapies for more than 6 months per year for any diagnosis, were excluded from the analysis (43 children).

The response rate was 72%, as 5180 parents out of the 7246 who signed parental consent forms have fully completed the questionnaire. After examination of univariate statistics to detect any anomalies in the distribution of variables, (especially outliers or missing values), aberrant values and duplicates (36 cases on the total), the total study sample in this analysis included 5144 secondary school children.

2.1. Measurement

Anthropometric measurements were conducted by sixteen health professionals, hired and trained for the purposes of this study. Children were measured by two trained members of the research team, using the same equipment and protocol. Body weight was measured to the nearest 100 g using a Tanita digital scale (Tanita BWB 800MA). Adolescents were weighed without shoes, with minimal possible clothing. Height was measured to the nearest 0.1 cm using a commercial stadiometer (Charder HM 200P Portstad). The Charderstadiometer was standardized against a Harpenden portable stadiometer. During the measurement of height, each adolescent was standing barefoot, keeping shoulders in a relaxed position, arms hanging freely, and head aligned to the Frankfort horizontal plane. Anthropometric measurements were taken three times, and the arithmetic mean of the three measurements was computed. Body weight and height were used one to calculate BMI, using the Quetelet'sequation, i.e., body weight (kg)/height^2 (m^2). BMI was calculated and subsequently adolescents were categorized according to International Obesity Task Force (IOTF) criteria [13] into the following four BMI categories: Underweight, Normal, Overweight and Obese. Both inter-rater and intra-rater reliability, measured with the intra-class correlation coefficients (ICC), yielded values greater than 0.97.

2.2. Questionnaires

Two structured questionnaires were developed and administered to the parents and students. Validity and reliability of the two questionnaires was tested and found to satisfy the principles of reliability [14]. In order to assess reliability, prior to initiation of the study, data were collected from 450 parents of children aged 12–15 and 250 adolescents aged 12–15 from the region of Attica. Cronbach's alpha (α) and ICC were used to test reliability. Cronbach's alpha and ICC showed acceptable reliability (α: 0.79 = 0.90 and ICC: >0.690–0.910). The factors addressed included socio-demographic characteristics, such as age, gender, geographic area (urban, semi urban, rural), nutrition and physical activity habits and perception, socioeconomic status (SES). SES index has a range between of 0–13, with higher values indicating higher SES of the family, as previously published by Moschonis et al., 2013 [15].

2.3. Statistical Analysis

Factor Analysis of Mixed Data

A mixed data factor analysis (FAMD) was attempted in order to reduce the number of variables. Factor Analysis of Mixed Data is a main component method dedicated to exploring data with both continuous and categorical variables. This factor analysis is suitable when the dataset includes both qualitative and quantitative variables. It can be seen roughly as a mix between Principal Component Analysis and Multiple Correspondence Analysis [16,17]. This ensures a balance between the influence of both continuous and categorical variables in the analysis.

The initial number of variables was 180. We have removed all items with a communality score less than 0.2 [18]. Items with low communality scores may indicate additional factors which could be explored in further studies by measuring additional items [19]. Any item which did not load above 0.3 on any factor was removed and the analysis was re-run. All retained factors had at least three items [20,21]. Items in the rotated factor matrix that cross-loaded on more than one factor were removed in turn, starting with the item with the highest ratio of loadings on the most variables with the lowest highest loading. Finally, 9 factors were retained with 32 variables that explain 59% of the total variance [22]. Results support the factorability of the correlation matrix.

Figure A1a (screeplot) and Figure A1b in Appendix A indicate respectively the percentages of inertia explained by each of the final 9 FAMD and the individual factor map.

Figure A2 indicates the first 15 well projected variables for the first two dimensions. As can be seen in Figure A2, eating habits (meals frequency) and fattening perceptions (five meals, skipping breakfast, eating frequently, eating light products), as well as socio-demographic characteristics (age, area, sex), have the most important contribution to the two first dimensions Variables related to body image (such as "I want to be thin" and "I deal with diets"), have the most important contribution to dimension 3. Perceptions for physical activity (such as self-evaluation on physical activity and efficiency of school's gym hours and breaks), midday and after meal snacks (cheese pie, bread and fruits after dinner) and drinks in breakfast (such as cocoa milk, and whole milk), had respectively the most important contribution to the dimensions 4, 5 and 6. Organized sports (such as football, dance and track and field sports) had the most important contribution to Dimension 7. Purchase criteria/choice of food (according to their price or their calories) and SES, had the most important contribution to Dimension 8. Sedentary behaviors combined with eating such as meals in front of PC per week, snack (salty) in front of PC/tv per week, snack (sweet) in front of PC (TV) per week, had the most important contribution to Dimension 9. Also, sex has a significant contribution on Dimension 2, 5 and 7, that supports our decision to analyze the 2 sexes separately in order to avoid the possible additional complexity in our model. Factors description is presented in Appendix A, Table A2.

Descriptive Statistics-Outcome

Descriptive statistics were calculated for the remained variables. Chi-square tests and t-student tests were used to test the homogeneity among boys and girls for each variable at significance level $\alpha = 5\%$.

Weight category was measured on an ordinal scale: the codification of the outcome variable is: 0 = Normal weight/underweight, 1 = Overweight, 2 = Obese.

Ordered logistic models

For ordered dependent variables Y, the ordered logit model is often the natural choice. In ordinal logistic regression, the odds of being at category j or lower is:

$$\frac{P(Y \leq j)}{P(Y > j)}; j = 1, \ldots, c-1; P(Y \leq c) = 1$$

The ordered logit model, however, features a very restrictive model assumption, the assumption of proportional odds, that is often rejected in empirical research.

The proportional odds assumption in this study implies that the distances between different BMI levels are the same. The generalized ordered logit model differs from the standard ordinal or proportional odds model in that it relaxes the proportional-odds assumption. It allows that the predictors may have different effects on the odds that the response is above a cut off point, depending on how the outcomes are dichotomized. The Partial Proportional Odds (PPO) model is preferred to the generalized ordinal logistic regression if some predictor variables violate the assumption and their effects are estimated freely across different categories of the ordinal response variable [23–25].

Firstly, univariate ordinal logit model was fitted and the Brant test was performed to evaluate the parallel assumption. This Brant test is used to compare the coefficients of beta from c-1 binary logits and gives a list of variables violated the parallel assumption. Constraints were imposed on the variables where the parallel assumption was not violated [23].

The variables found, by use of univariate analysis, to be associated with the outcome variable at the $p < 0.20$ level, were included in the initial models to determine which factors were independent predictors of the outcome variable in the study subjects. All the ordinal logistic models were estimated via Maximum Likelihood Estimation (MLE) technique. ML estimates are values of the parameters having the ML of producing the observed sample [25]. The likelihood equations lead to the unknown parameters in a non-linear function. The ordinal logistic regression model was fitted to the observed responsesusing the maximum likelihood approach. In general, the method of maximum likelihood produces values of the observed probability values. According to the Brant test, parallel lines assumption was significantly violated for two variables in boys' model and for four variables in girls' model. Subsequently, PPO and generalized ordered logit model (GOLM) were fitted to the data. Finally, a comparison of the multivariate models was made [24].

The results were recorded as frequencies (N) and percentages, means and standard deviations (SD), odds ratios (OR) with 95% confidence intervals (CI), and p values. Hence, OR > 1 indicate that higher category values make it more likely that the respondent will be in a higher category than the current one, while OR < 1 indicate that higher category values on the predictor increase the likelihood of being in the current or a lower category.

All analyses were stratified by gender. R language (packages factorMiner, factorExtra) as well as Stata 14.0 software were used.

3. Results

3.1. Sample Characteristics

Sample characteristics followed by homogeneity tests, (α = 5%), between sexes are given on Table A3 in Appendix A for all variables included in final models. Results for the rest of variables are given on Table A4 in Appendix A). The prevalence of overweight and obesity was 24.8% and 6.8% respectively. Boys were 2.9 (95%CI: 2.592–3.328) times more likely to be overweight/obese than girls.

Statistically significant differences were observed among boys and girls in their self-evaluation in relation to physical activity with girls being significantly less active than boys ($p < 0.001$) and in relation to the perception regarding efficiency of school's gym hours and breaks ($p = 0.001$). Also, boys participated more frequently than girls in outdoor sport activities such as track and field ($p = 0.037$). Girls seem to have a better level of knowledge in relation to eating habits, such as their opinion on "eating five meals per day" ($p < 0.001$), their agreement to "skipping breakfast is fattening" ($p < 0.001$) and the consumption of cheese pie at breakfast ($p < 0.001$). Significant differences were observed in fruit after dinner consumption that is more frequent in boys ($p = 0.023$). Results are in the same direction in cocoa milk consumption at breakfast ($p < 0.001$) and in frequency in dinner consumption ($p < 0.001$). Also, girls seem to have greater involvement with diets ($p < 0.001$) and to buy more frequently food products according to their calories ($p < 0.001$). It seems that boys are less concerned with their body image ("I'm scared to get overweight <0.001", "I want to be thin": $p < 0.001$).

3.2. Results of Partial Proportional Odds Models

As can be seen on Table A5 in Appendix B, Partial proportional odds (PPO) models presented better performance for both sexes. The model which represented the best fit according to Akaike's Information Criterion (AIC) and Bayesian Information Criterion (BIC) is PPO model in both sexes as it has the smallest AIC and BIC and it is also more parsimonious. Results are presented and interpreted for the significant predictors in univariate analyses. The variables associated with the outcome at the 5% significance level were maintained in the final models Table A6 in Appendix B presents the data for underweight/normal weight children and compares them with data from children with overweight/obesity. Similarly, the second panel, (Table A7 in Appendix B), compares children with obesity with all other BMI categories.

3.2.1. Partial Proportional Odds Models (PPOM): Boys

Predictors that do not violate the parallel line assumption

Holding the other predictors constant, the increase in frequency of cocoa milk consumption in breakfast by one unit was negatively associated with the odds (95% OR: 0.314, 95% CI: 0.125–0.792) to be in higher BMI categories, from underweight/normal weight to overweight/obese or from all other categories to obese)

Track and field sports seem to be a protective factor for obesity: Boys who regularly took part in track and field training for at least 2–3 times per week were 0.454 times (95%CI:

0.239–0.864) less likely to be in higher BMI categories, compared with boys who did not participate in track and field sports.

Dealing with diets was positively associated with the likelihood of being in a higher BMI category. Boys who never followed any diet were 0.203 (95% CI: 0.084–0.592) times less likely to move to higher categories in contrast to those who usually follow diets.

The increase of the frequency of afternoon meal per week by one unit decreased the odds to move from normal weight/underweight to higher BMI categories or from all other BMI categories to obesity by 0.203 times (95%CI: 0.088–0.468).

As compared to a boy who is always concerned with the desire to become thinner, a boy who was sometimes/rarely concerned with the desire to become thinner is 0.272 times (95% CI: 0.159–0.596) less likely to be in higher BMI categories. As opposed to a boy who was always concerned with the desire to become thinner, a boy who is never concerned with the desire to become thinner was 0.246 times (95% CI: 0.149–0.496) less likely to be in higher BMI categories, holding the other predictors constant.

As compared to a boy who is "always scared", a boy who is "rarely scared" is 2.504 times more likely to be in overweight or obese status, (95% CI: 1.242–5.048). As compared to a boy who is "always scared", a boy who is "never scared" was 2.070 times (95% CI: 1.118–3.831) more likely to be in overweight or obese status, holding the other predictors constant.

The subjective estimate of the level of physical activity had a significant effect among both binary models. A boy who characterized himself as quite/very active was 0.691 times (95% CI: 0.550–0.868) less likely to be in higher BMI categories as compared to a boy who did not characterize himself as quite/very active.

The daily consumption of cheese pie at brunch increased the odds to be in higher BMI categories by 4.465 times (95% CI: 1.567–10.724) in contrast to those who never or rarely ate cheese pie at breakfast.

A boy who agreed with the statement that "eating frequently without order fattens", as compared to a boy who strongly disagreed/disagreed with this, was 0.508 (95% CI: 0.275–0.940) times less likely to be in higher BMI categories, from under-weight/normal weight to overweight/obese or from other categories to obese, holding all other factors constant.

Eating bread "sometimes" as compared to "never" decreased the odds to be in higher BMI categories by 0.453 times (95% CI: 0.274–0.747) in both BMI comparisons, holding the other predictors constant.

Predictors which violated the parallel regression assumption

A boy who agreed/strongly agreed with the perception that "light products fatten was 1.902 times (95% CI: 1.139–3.175) more likely to be in higher BMI categories from underweight/normal to overweight/obese as compared to a boy who did not agree/strongly disagree with this perception. The odds ratio became larger when the final binary model was used to compare obese with the other BMI categories. Moreover, a boy who strongly agreed/agreed with this perception in the final comparison (obese versus other categories) increased the odds to be in the higher BMI category by 3.815 (1.927–7.554) times as compared to a boy who did not agree/strongly disagree with this perception.

A boy who ate often (3–4 times per week) fruit after diner was by 0.440 times (95% CI: 0.195–0.988) less likely to be in a higher BMI category as compared to a boy who never ate fruit after diner. This predictor becomes significant only in the comparison among obese and lower BMI categories.

3.2.2. Partial Proportional Odds Models (PPOM): Girls

Predictors which do not violate the parallel line assumption

A girl who characterized herself as quite/very active was 0.714 (95% CI: 0.582–0.877) times less likely to be in higher BMI categories as compared to a girl who did not characterize herself as active, from underweight/normal weight to overweight/obese or from other categories to obese, holding all other factors constant.

Also, higher values of the variable "dinner frequency" were related with lower values of BMI categories. In terms of odds ratio, the increase in frequency of this variable was negatively associated with the odds (OR: 0.863, 95% CI: 0.748–0.997) of being to a higher BMI category, from underweight/normal weight to overweight/obese or from other categories to obese, holding all other factors constant.

Increased frequency of eating bread ("often/always" as compared to "never") at brunch, decreased the odds to be in higher BMI categories by 0.382 times (95% CI: (0.157–0.932), from underweight/normal weight to overweight/obese or from other categories to obese, holding all other factors constant.

Considering that five meals per day were good/very good (as opposed to "bad/very bad"), decreases the odds to be in higher BMI categories by 0.241 times (96% OR: 0.079–0.735) from underweight/normal weight to overweight/obese or from other categories to obese, holding all other factors constant.

A girl who considered that the hours of physical activity in school classes and breaks are adequate in order to be physically active was 2.509 (95% CI: 1.338–4.704) times more likely to be in higher BMI categories as opposed to a girl who did not agree/strongly disagree with that.

Regular breakfast consumption seems to have a protective effect for obesity. In terms of odds ratio, the increase in frequency of this variable by one unit was negatively associated with the odds (OR: 0.537, 95% CI: 0.408–0.711) of being to a higher BMI category, from underweight/normal weight to overweight/obese or from other categories to obese, holding all other factors constant.

Considering that "skipping breakfast fattens" seems to have a protective effect against obesity. A girl who agreed that skipping breakfast consumption is fattening as opposed to a girl who did not agree/strongly disagree with that, was 0.241 (95% CI:0.078–0.734) times less likely to belong to higher BMI categories, holding the other predictors constant.

A girl who was usually/often concerned with the desire to become thinner was 0.641 times (95% CI: 0.491–0.836) less likely to be classified in a higher BMI category as compared to a girl who was always concerned with this desire. Girls who are some-times or rarely concerned with the desire to become thinner were 0.476 times (95% CI: 0.351–0.646) less likely to be classified in a higher BMI category in comparison to girls who were always concerned with this desire. Also, girls who were never concerned with the desire to become thinner were 0.315 times (95% CI: 0.136–0.271) less likely to be classified in a higher BMI category when compared to girls who were always concerned with this desire.

Girls who were "scared of the idea of becoming obese" (from often through usually) were less likely to move to higher categories as compared to girls who are never "scared of the idea of becoming obese, from underweight/normal weight to overweight or from other categories to obesity": As compared to a girl who is "always scared", a girl who is "rarely scared" is 3.829 times more likely to be in overweight or obese status, (95% CI: 2.080–7.047). As compared to a girl who is "always scared", a girl who is "never scared" is 2.438 times (95% CI: 1.305–4.354) more likely to be in overweight or obese status, holding the other predictors constant.

Predictors which violated the parallel regression assumption

Geographic area is a significant predictor only in the second binary model, when comparing obesity with other BMI categories. Girls who live in an urban area were 0.537 times (95% CI: (0.408–0.711)) less likely to be in the obesity category as opposed to girls who live in a rural area, holding the other predictors constant.

Age was negatively associated with the likelihood of being in a higher BMI category only when comparing underweight/normal weight with higher BMI categories. An age increase by 1 year, decreased the likelihood that a girl was classified in a higher BMI category by 0.668 times (95% CI: 0.584–0.813), holding the other predictors constant.

Girls who selected their foods according to their caloric content were 2.871 (95% CI: 1.042–7.901) times more likely to be in higher BMI categories than those who do not consider this criterion as important. This variable was significant, only in the final comparison (obesity versus other BMI categories).

Girls who drank whole milk at breakfast on a daily basis, were 2.483 (95% CI: 1.088–5.668) times more likely to be in obesity category than those who never drank whole milk at breakfast. This variable was significant, only in the final comparison (obesity versus other BMI categories).

4. Discussion

In the present study we addressed habits and beliefs that possibly lead to certain behaviors and choices in regards to eating and physical activity habits. It has been shown in previous research that a number of nutrition habits as well as sedentary activities are correlated with a positive increase of BMI [4]. Adolescents receive a large number of positive and negative messages from parents, teachers, caregivers and coaches regarding what consists a healthy lifestyle. Depending on their age, sex, intelligence, social and family environment they integrate in their beliefs a variable mixture of what they have been taught, and their thinking most likely reflects on their behavior (attitude). Boys and girls internalize stimuli in a different way and may react in distinct patterns.

In the representative sample of adolescents attending high schools throughout Greece, a number of differences among the two sexes were appreciated in regards to their habits, beliefs and fears concerning the factors that contribute to overweight and obesity. These beliefs had to do with what was more important in choosing the right food or avoid the unhealthy food i.e., calories, homemade or commercially available, the timing and number of meals during the day. The fear of obesity and the desire to lose weight or achieve a thinner body figure were also questioned. The subjective judgment of the level of activity and degree of physical fitness was addressed

The use of statistical tests and models has revealed the importance of a constellation of factors that correlate with higher BMI that are sex dimorphic. Girls seem to have greater involvement with diets and to buy more frequently food products according to their calories and are more concerned with their body image. Whilst avoidance of obesity is considered a healthy approach, inappropriate dieting and weight-loss behaviors known to accompany fear of fatness among adolescents, may pause a serious health risk [21]. It is possible that girls who have a desire to become thinner have a tendency to follow stricter diets for a short period of time and are at higher risk of emotional eating. Females are also more prone than boys to develop eating disorders [22].

Regarding their attitude towards dietary habits the notion that skipping breakfast is preventing for overweight was revealed to be a risk factor for obesity and the same applies for the concept that food choice according to their calorie content, is an important practice in order to halt BMI increase. It is anticipated that the attitude that skipping breakfast supports weight control is followed by omitting breakfast on a regular basis. The importance of breakfast intake on a daily base has emerged as an important factor preventing obesity, in several cross-sectional studies but not in cohort studies as it is published in a recent meta-analysis The risk of obesity in children and adolescents who skipped breakfast was 43% greater than those who ate breakfast regularly.

A possible explanation of the negative effect of food choices based on calorie content is that consumers frequently underestimate the caloric content of foods [26]. Another important factor is that it has been shown that paying attention only to caloric content does not assure the healthier choice as far as the content of trans-fat, carbohydrates, sugars, sodium and fiber that may not be optimal. Of interest is recent study that reports on the importance of the side where the label is placed and the impact that labeling has on consumer's choice. They demonstrated that the label that has a positive statement such as healthy choice has stronger effect than a negative statement as high calorie food [27].

On the other hand a protective effect was elucidated for the impression that the consumption of five meals per day is a good practice. Girls who have the impression that consuming 5 meals per day, is a healthy practice have a higher possibility of applying this habit and also higher chance of having more family meals. Recent meta-analysis have demonstrated a significant relationship between frequent family meals and better nutritional health-in younger and older children, across countries and socioeconomic groups [28]. It can also be contemplated that those girls make healthier choices of small meals or snacks and avoid frequent snacking or poor snack choices [29].

Referring to their judgment as to the adequacy of the time spent for physical activity in school as part of the physical education classes combined with the recreational activities and sports during school intermissions, a negative correlation was recognized. Adolescent girls who assume that this level of physical activity is appropriate as a daily standard of activity have higher chance of being in the higher level of BMI. This belief most likely leads to considerable inactivity during their leisure time during after school hours. Low levels of physical activity during adolescence are considered a global burden [30] and beliefs play an important role.

The subjective impression of the level of physical activity reflected to their BMI status as girls who considered themselves as being active or very active had lower chances to be in higher BMI categories than girls who do not characterize themselves as active. Again it is reasonable to contemplate that their self-judgment reflects on their involvement in sport activities.

Concerning their habits, girls who eat breakfast and dinner regularly have lower odds of obesity. To the same direction is the impact of consuming bread as part of brunch, especially for girls. This finding highlight the importance of eating breakfast as it was already stated but also the importance of having dinner in the context of having 5 meals per day.

Another factor that had a significant relation in a negative manner was the age. As girls move to higher class in high school had lower odds of being in the overweight/obese category. Specifically the increase of the age by 1 year decreases by 0.621 times the likelihood that a girl moves from underweight/normal weight to a higher BMI level. The impact of age can possibly be explained with the correlation that was noted that the desire to avoid overweight has a protective effect. As girls get older they have greater preoccupation with their body image and the fear obesity may play a stronger role.

In boys, concerning their beliefs and attitudes regarding what is healthy and what helps them to prevent overweight and obesity, it was elucidated that boys who think that unlimited snacking is related to a tendency to obesity were less likely to be overweight and obese. Meals and snacks are quite different in terms of way of preparation and setting in which they are consumed. It is most likely that these boys avoid an unordered way of eating and snacking throughout the day and thus attain a healthier body size. Recent study has shown that parents pay less attention and effort in preparing snacks as compared to meals and they are more prone to offer unhealthy snacks than unhealthy meals. Furthermore, they reported that this observation holds true for normal weight as well as overweight or obese children. In the same study differences were appreciated in the way snacks were treated among adolescent boys and girls with normal and increased BMI. It is notable that a greater percentage of non-overweight youth (both boys and girls) reported the consumption of fruits and vegetables as snacks, and boys, those of higher weight status were less likely than girls to eat foods prepared at home as snacks [31].

Boys who were preoccupied with diets and different types of dieting they were more likely to belong to the obesity group. This finding may be consistent with assumption that in order to lose weight or to maintain a healthy weight someone should follow a restrictive diet. This notion though may lead to a vicious cycle as restrictive diets have been associated with short term weight loss but long term aggravation of BMI. Furthermore, restrictive diets are not recommended during childhood or adolescence [32]. A study from Brazil reported that adolescents with poor self-image and higher BMI had a higher trend to follow restrictive diets, with no sex predilection [33].

The perception that light products fatten was proven to be a risk factor that increases the odds of being in the obese group. This viewpoint most likely prohibits them from including light products to their daily nutrition program and rather uses other foods that conceivably are more calories dense. To our knowledge there are no similar reports in the literature. Similarly, the daily consumption of whole milk in girls increases the odds to be to obesity category.

Regarding boys attitude towards "thinness", results are in the same direction as in girls, although boys are less concerned with their body image than girls. Remarkable is that boys and girls who are indifferent of the status of obesity, "they do not have a fear of becoming obese", have higher tendency to belong to the higher BMI group, whereas the opposite is true if they don't have any desire of being thin. Recent study has revealed that adolescents have developed phobias as a result of being discriminated [34].

Self-assessment of the level of physical activity has a negative correlation with BMI category. The higher the impression of the level of physical activity the less the possibility to belong to the obesity group. This finding is in line with the observation in girls that underlines that adolescents can accurately estimate their level of activity and reflects their real-life level of activity.

Regarding boys' nutritional habits several aspects are in line and support the importance of the having 5 meals a day in order to maintain a normal BMI. Boys who used to drink milk with cocoa for breakfast, have an afternoon snack, eat dinner, and/or have a fruit after dinner tend to be in the group of normal weight. It is of interest the finding that consumption of milk with cocoa has a protective effect. Similar findings for the protective effect of milk consumption in adolescent boys against obesity were reported by Murphy et al. [35]. The increased frequency of eating dinner was negatively associated with the odds of being in a higher BMI category. Eating bread for brunch or midday snack has a protective effect being a healthier choice compared with alternatives such as pies, cakes, and biscuits. On the other hand eating daily cheese pie for breakfast is a choice that increases the odds to be in the higher BMI group. This variable remains significant in the multivariate model for boys. Cheese pie is a high fat, high carbohydrate choice very popular among Greeks.

In regards to physical activity, boys who are involved in track and field sports had greater possibility of being in the normal weight group. Involvement in organized physical activity has been shown to be a protective affect for the development of obesity [36,37], however there is no clear impression as to what type of sport activity has a stronger effect. Track and field sports are more widely followed in Greece and this is reflected in the present study.

In regards to area of residence, living in a rural area remains significantly associated with obesity in the final models only for girls. The sociocultural differences, the differences in lifestyle habits and the lack of infrastructure in rural areas [36], that preclude the access of adolescents to gyms and sports facilities seems to have a more serious impact on the weight of girls than boys.

A limitation of the present study is the cross-sectional design which does not allow for causality conclusions and the self-reporting of information regarding sports participation and diet habits which is a source of bias. Longitudinal data are necessary to further unravel the complex interplay between the outcome and the above mentioned covariates. Strong points of the study are the large representative sample, the nationwide participation that increases the external validity of this study.

The current data support the hypothesis that beliefs and habits play an important and the perception role towards the development of obesity, however different factors may be protective as well as risk factors among the two genders. As was explicitly analyzed in the results section distinctive risk or protective factors emerged for the girls and boys. Regarding their impressions, the fear of obesity was protective for girls and for boys, whereas preoccupation with diets is a risk factor for obesity for both sexes. More healthy choices in mid-day snacks-such as bread-and frequent meals are protective factors for both sexes Gender dimorphic factors were recognized and these are the choice of food based on the calorie content for girls, frequent snacking for boys. Also, daily whole milk consumption at breakfast is associated with obesity in girls—although this consumption is more frequent for boys-, and high fat products consumption at breakfast that is more frequent for boys are related to increased risk for obesity for boys. On the other hand, regular cocoa milk consumption that is more frequent in boys than girls, seems to have a protective effect against obesity only for boys. Also girls seem to be more vulnerable to some sociodemographic factors such as age and geographic area. It is known that, beyond the biological differences and differences due to society or culture including food choices and dietary concerns, the levels of resting energy expenditure and energy requirements are different between girls and boys and the results of this study support these differences [38].

Regarding physical activity habits and perceptions, sex differences in engage in outdoor sport activities is evident in our study and this more frequent participation of boys emerges in this study as a protective factor against obesity as well [30,36].

A theoretical implication of these differences is that exposure to different role models, family dynamics as well as exposure to advertisements may affect the way children and adolescents appreciate weight status and factors correlating with weight control.

A practical implication is that the way doctors, parents and teachers approach children and adolescents promoting the healthy habits is of paramount importance as it can lead to negative or positive behaviors. An important finding of the present study is that the preoccupation with diets and dieting emerges as a risk factor for overweight and obesity. The tentative message is that positive role modeling and early education regarding healthy choices is desirable. Trying to understand more what the children think and criticize less could be helpful in helping them internalize health perceptions and follow healthy habits. The search for the perfect diet can have the opposite effect on BMI and this applies to both genders. Furthermore, the adherence to a five-mealplan per day has a protective effect and can prevent the development of obesity.

As public health measures are concerned, applying a prevention plan that includes psychological assessment and intervention taking into consideration the developmental differences of boys and girls as well as their perceptions which should be appreciated. Furthermore, ministry of education can implement measures for elementary schools on a regular basis and not as an intervention project of short duration taking into consideration the aspects of self-image, fear of obesity, preoccupation with dieting and diets. Having breakfast and mid-day snack at school together with the teachers routinely, will support the five meal plan per day.

Further research projects can address on a longitudinal basis, in prospective studies, the effect of alleviation of barriers on adoption of healthy life style habits considering the different needs of both sexes.

5. Conclusions

This study provides additional evidence that nutrition and physical activity habits and perceptions are important factors to prevent overweight/obesity in both sexes. Also, this analysis indicates that a number of perceptions and attitudes that correlate with obesity are sex dimorphic. A better understanding of trends in boys and girls nutrition habits and physical activity patterns within different weight status, seems to be a priority.

Interventions should be tailored according to sex in order to support adolescents to maintain healthy life style habits

Author Contributions: V.C., D.K., G.C.B., E.V., T.P., Y.M., F.K., A.H. and S.M. contributed to the methodology. V.C. led the formal analysis, data analysis and the writing of the manuscript with the contribution and input from all authors. All authors critically reviewed and approved the final version of the manuscript for publication. E.V. has contributed on Project administration and on writing-review & editing. S.M. has contributed on Project administration. All authors have read and agreed to the published version of the manuscript.

Funding: This research was part of the "Hellenic National Action Plan for the Assessment, Prevention and Treatment of childhood obesity. Actions for exercise and physical activity". (MIS 301205) which was co-financed by the European Union (European Social Fund—ESF) and Greek national funds through the National Strategic Reference Framework (NSRF). The funding body/bodito prevent es had approved the design of the study and supervised that the methodology and timetable were followed as planned. They had no involvement in the collection, analysis, and interpretation of data or in writing of the manuscript.

Institutional Review Board Statement: The study was conducted according to the guidelines of the Declaration of Helsinki, and approved by the Greek Ministry of National Education and the Greek Ministry of Health and the Hellenic Data Protection Authority.

Informed Consent Statement: Informed consent was obtained from all subjects involved in the study.

Data Availability Statement: The data presented in this study are available on request from the corresponding author.

Acknowledgments: The authors are indebted to all research team members, as well as to the parents/caregivers and children for their participation in the study.

Conflicts of Interest: The authors declare no conflict of interest.

Appendix A

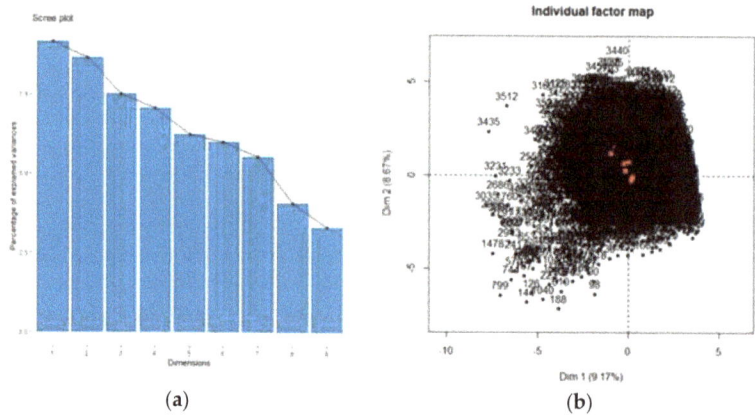

Figure A1. (a,b) Scree plot for each of the first 9 FAMD dimensions and individual factor map.

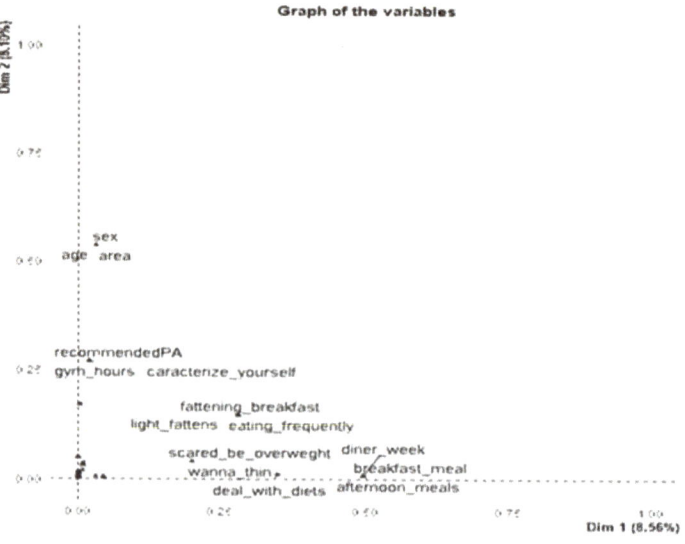

Figure A2. The first 15 well projected variables for the first two dimensions.

Table A1. Regions and Prefectures included in the sample.

Regions	Prefectures	% of Sample
Eastern Macedonia Thrace	Drama	1.10
	Evros	1.10
	Kavala	1.10
	Xanthi	1.10
	Rodopi	1.10
Central Macedonia	Thessaloniki (2 regional units)	10.40
	Imathia	1.10
	Kilkis	1.10
	Pella	1.10
	Pieria	1.10
	Serres	2.20
	Halkidiki	1.10
Western Macedonia	Kastoria	1.10
	Kozani	2.20
	Florina	1.10
Epirus	Arta	1.10
	Thesprotia	1.10
	Ioannina	2.20
	Preveza	1.10
Thessalia	Magnesia	2.00
	Larissa	2.70
	Trikala	1.50
Ionian Islands	Zakynthos	1.00
	Corfu	1.10
	Kefallinia	1.00
Western Greece	Aetoloakarnania	2.50
	Ahaia	3.20
	Viotia	1.80
	Evia	2.00
	Fthiotida	1.70
Attiki	Athens (6 regional units)	20.80
	Piraeus	6.30
Peloponnese	Argolida	1.10
	Arkadia	1.10
	Corinthos	1.10
	Laconia	1.10
	Messenia	2.20
North Aegean	Lesvos	1.10
	Samos	1.10
	Chios	1.10
South Aegean	Cyclades (Samos, Santorini)	2.20

Table A1. Cont.

Regions	Prefectures	% of Sample
	Dodecanese (Rhodes, Kastelorizo)	2.20
Crete	Heraklion	2.60
	Lasithi	1.00
	Rethymno	1.00

Table A2. Factors extracted by Factor Analysis of Mixed Data and variables description.

Compounds	Eigenvalues	% Cumulative Variance	Description	Variable Labels	Variable Names
comp 1	3.85	9.167	Meals frequency and perceptions of fattening	Number of afternoon meals/week	afternoon_meals
				Frequency of dinner meals per week	diner_week
				Frequency of breakfast consumption per week	breakfast_meal
				Eating 5 meals per day is:	five_meals_per_day
				Eating frequently (without order) fattens	eating_frequently
				Skipping breakfast fattens	fattening_breakfast
				Eating light products fattens	light_fattens
comp 2	3.643	17.839	Sociodemographic factors	Age	age
				Area	area
				Sex	sex
Comp 3	3.155	25.45	Body images and behaviors against obesity and fattening	I want to be thin	wanna_be_thin
				I deal with diets	deal_with_diets
				I'm scared to be overweight	scared_be_overweght
Comp 4	2.969	32.55	Perceptions about physical activity	Self evaluation of physical activity	caracterize_yourself
				The recommended physical activity is 1 h	recommendedPA
				The gym hours and breaks at school are enough to be physically active	gym_hours
Comp 5	2.613	38.6	Foods/snacks eaten at meals and after meals	Bread at brunch	bread_brunch
				Cheese pie at breakfast	pie_cheese
				Fruit after diner	fruit_afterdiner
Comp 6	2.517	44.6	Drinks consumed for breakfast	Whole milk at breakfast per week	whole_milk
				Cocoa milk at breakfast per week	cocoa_milk
				Fresh juice per week	freshjuice
Compound 7	2.319	50.31	Organized physical activity	Football per week	football
				Basket per week	basket
				Track and field per week	track_field
				Dance per week	danse_week
Comp 8	1.703	54.71	Purchase criteria/choice of food and socioeconomic status	Buying products according to their price	importance_of_low_cost
				Buying products according to their calories	count_calories
				ses	ses
comp 9	1.583	58.51	Sedentary behaviors and eating	Meals in front of PC per week	pc_food
				Snack (salty) in front of PC/tv per week	tv_snack
				Snack (sweet) in front of pc(TV) per week	pc_snack

Table A3. Descriptive statistics and statistical tests ($\alpha = 5\%$) by sex, for significant variables on multivariate models.

Variables (Codes)	Boys N = 2527 (49.00) N (%)	Girls N = 2617 (51.00) N (%)	p-Value [1]
BMI			
Underweight/Normal Weight (0)	1574 (62.3)	1824 (69.7)	<0.001
Overweight (1)	661 (26.2)	574 (21.9)	
Obese (2)	209 (8.2)	130 (5.0)	
Missing	83 (3.3)	89 (3.4)	
Area			
Rural (0)	610 (24.1)	633 (24.2)	0.753
Semi urban (1)	462 (18.3)	492 (18.8)	
Urban (2)	1455 (57.6)	1492 (57.0)	
Track and field per week			
Never (0)	1699 (67.2)	1809 (69.1)	0.037
1 time (1)	319 (12.6)	271 (10.4)	
At least 2–3 times (2)	342 (13.6)	341 (13.0)	
Missing	167 (6.6)	196 (7.5)	
Characterize yourself in relation to physical activity			
No active/Not much either a little (1)	606 (24.0)	1067 (40.8)	<0.001
Quite/very active (2)	1921 (76.0)	1550 (59.2)	
The gym hours and breaks at school are enough for me to be physically active			
Strongly disagree/disagree (0)	1176 (46.5)	1300 (49.7)	0.001
Undecided (1)	559 (22.1)	628 (24.0)	
Agree/strongly agree (2)	740 (29.3)	647 (24.7)	
Missing	52 (2.1)	42 (0.6)	
Eating cheese pie at breakfast			
Never/rarely (0)	1439 (56.9)	1764 (67.4)	<0.001
Sometimes/often (1)	847 (33.5)	629 (24.0)	
Daily (2)	68 (2.8)	29 (1.1)	
Missing	173 (6.8)	195 (7.5)	
I deal with diets			
Always (0)	64 (2.5)	111 (4.2)	<0.001
Sometimes/often (1)	243 (9.6)	337 (12.9)	
Rarely (2)	608 (24.1)	798 (30.5)	
Never (3)	1529 (60.5)	1299 (49.6)	
Missing	83 (3.3)	72 (2.8)	
I am scared to get overweight			
Always (0)	1065 (42.1)	1463 (55.9)	<0.001
Sometimes/often (1)	681 (26.9)	623 (23.8)	
Rarely (2)	440 (17.4)	345 (13.2)	
Never (3)	272 (10.9)	134 (5.1)	
Missing	69 (2.7)	52 (2.0)	

Table A3. Cont.

Variables (Codes)	Boys N = 2527 (49.00) N (%)	Girls N = 2617 (51.00) N (%)	p-Value [1]
I want to be thin			
Always (0)	453 (17.9)	762 (29.1)	<0.001
Sometimes/often (1)	476 (18.8)	567 (21.7)	
Rarely (2)	634 (25.1)	610 (23.3)	
Never (3)	894 (35.4)	632 (24.1)	
Missing	70 (2.8)	46 (1.8)	
Drinking whole milk at breakfast			
Never/rarely	732 (29.0)	876 (33.5)	<0.001
Sometimes/Often	648 (25.6)	606 (23.2)	
Daily	933 (36.9)	912 (34.8)	
Missing	214 (8.5)	223 (8.5)	
Eating bread at brunch			
Never	635 (25.1)	643 (24.6)	0.079
Sometimes	1071 (42.4)	1201 (45.9)	
Often/always	629 (24.9)	607 (23.2)	
Missing	192 (7.6)	166 (6.3)	
Eating fruit after dinner			
Never	608 (24.0)	701 (26.8)	0.023
1–2 times	675 (26.7)	734 (28.0)	
3–4 times	553 (21.9)	507 (19.4)	
>4 times	623 (24.7)	610 (23.3)	
Missing	68 (2.7)	65 (2.5)	
Buying products according to their calories			
Not or little important	833 (33.0)	732 (28.0)	<0.001
Enough Important	726 (28.7)	610 (23.3)	
Very Important	858 (34.0)	1198 (45.8)	
Missing	110 (4.4)	77 (2.9)	
Eating five meals per day is			
Very bad/bad	338 (13.4)	221 (8.4)	<0.001
Neither good or bad	560 (22.2)	519 (19.8)	
Good/very good	1540 (60.9)	1813 (69.4)	
Missing	89 (3.5)	64 (2.4)	
Eating light products is fattening			
Strongly disagree/disagree	1137 (45.0)	1220 (46.6)	0.574
Undecided	781 (30.9)	805 (30.8)	
Agree/Strongly agree	506 (20.0)	503 (19.2)	
Missing	103 (4.1)	89 (3.4)	
Skipping breakfast is fattening			
Strongly disagree/disagree	1501 (59.4)	1386 (53.0)	<0.001
Undecided	449 (17.8)	446 (17.0)	

Table A3. Cont.

Variables (Codes)	Boys N = 2527 (49.00) N (%)	Girls N = 2617 (51.00) N (%)	p-Value [1]
Agree/strongly agree	485 (19.2)	722 (27.6)	
Missing	92 (3.6)	63 (2.4)	
Frequency of breakfast consumption per week	3.82 (1.37)	3.76 (1.43)	0.102
Frequency of dinner meals per week	4.03 (1.13)	3.80 (1.23)	**<0.001**
Number of afternoon meals/week	3.56 (1.26)	3.57 (1.28)	0.839
Cocoa milk for breakfast per week	3.82 (1.26)	1.71 (1.20)	**<0.001**
Age	13.55 (0.94)	13.54 (0.94)	0.845

[1] The Chi-square test was used to calculate the p-value. Descriptive statistics and statistical tests ($\alpha = 5\%$) by sex (continuous variables). Bold: The t-student was used to calculate the p-value.

Table A4. Descriptive statistics and statistical tests ($\alpha = 5\%$) by sex for no significant variables on multivariate models.

Variables (Codes)	Boys N = 2527 (49.00) Boys	Girls N = 2617 (51.00) Girls	p-Value [1]
The recommended physical activity is 1 h			
Strongly disagree/disagree (0)	356 (14.1)	221 (8.4)	<0.001
Undecided (1)	1256 (49.7)	1344 (51.4)	
Agree/strongly agree (2)	831 (32.9)	984 (37.6)	
Missing	84 (3.3)	68 (2.6)	
Buying products according to their price			
Not or little important (0)	1828 (72.3)	2154 (82.3)	<0.001
Enough Important (1)	401 (15.9)	255 (9.7)	
Very Important (2)	199 (7.9)	133 (5.1)	
Missing	99 (3.9)	75 (2.9)	
Football per week			
Never (0)	763 (30.1)	2027 (77.5)	<0.001
1 time (1)	328 (13.0)	361 (13.8)	
At least 2–3 times (2)	1414 (56.0)	219 (8.3)	
Missing	22 (0.9)	10 (0.4)	
Basket per week			
Never (0)	862 (34.1)	1445 (55.2)	<0.001
1 time (1)	600 (23.7)	429 (16.4)	
At least 2–3 times (2)	754 (29.9)	291 (11.1)	
Missing	311 (12.3)	452 (17.3)	
Dance per week			
Never (0)	1824 (72.2)	936 (35.8)	<0.001
1 time (1)	222 (8.8)	547 (20.9)	
At least 2–3 times (2)	86 (3.4)	768 (29.3)	
Missing	395 (15.6)	366 (14.0)	
Meals in front of PC per week	2.32 (1.087)	2.06 (1.066)	**0.015**
Snack (salty) in front of PC per week	1.990 (1.056)	1.910 (1.092)	**<0.001**
Snack (sweet) in front of TV per week	1.980 (1.079)	2.480 (1.054)	**<0.001**
SES	6.330 (1.841)	6.870 (0.900)	**<0.001**
Fresh juice per week	3.140 (1.315)	3.040 (1.310)	**0.008**

[1] The Chi-square test was used to calculate the p-value. Bold: The t-student was used to calculate the p-value.

Appendix B

Table A5. Log–likelihood and likelihood ratio estimates.

	Partial Proportional Odds Model PPOM		Generalized Ordered Logit Model GOLM	
	Boys	Girls	Boys	Girls
Log Likelihood (null)	−886.01	−708.56	−886.01	−708.56
Log Likelihood (model)	−599.02	−540.91	−585.40	−536.60
Likelihood Ratio chi2	573.96	335.38	580.60	339.44
p-value	<0.001	<0.001	<0.001	<0.001
Akaike's Information Criterion	1442.06	1237.82	1455.30	1244.71
Bayesian Information Criterion	2046.29	1619.05	2064.45	1616.08

Table A6. Maximum likelihood estimates of Partial proportional odds model (overweight/obese versus other BMI categories).

Predictors	$p > \lvert z \rvert$		Odds Ratio (95% CI)	
Overweight/Obese Versus other BMI Categories				
Characterize yourself in relation to physical activity	Boys	Girls		
Quite/very active	0.001	0.001	0.691(0.550–0.868)	0.714(0.582–0.877)
I think eating frequently (without order) is fattening				
Undecided	0.845	NS [1]	0.938 (0.294–1.166)	NS
Strongly agree / agree	0.031	NS	0.508 (0.275–0.940)	NS
Eating bread for brunch				
Sometimes/Rarely	0.002	0.065	0.453 (0.274–0.747)	0.468 (0.209–1.048)
Often/always	0.236	0.034	0.573 (0.228–1.439)	0.382 (0.157–0.932)
Eating five meals per day is				
Neither good or bad	0.493	0.232	1.198 (0.716–2.000)	1.376 (0.815–2.323)
Good/very good	0.384	0.012	1.231(0.771–1.966)	0.241(0.079–0.735)
Area	Boys	Girls	Boys	Girls
Semi-urban	0.972	0.293	1.009 (0.601–1.697)	0.767 (0.468–1.257)
Urban	0.327	0.387	0.816 (0.544–1.225)	0.837(0.560–1.252)
Frequency of breakfast consumption per week	0.373	<0.001	0.849 (0.359–2.011)	0.537 (0.408–0.711)
Frequency of dinner meals per week	0.089	0.045	0.955 (0.845–1.195)	0.863 (0.748–0.997)
Eating cheese pie (breakfast)				
Sometimes/often	0.402	0.072	1.204 (0.780–1.860)	0.810 (0.644–1.019)
Daily	0.005	0.081	4.465 (1.567–10.724)	0.319 (0.088–1.153)
I am scared to get overweight				
Sometimes/often	0.080	0.365	1.669 (0.941–2.959)	1.455 (0.890–2.379)
Rarely	0.010	<0.001	2.504 (1.242 5.048)	3.829 (2.080–7.047)
Never	0.021	0.005	2.070 (1.118–3.831)	2.438(1.305–4.554)
I want to be thin				
Usually/often	0.005	0.001	0.445 (0.251–0.788)	0.641(0.491–0.836)
Sometimes/rarely	<0.001	<0.001	0.272 (0.159–0.596)	0.476 (0.351–0.646)
Never	<0.001	<0.001	0.246 (0.149–0.496)	0.315 (0.136–0.271)

Table A6. Cont.

Predictors	$p > |z|$		Odds Ratio (95% CI)	
Overweight/Obese Versus other BMI Categories				
Frequency of track and field per week				
1 time per week	0.704	0.140	0.909(0.555–1.488)	0.669(0.392–1.141)
At least 2–3 times/week	0.016	0.437	0.454(0.239–0.864)	0.777 (0.412–1.468)
Cocoa milk for breakfast per week	0.014	NS	0.314 (0.125–0.792)	NS
I deal with diets				
Sometimes/often	0.581	0.878	0.718(0.22198–2.325)	1.071 (0.444–2.582)
Rarely	0.858	0.551	0.901 (0.288–2.819)	1.324(0.526–3.331)
Never	0.018	0.377	0.258(0.084–0.592)	1.324(0.526–3.331)
Number of afternoon meals/week	<0.001	0.311 (0.809–1.947)	0.203 (0.088–0.468)	1.255(0.809–1.947)
Eating light products is fattening				
Undecided	0.392	NS	1.307 (0.708–2.415)	NS
Agree /Strongly agree	<0.001	NS	1.902 (1.139–3.175)	NS
Skipping breakfast is fattening				
Undecided	0.384	0.013	1.231 (0.771–1.966)	1.376 (0.815–2.323)
Agree/strongly agree	0.493	0.232	1.197(0.716–2.000)	0.241(0.078–0.734)
The gym hours and breaks at school are enough for me to be physically active				
Undecided	NS	0.121	NS	0.352 (0.699–2.154)
Agree/strongly agree	NS	0.004	NS	2.509(1.338–4.704)
Age		<0.001	NS	0.668(0.548–0.813)
Drinking whole milk at breakfast				
Sometimes/often	0.244	0.467	0.394 (0.798–2.422)	0.895 (0.508–1.578)
Daily	0.247	0.187	0.725 (0.451–1.168)	0.765 (0.486–1.204)
Buying products according to their calories				
Enough Important	NS	0.041	NS	2.871 (1.042–7.901)
Very Important	NS	0.810	NS	0.926 (0.495–1.731)
Eating fruit after dinner				
1–2 times	0.560	0.712	0.919 (0.585–1.441)	1.151 (0.717–1.849)
3–4 times	0.803	0.997	1.001 (0.616–1.626)	1.071 (0.625–1.836)
>4 times	0.352	0.232	0.679(0.360–1.281)	0.727 (0.539–1.848)

[1] Non Significant in univariate analysis.

Table A7. Maximum likelihood estimates of Partial proportional odds model (obese versus other BMI categories).

Predictors	$p > |z|$		Odds Ratio (95% CI)	
	Obese Versus other BMI Categories			
Characterize yourself in relation to physical activity				
Quite/very active	0.001	0.004	0.691 (0.550–0.868)	0.714 (0.582–0.877)
I think eating frequently (without order) is fattening				
Undecided	0.845	NS	0.938 (0.294–1.166)	NS
Strongly agree/agree	0.031	NS	0.508 (0.275–0.940)	NS
Eating bread for brunch				
Sometimes	0.002	0.065	0.453 (0.274–0.747)	0.468 (0.209–1.048)
Often/always	0.236	0.034	0.573 (0.228–1.439)	0.382 (0.157–0.932)
Eating five meals per day is				
Neither good or bad	0.493	0.232	1.198 (0.716–2.000)	1.376 (0.815–2.323)
Good/very good	0.384	0.012	1.231 (0.771–1.966)	0.241 (0.079–0.735)
Area	Boys	Girls	Boys	Girls
Semi-urban	0.972	0.293	1.009 (0.601–1.697)	0.767 (0.468–1.257)
Urban	0.327	0.005	0.816 (0.544–1.225)	0.332 (0.154–0.712)
Frequency of breakfast consumption per week	0.373	<0.001	0.849 (0.359–2.011)	0.537 (0.408–0.711)
Frequency of dinner meals per week	0.089	0.045	0.955 (0.845–1.195)	0.863 (0.748–0.997)
Eating cheese pie (breakfast)				
Sometimes/often	0.402	0.072	1.204 (0.780–1.860)	0.810 (0.644–1.019)
Daily	0.005	0.081	4.465 (1.567–10.724)	0.319 (0.088–1.153)
I am scared to get overweight				
sometimes/often	0.080	0.365	1.669 (0.941–2.959)	1.455 (0.890–2.379)
rarely	0.010	<0.001	2.504 (1.242–5.048)	3.829 (2.080–7.047)
Never	0.021	0.005	2.070 (1.118–3.831)	2.438 (1.305–4.554)
I want to be thin				
Usually/often	0.005	0.001	0.445 (0.251–0.788)	0.641 (0.491–0.836)
Sometimes/rarely	<0.001	<0.001	0.272 (0.149–0.496)	0.476 (0.351–0.646)
Never	<0.001	<0.001	0.246 (0.149–0.496)	0.315 (0.136–0.271)
Frequency of track and field per week				
1 time per week	0.704	0.140	0.909 (0.555–1.488)	0.669 (0.392–1.141)
At least 2–3 times/week	0.016	0.437	0.454 (0.239–0.864)	0.777 (0.412–1.468)
Cocoa milk for breakfast per week	0.014	NS	0.314 (0.125–0.792)	NS
I deal with diets				
Sometimes/often	0.581	0.878	0.718 (0.22198–2.325)	1.071 (0.444–2.582)
Rarely	0.858	0.551	0.901 (0.288–2.819)	1.324 (0.526–3.331)
Never	0.018	0.377	0.258 (0.084–0.792)	1.324 (0.526–3.331)
Number of afternoon meals/week	<0.001	0.311 (0.809–1.947)	0.203 (0.088–0.468)	1.255 (0.809–1.947)
Eating light products is fattening				
Undecided	0.392	NS	1.307 (0.708–2.415)	NS
Agree/Strongly agree	<0.001	NS	3.815 (1.927–7.554)	NS

Table A7. Cont.

Predictors	p > |z|		Odds Ratio (95% CI)	
	Obese Versus other BMI Categories			
The gym hours and breaks at school are enough for me to be physically active				
Undecided	NS	0.121	NS	0.352 (0.699–2.154)
Agree/strongly agree	NS	0.004	NS	2.509 (1.338–4.704)
Drinking whole milk at breakfast				
Sometimes/often	0.244	0.467	0.394 (0.798–2.422)	0.895 (0.508–1.578)
Daily	0.247	0.031	0.725 (0.451–1.168)	2.483 (1.088–5.668)
Age	NS	0.861	NS	0.967 (0.663–1.410)
Buying products according to their calories				
Enough Important	NS	0.203	NS	1.478 (0.810–2.697)
Very Important	NS	0.810	NS	0.926 (0.495–1.731)
Eating fruit after dinner				
1–2 times	0.560	0.712	0.919 (0.585–1.441)	1.151 (0.717–1.849)
3–4 times	0.047	0.997	0.440 (0.196–0.988)	1.071 (0.625–1.836)
>4 times	0.352	0.232	0.679 (0.360–1.281)	0.727 (0.539–1.848)

References

1. Golden, N.H.; Schneider, M.; Wood, C.; Daniels, S.; Abrams, S.; Corkins, M.; De Ferranti, S.; Magge, S.N.; Schwarzenberg, S.; Critch, J.; et al. Preventing obesity and eating disorders in adolescents. *Pediatrics* **2016**, *138*. [CrossRef] [PubMed]
2. WHO. *World Health Organization Report of the Commission on Ending Childhood Obesity*; WHO: Geneva, Switzerland, 2017.
3. Spinelli, A.; Buoncristiano, M.; Kovacs, V.A.; Yngve, A.; Spiroski, I.; Obreja, G.; Starc, G.; Pérez, N.; Rito, A.I.; Kunešová, M.; et al. Prevalence of severe obesity among primary school children in 21 European countries. *Obes. Facts* **2019**, *12*, 244–258. [CrossRef]
4. Kumar, S.; Kelly, A.S. Review of Childhood Obesity: From Epidemiology, Etiology, and Comorbidities to Clinical Assessment and Treatment. *Mayo Clin. Proc.* **2017**, *92*, 251–265. [CrossRef]
5. Campbell, M.K. Biological, environmental, and social influences on childhood obesity. *Pediatr. Res.* **2016**, *79*, 205–211. [CrossRef]
6. Magge, S.N.; Goodman, E.; Armstrong, S.C. The Metabolic Syndrome in Children and Adolescents: Shifting the Focus to Cardiometabolic Risk Factor Clustering. *Pediatrics* **2017**, *140*, e20171603. [CrossRef]
7. Tirosh, A.; Shai, I.; Afek, A.; Dubnov-Raz, G.; Ayalon, N.; Gordon, B.; Derazne, E.; Tzur, D.; Shamis, A.; Vinker, S.; et al. Adolescent BMI Trajectory and Risk of Diabetes versus Coronary Disease. *N. Engl. J. Med.* **2011**, *364*, 1315–1325. [CrossRef]
8. Govindan, M.; Gurm, R.; Mohan, S.; Kline-Rogers, E.; Corriveau, N.; Goldberg, C.; Du Russel-Weston, J.; Eagle, K.A.; Jackson, E.A. Gender differences in physiologic markers and health behaviors associated with childhood obesity. *Pediatrics* **2013**, *132*, 468–474. [CrossRef] [PubMed]
9. Bartholdy, S.; Allen, K.; Hodsoll, J.; O'Daly, O.G.; Campbell, I.C.; Banaschewski, T.; Bokde, A.L.W.; Bromberg, U.; Büchel, C.; Quinlan, E.B.; et al. Identifying disordered eating behaviours in adolescents: How do parent and adolescent reports differ by sex and age? *Eur. Child Adolesc. Psychiatry* **2017**, *26*, 691–701. [CrossRef]
10. Trompeter, N.; Bussey, K.; Hay, P.; Griffiths, S.; Murray, S.B.; Mond, J.; Lonergan, A.; Pike, K.M.; Mitchison, D. Fear of negative evaluation among eating disorders: Examining the association with weight/shape concerns in adolescence. *Int. J. Eat. Disord.* **2019**, *52*, 261–269. [CrossRef] [PubMed]
11. Barstad, L.H.; Júlíusson, P.B.; Johnson, L.K.; Hertel, J.K.; Lekhal, S.; Hjelmesæth, J. Gender-related differences in cardiometabolic risk factors and lifestyle behaviors in treatment-seeking adolescents with severe obesity. *BMC Pediatr.* **2018**, *18*. [CrossRef]
12. Wang, V.H.; Min, J.; Xue, H.; Du, S.; Xu, F.; Wang, H.; Wang, Y. Factors contributing to sex differences in childhood obesity prevalence in China. *Public Health Nutr.* **2018**, *21*, 2056–2064. [CrossRef]
13. Cole, T.J.; Lobstein, T. Extended international (IOTF) body mass index cut-offs for thinness, overweight and obesity. *Pediatr. Obes.* **2012**, *7*, 284–294. [CrossRef]

14. Carayanni, V.; Vlachopapadopoulou, E.; Psaltopoulou, T.; Koutsouki, D.; Bogdanis, G.; Karachaliou, F.; Manios, Y.; Kapsali, A.; Papadopoulou, A.; Hatzakis, A.; et al. Validity and Reliability of Three New Instruments for Parents and Children Assessing Nutrition and Physical Activity Behaviors, Environment and Knowledge and Health in Childhood and Adolescence in Greece During the Economic Recession: Data from the National Action Plan for Public Health (MIS301205). *Value Health* **2016**, *19*, A395. [CrossRef]
15. Moschonis, G.; Mavrogianni, C.; Karatzi, K.; Iatridi, V.; Chrousos, G.P.; Lionis, C.; Manios, Y. Increased physical activity combined with more eating occasions is beneficial against dyslipidemias in children. The Healthy Growth Study. *Eur. J. Nutr.* **2013**, *52*, 1135–1144. [CrossRef]
16. Escofi, B.; Pagès, J. *Cours et Études de cas Analyses Factorielles Simples et Multiples*; Dunod: Paris, France, 2008.
17. Husson, F.; Lê, S.; Pagès, J. *Exploratory Multivariate Analysis by Example Using R*; CRC Press: Boca Raton, FL, USA, 2010; ISBN 97814398358.
18. Pagès, J.; Husson, F. Multiple factor analysis: Presentation of the method using sensory data. *Mathe-Matical Stat. Methods Food Sci. Technol.* **2014**, *87*, 102.
19. Child, D. The Essentials of Factor Analysis—Google Books. Available online: https://www.bloomsbury.com/uk/the-essentials-of-factor-analysis-9780826480002/ (accessed on 1 February 2021).
20. Costello, A.B.; Osborne, J. Best practices in exploratory factor analysis: Four recommendations for getting the most from your analysis. *Res. Eval. Pract. Assess. Res. Eval.* **2005**, *10*, 7. [CrossRef]
21. Roberts, L.D.; Koulman, A.; Griffin, J.L. Towards metabolic biomarkers of insulin resistance and type 2 diabetes: Progress from the metabolome. *Lancet Diabetes Endocrinol.* **2014**, *2*, 65–75. [CrossRef]
22. Ruiz, L.D.; Zuelch, M.L.; Dimitratos, S.M.; Scherr, R.E. Adolescent Obesity: Diet Quality, Psychosocial Health, and Cardiometabolic Risk Factors. *Nutrients* **2020**, *12*, 43. [CrossRef]
23. Xing, L. *Applied Ordinal Logistic Regression*; Sage Publications: Thousand Oaks, CA, USA, 2016; ISBN 978-1-4833-1975-9.
24. Hilbe, J.M. *Logistic Regression Models (Chapman & Hall/CRC Texts in Statistical Science)*; CRC Press: Boca Raton, FL, USA, 2011.
25. Kassie, G.W.; Workie, D.L. Determinants of under-nutrition among children under five years of age in Ethiopia. *BMC Public Health* **2020**, *20*, 1–11. [CrossRef]
26. Block, J.P.; Condon, S.K.; Kleinman, K.; Mullen, J.; Linakis, S.; Rifas-Shiman, S.; Gillman, M.W. Consumers' estimation of calorie content at fast food restaurants: Cross sectional observational study. *BMJ* **2013**, *346*, 1–10. [CrossRef] [PubMed]
27. Manippa, V.; Giuliani, F.; Brancucci, A. Healthiness or calories? Side biases in food perception and preference. *Appetite* **2020**, *147*, 104552. [CrossRef]
28. Dallacker, M.; Hertwig, R.; Mata, J. The frequency of family meals and nutritional health in children: A meta-analysis. *Obes. Rev.* **2018**, *19*, 638–653. [CrossRef]
29. Marangoni, F.; Martini, D.; Scaglioni, S.; Sculati, M.; Donini, L.M.; Leonardi, F.; Agostoni, C.; Castelnuovo, G.; Ferrara, N.; Ghiselli, A.; et al. Snacking in nutrition and health. *Int. J. Food Sci. Nutr.* **2019**, *70*, 909–923. [CrossRef]
30. Ramires, V.V.; Dumith, S.C.; Gonçalves, H. Longitudinal association between physical activity and body fat during adolescence: A systematic review. *J. Phys. Act. Health* **2015**, *12*, 1344–1358. [CrossRef]
31. Loth, K.A.; Tate, A.D.; Trofholz, A.; Fisher, J.O.; Miller, L.; Neumark-Sztainer, D.; Berge, J.M. Ecological momentary assessment of the snacking environments of children from racially/ethnically diverse households. *Appetite* **2020**, *145*, 104497. [CrossRef]
32. Styne, D.M.; Arslanian, S.A.; Connor, E.L.; Farooqi, I.S.; Murad, M.H.; Silverstein, J.H.; Yanovski, J.A. Pediatric obesity-assessment, treatment, and prevention: An endocrine society clinical practice guideline. *J. Clin. Endocrinol. Metab.* **2017**, *102*, 709–757. [CrossRef]
33. De Cássia Ribeiro-Silva, R.; Fiaccone, R.L.; da Conceição-Machado, M.E.P.; Ruiz, A.S.; Barreto, M.L.; Santana, M.L.P. Body image dissatisfaction and dietary patterns according to nutritional status in adolescents. *J. Pediatr.* **2018**, *94*, 155–161. [CrossRef]
34. Kohlmann, C.W.; Eschenbeck, H.; Heim-Dreger, U.; Hock, M.; Platt, T.; Ruch, W. Fear of being laughed at in children and adolescents: Exploring the importance of overweight, underweight, and teasing. *Front. Psychol.* **2018**, *9*, 1–15. [CrossRef]
35. Murphy, M.M.; Douglass, J.S.; Johnson, R.K.; Spence, L.A. Drinking flavored or plain milk is positively associated with nutrient intake and is not associated with adverse effects on weight status in US children and adolescents. *J. Am. Diet Assoc.* **2008**, *108*, 631–639. [CrossRef]
36. Bengoechea, E.G.; Sabiston, C.M.; Ahmed, R.; Farnoush, M. Exploring links to unorganized and organized physical activity during adolescence: The role of gender, socioeconomic status, weight status, and enjoyment of physical education. *Res. Q. Exerc. Sport* **2010**, *81*, 7–16. [CrossRef] [PubMed]
37. Carayanni, V.; Vlachopapadopoulou, E.; Koutsouki, D.; Bogdanis, G.C.; Psaltopoulou Manios, Y.T.; Karachaliou, F.; Hatzakis, A.; Michalacos, S. Effects of Body Mass Index (BMI), demographic and socioeconomic factors on organized physical activity (OPA) participation in children aged 6-15 years: A cross-sectional study comparing primary and secondary school children in Greece. *BMC Pediatrics* **2020**, *20*, 1–11. [CrossRef]
38. Sweeting, H.N. Gendered dimensions of obesity in childhood and adolescence. *Nutr. J.* **2008**, *7*, 1–14. [CrossRef]

MDPI
St. Alban-Anlage 66
4052 Basel
Switzerland
Tel. +41 61 683 77 34
Fax +41 61 302 89 18
www.mdpi.com

Children Editorial Office
E-mail: children@mdpi.com
www.mdpi.com/journal/children